# MOSBY'S

# CEN®

# Examination
# REVIEW

## THIRD EDITION

# MOSBY'S

# CEN®

# Examination
# REVIEW

## THIRD EDITION

## Reneé Semonin Holleran
RN, PhD, CEN, CCRN, CFRN
Chief Flight Nurse, University Air Care
Emergency Clinical Nurse Specialist
University of Cincinnati Hospital
Cincinnati, Ohio

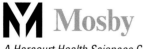 Mosby

*A Harcourt Health Sciences Company*

St. Louis   London   Philadelphia   Sydney   Toronto

*Vice-President, Nursing Editorial Director:* Sally Schrefer
*Executive Editor:* June Thompson
*Managing Editor:* Lisa Potts
*Developmental Editor:* Billi Sharp
*Project Manager:* John Rogers
*Editing and Production:* Clarinda Publication Services
*Designer:* Kathi Gosche
*Cover Art:* Kathi Gosche

Mosby, Inc.
*A Harcourt Health Sciences Company*
11830 Westline Industrial Drive
St. Louis, Missouri 63146


Printed in the United States of America

**Library of Congress Cataloging-in-Publication Data**

Holleran, Reneé Semonin.
    Mosby's CEN examination review / Reneé Semonin Holleran.—3rd ed.
        p. cm.
    Includes bibliographical references and index.
    ISBN 0-323-01234-5 (alk. paper)
    1. Emergency nursing—Examinations, questions, etc.   I. Title.
    RT120.E4 H65 2000
    610.73′61′076—dc21                                                                    00-041574


00  01  02  03  04  CL/MVY  9  8  7  6  5  4  3  2  1

*This book is dedicated first to my family—*
*Micke, Erin, Sara, and my mother and my work family at University Air Care and University Hospital.*
*Second, I dedicate this book to all those who practice or have practiced emergency and flight nursing.*

*I would particularly like to recognize two of my friends—*
*Sandy Sigman, a flight nurse who lost her life caring for patients, and*
*Cece Paige, an emergency nurse who dedicated her life to emergency care.*

*As I have come to find, nursing is a way of life.*

# Foreword

## TAKING THE CERTIFIED EMERGENCY AND FLIGHT NURSE EXAMINATIONS

The Board of Certification first offered the emergency nursing certification examination in July 1980 for Emergency Nursing. The registered nurse who passes this test is designated as a certified emergency nurse, or CEN®.

The certification examination for flight nursing was first offered in July 1993. This examination was created through a collaboration between the National Flight Nurses Association (NFNA) and the Board of Certification for Emergency Nursing. The registered nurse who passes this test is designated as a certified flight nurse, or CFRN.

Certification is a process whereby qualifications are validated and the knowledge for practice in a defined functional or clinical area of nursing is measured. The purpose of both the CEN® and CFRN examinations is to provide a method of measuring competency in the attainment and application of emergency and flight nursing.

CEN® and CFRN are now only available through computer testing. Although this may pose a challenge to some, the advantages include the ability to offer the tests in more locations and more frequently than was done in the past. The examinations are offered in other nations such as Australia and New Zealand.

There are several ways to prepare for the CEN® or CFRN examination. The following test-taking strategies may help you to improve your test-taking skills and increase your test scores.

1. Obtain a *CEN®* or *CFRN Examination Handbook* as soon as possible. The handbook contains the necessary information about the CEN® or CFRN examination (dates, deadlines, application forms, fees, and so on). You are responsible for knowing its content. After reading this handbook, you will know exactly what is expected of you, and this knowledge will help bolster your confidence.

   Single copies of the *CEN®* or *CFRN Examination Handbook* and applications may be obtained from the BCEN at 915 Lee Street, Des Plaines, IL 60016 or at the ENA web site www.ena.org and the ASTNA Web site www.astna.org

   Members of the Emergency Nurses Association (ENA) and the Air and Surface Transport Nurses Association (ASTNA) receive a discount on the examination fee. One of the other important benefits of membership in these associations is the availability of journals, conferences, and resources to prepare for both examinations and remain up to date on all the information and changes that affect our practice. Information about membership is available on both associations' Web sites.

2. Prepare for the examination a few months before the test date. Set aside an hour or two a few days each week to review the major content areas of the examination. Review *Mosby's Emergency and Transport Nursing Review,* the *Emergency Nursing Core Curriculum,* and the *Flight Nursing Core Curriculum.* Carefully review the questions in this book until you are able to answer most of them correctly. Other sources of information include *Journal of Emergency Nursing; AirMed; Air Medical Journal; Sheehy's Emergency Nursing Principles and Practice* and *Flight Nursing Principles and Practice.*

   Consider taking a CEN® or CFRN examination review course and ask yourself the following questions: Will this course actually help me to pass the examination? Who are the faculty? Are the faculty members CENs or CFRNs? What are the objectives of the course? Is the course accredited? Most of these courses help you to identify your learning needs. They are not a substitute for studying. Talk to your nursing colleagues who are CENs or CFRNs. Ask what worked for them in preparing for the examination and if they have any suggestions.

   Review advanced cardiac life support (ACLS), pediatric advanced life support (PALS), and flight nurse advanced trauma course (FNATC) courses or become recertified. (See Chapter 1 for suggestions for additional courses and references.) Because many questions on the examination come directly from these standards of care, it is important that you know these standards. Concentrate on those areas you have identified as areas of weakness. If, for example, your knowledge or understanding of arterial blood gases (ABGs) is lacking, concentrate on this subject for a few days. Read a chapter on respiratory physiology from a pathophysiology text. Copy and read journal articles on ABGs. Practice ABG interpretation on each of your patients who have ABGs drawn. Discuss your findings with another nurse or physician. Applying principles to the clinical setting is the best way for most nurses to learn. Remember, the key here is to study but also to keep your studying clinically focused.

It may help to keep your review materials handy, especially at work, so that you can review material during slower times in the emergency department. You might read appropriate emergency care journals to break the monotony and increase your knowledge base. It may also help to keep a simple log on how much time you spend reviewing (even if it is only 10 minutes between appointments). After a while you may be surprised to see how much unscheduled time you have accumulated in studying for this examination. This also helps to boost self-confidence.

Another useful way to review information in preparation for the CEN® and CFRN examinations is to use the Internet. Over the past few years, the access to information on the Internet has become easier. In addition, many medical and nursing journals are available on line. The Centers for Disease Control and Prevention provides guidelines, research, and pertinent bulletins on-line. Both the Emergency Nurses Association (ENA) and the Air and Surface Transport Nurses Association have Web sites as previously noted. Nicoll, editor of *Computers in Nursing*[1] has written a particularly useful guide to get started using the Internet. "Surfing the Web" also provides you with the opportunity to practice your computer skills.

One more point about spending time preparing for the CEN® or CFRN examination: because the examination is based on current emergency and transport nursing practice, it is important that you think about how many hours you have worked in the emergency department or how much transport time you have accrued. Full-time employment works out to be about 2,080 hours per year; part-time employment is about 1040 hours per hear. The best way to prepare yourself for this examination is to have at least 2 years of current emergency or flight or transport nursing experience, so you may have already spent thousands of hours in preparation. You may know more than you think; but, nonetheless, be prepared.

The current CEN® examination is based on six components:
  I. Clinical pathophysiology by system
 II. Patient care management
III. Environment and toxicology
 IV. Shock/multisystem trauma
  V. Medical
 VI. Professional issues

The current CFRN examination is based upon five components:
  I. Pathophysiology by system
 II. Multisystem emergencies
III. Patient management
 IV. Safety issues
  V. Professional issues

If you have not tested well in the past, or if you have not taken a test in several years, consider taking the practice tests from other review books. The current edition of this book provides you with an opportunity to practice taking the test on a computer. If you have limited exposure to computer testing, it is a good idea to practice "clicking." *Both examinations will now allow you to skip questions and return back to them. Again, if you are not familiar with doing that on a computer, practice!*

3. Be sure to get a good night's sleep the night before the test. Do not take alcohol or drugs to help you sleep because they will affect your performance the following day. Eat a good but light breakfast to "feed your brain" as well as your stomach.

4. As you begin to take the test, remember to relax. Anxiety will prevent you from doing a good job. Do not let brief and needless anxiety affect your knowledge of emergency or transport nursing. Your skills are tested every day with human lives; sitting down to take an examination is the easy part of an emergency or transport nurse's job.

5. Remember a cardinal rule for test taking: always keep the first answer you choose. Do not go back and change an answer unless you are certain the new one is correct. Do not overlook key words such as *early, late, except, not, immediate,* or *nursing intervention.* There is usually no pattern to the answers on a test. Do not select *B* simply because you have not answered *B* for the last 10 questions.

Beware of answer choices that contain qualifiers such as *always, never, all,* or *every.* These are blanket terms, and we know that in nursing nothing is ever 100% certain. Answers that contain these words can usually, but not always, be considered false.

What if you come to a question that confuses you? First of all, it cannot be overemphasized how clinically oriented these examinations are. Imagine yourself in that particular clinical situation. What would you do? You may be surprised at how automatically some answers to confusing questions will come to you if you put yourself in the clinical setting. And remember, who is better at sorting out confusion than an emergency or transport nurse?

If you come to a question that you cannot answer, return to it later. The new examination will allow you to skip questions and return to them. However, it might be a good idea to write down the number of the question skipped because you no longer have a written examination in front of you, and the screens will change. Perhaps another question on the test may give you a clue to the correct answer. Narrow your choices to a question by eliminating the obviously wrong answers. Each test is now composed of 175 questions, and you will receive your score at the test site.

Finally, we wish you well. It is a big commitment to work toward becoming a CEN® or CFRN. Congratulations on putting forth the effort. We hope that these suggestions will make taking the examination a more positive experience. The time you invest in studying will pay off. Good luck!

**Terry Matthew Foster**
**Reneé Semonin Holleran**

**REFERENCES**

1. Nicoll LH: *Nurses' guide to the Internet*. Philadelphia, 1998, Lippincott.
2. CEN® and CFRN News. In *J Emerg Nurs* 26(1):37A, 2000.
3. *Handbook for CEN examination,* Des Plaines, IL, Board of Certification.
4. *Handbook for CFRN Examination,* Des Plaines, IL, Board of Certification.

# Preface

There are some major and minor changes in this edition. First, part of the title. Flight nursing has expanded its horizons to include all aspects of patient transport. The National Flight Nurses Association (NFNA) has changed its name to the Air and Surface Transport Nurses Association (ASTNA). Most have us have been providing both ground and air transport for most of our careers. The change to transport nursing provides a broader framework to the concept of patient care during the transport process.

Second, there has been explosion of knowledge in selected areas of emergency nursing practice, including the management of acute myocardial infarction, shock, and stroke. As we continue to uncover the pathophysiology of disease, our care becomes more focused on controlling the disease process and preventing additional injury.

Finally, this edition is based on both the Emergency Nursing Core Curriculum[1] and the Flight Nursing Core Curriculum.[2] I have tried to include both "book" and practice examples of all the information we must possess to practice competent and safe emergency and transport nursing practice.

## EMERGENCY AND TRANSPORT NURSING AND CERTIFICATION

The practice of emergency and transport nursing requires possessing a unique body of knowledge. The emergency nurse has to be a specialist who practices in complex situations requiring a great deal of knowledge about many things. Transport nurses need to be able to modify their care to practice in different environments both inside and outside of the hospital. Emergency and transport nurses confront a variety of patient care situations and essentially must be prepared for anything.

Both the Emergency Nursing Standards of Care and the Standards of Flight Nursing Practice state that emergency and flight nurses need to obtain and maintain the knowledge necessary to provide safe and competent care to the patients for whom they are responsible. By achieving emergency or flight nursing certification and through continuing education, nurses may gain the knowledge necessary for practicing competent nursing.

Emergency and transport nursing are specialties in the nursing profession. As professionals, nurses have an obligation to the people they care for to define the distinctive aspects of their specialty. Once this is identified, nurses need to be accountable for what they profess.[3] Accountability is achieved through the adoption of standards of practice, a code of ethics, research, and certification.[3]

Two specific goals of certification include ensuring consumer access to care and consumer and provider protection.[3] Certification can provide consumer access to care by demonstrating that nurses have gained a certain body of knowledge to practice in a specific role,[4,5] for example, certification for nurse-midwives and for pediatric nurse practitioners.

Research has also demonstrated that certified nurses have higher self-esteem, strive for personal achievement, demonstrate a higher level of planning, evaluation, collaboration and willingness to teach, and are more likely to pursue professional growth.[5]

Certification can provide protection for both the consumer and the provider of nursing care by allowing only qualified individuals to be involved in specialized nursing practice. For example, emergency and flight nurses who have achieved the Certification in Emergency Nursing (CEN®) or Certification in Flight Nursing (CRFN) have demonstrated the knowledge necessary to practice emergency or flight nursing.

## THE NURSING PROCESS

The certification examinations given by the Board of Certification for Emergency Nursing for both the emergency nurse and flight nurse are based on the nursing process.[6,7,8] The nursing process is a problem-solving approach that nurses use to assess patients, identify patient needs and problems, plan and provide care for patients, and evaluate the outcomes of the care. The components of the nursing process include assessment (data collection), analysis (nursing diagnosis/collaborative problems), intervention (independent and collaborative), and evaluation (expected outcomes).[7] It is important to remember that patient care in the prehospital and emergency environment involves collaboration. The nursing process provides the nurse with a framework to identify patient problems, provide collaborative care interventions, and evaluate their effectiveness.

### Assessment

Assessment begins with data collection, which includes both subjective and objective information. Patient assessment in both the prehospital environment and the emergency department generally is episodic, focused, and brief. Current and past medical history, social support, and past care experiences can provide key clues in identifying the health needs of the patient.[6,7,8]

### Analysis

The analysis component of the nursing process summarizes the data collected during the patient assessment. Both specific nursing as well as collaborative patient problems are identified. Based on this summary, the emergency or transport nurse determines the patient's potential or actual health problems.[6] Nursing diagnosis are used as a means of identifying the patient's potential or actual health care problems and as a framework on which nurses can base their interventions and evaluate the effectiveness of these interventions. The North American Nursing Diagnosis Association (NANDA) has identified over 100 nursing diagnoses. Research continues on the development of even more. Several sources for nursing diagnoses include their definitions, defining characteristics, and related findings. Useful texts containing nursing diagnoses and their application to clinical nursing practice are included in several of the References and/or Additional Readings sections, which are located at the end of each chapter.

Even though the analysis component of the nursing process generally uses nursing diagnoses, patient care in the prehospital and emergency department is a collaborative process. In the fifth edition of the *Emergency Nursing Core Curriculum,* the analysis section includes not only differential nursing diagnoses but also a list of patient problems that are approached collaboratively.

### Intervention

Interventions are specific nursing and collaborative measures taken to meet the patient's potential or actual health care needs. Emergency and transport nursing interventions can be either independent or collaborative. Independent nursing interventions are based on

specific practice parameters established by the nursing profession. In addition, the state nursing practice acts in the states where nurses practice also prescribe the specific interventions that nurses may initiate.[3] Collaborative interventions include care provided by other health care personnel, along with the emergency nurse, including physicians, social workers, and prehospital care personnel.

### Evaluation/Expected Outcomes

The final component of the nursing process is evaluation/expected outcomes. The function of evaluation is to examine whether the interventions performed by the emergency or transport nurse, either independently or collaboratively, have been effective. The effectiveness of independent and collaborative emergency or flight nursing care can be evaluated using several methods. These include attainment of patient goals, total quality improvement, chart audits, and direct observation of the patient's response to interventions and achievement of expected outcomes.[3-8]

## HOW TO USE THIS BOOK

The immense scope of emergency and transport nursing practice makes it difficult for any one text to contain all aspects of these nursing specialties. In addition, it is difficult for any one text, journal, or periodical to keep abreast of all the nursing, medical, and societal changes that occur of which the emergency and flight nurse must be aware. Perhaps this is one of the reasons why many of us practice in the prehospital emergency environments—new challenges always await us. Since emergency and transport nurses are either men or women, the exclusive use of the pronouns *his, her, he* or *she* has been avoided.

The third edition of this book follows both the *Emergency Nursing Core Curriculum* and *Flight Nursing Core Curriculum.* Questions were developed using the content outlines for both examinations. Each chapter contains a review outline, questions and answers, and references. The new addition of this book is a disk that you may use to practice answering questions on the computer. Unlike the real examination, you can immediately look the answers up to confirm your correct answer or explore why the answer is wrong.

This book was written by practicing emergency and flight and transport nurses. We all practice in various emergency departments and transport programs, including community and inner-city facilities and private and hospital-based programs. We hope this diversity helps all of you in reviewing the knowledge base of emergency and flight nursing. We also hope it reflects our pride as emergency, flight, and transport nurses. We welcome your comments for future editions.

I would like to take this opportunity to thank all the contributors to the first and second editions of this book. This third edition would not have been possible without all your work.

At Mosby, Inc. I would like to thank Managing Editor Lisa Potts and Developmental Editor Billi Sharp for all their help and support of this project. Many thanks also to the production and design teams at Mosby.

**Diana James Demling, RN, BSN, CEN, CCRN, NEMT-P**
Flight Nurse, University Air Care
University of Cincinnati Hospital
Cincinnati, OH

**Mike Epperson, RN, BSN, CFRN**
Flight Nurse, Life Flight
University of California—San Diego
San Diego, California

**Terry Foster, RN, CEN, CCRN**
Clinical Director Nursing Association
Mercy Hospital
Cincinnati, Ohio;
Staff Nurse, Emergency Department
St. Elizabeth Medical Center
Covington, Kentucky

**Mary Ann Neihaus O'Toole, RN, MSN, CEN**
Staff Nurse
Emergency Department, Coronary Care Unit
University of Cincinnati Hospital
Cincinnati, Ohio

**Mike Rouse, RN, BSN, CFRN**
Flight Nurse, University Air Care
University of Cincinnati Hospital
Cincinnati, Ohio

**Jane Swaim, RN, MS**
Administrator, Patient Care Services
University of Cincinnati Medical Center
Associate Dean, Clinical Affairs
University of Cincinnati College of Nursing
Cincinnati, Ohio

**Nancy Peter Von Rotz, RN, MSN, CCRN**
Flight Nurse, University Air Care
University of Cincinnati Hospital
Cincinnati, Ohio

**Janet M. Williams, RN, BSN, CEN**
Flight Nurse, University Air Care
University of Cincinnati Hospital
Cincinnati, Ohio

**Cheryl Wraa, RN, BSN, CFRN**
President-Elect, National Flight Nurses Association
Flight Nurse, Life Flight
University of California—Davis
Sacramento, California

**REFERENCES**

1. Jordan K, editor: *Emergency nursing core curriculum,* ed 5, Philadelphia, 2000, WB Saunders.
2. Krupa D, editor: *Flight nursing core curriculum,* Park Ridge, 1997, Road Runner Press.
3. Bulechek GM, Maas ML: Nursing certification: a matter for the professional organization. In McCloskey JC, Grace HK, editors: *Current issues in nursing,* ed 3, St Louis, 1990, Mosby.
4. Manton A: Certification. In Newberry L, editor: *Sheehy's Emergency nursing: principles and practice,* ed 4, St Louis, 1998, Mosby.
5. Redd ML, Alexander JW: Does certification mean better performance? *Nurs Manage* 28(2):45-50, 1997.
6. Kidd P: Defining nursing process categories in the emergency nursing certification examination, *J Emerg Nurs* 16:78A, 1990.
7. Twedell D: Nursing process: assessment and priority setting. In Jordan K, editor: *Emergency nursing core curriculum,* ed 5, Philadelphia, 2000, WB Saunders.
8. Hepp H: *Standards of flight nursing practice,* St Louis, 1995, Mosby.

# Contents

# MOSBY'S

# CEN®

# Examination
# REVIEW

## THIRD EDITION

# Part One

# EMERGENCY NURSING

# Chapter 1

# Emergency and Transport Nursing Education

## REVIEW OUTLINE

I. Emergency nursing education
- A. Knowledge in
    1. Pediatrics
    2. Obstetrics
    3. Medicine
    4. Cardiology
    5. Trauma
    6. Oncology
    7. Infectious diseases
    8. Psychosocial issues
    9. General patient management
    10. Safety issues (personal, environmental)
- B. Collaborative care with other health care providers
- C. Crisis intervention and stress management skills
- D. Demonstrated competency in management of equipment used in the emergency department
- E. Prehospital care environment
- F. Disaster preparation and response
- G. Weapons of mass destruction and effect: nuclear, biological, chemical
- H. Management of violence
- I. Reimbursement issues, managed care, health care reform
- J. Legal and ethical issues
- K. Triage
- L. Adult education principles
- M. Patient education principles: adult, child, and community
- N. Illness and injury prevention strategies
- O. Professional behaviors
    1. Autonomy
    2. Critical thinking
    3. Leadership
    4. Delegation
    5. Collaborative roles
- P. Emergency nursing standards

- Q. Advanced practice roles
    1. Advanced practice nurse (APN)
    2. Clinical nurse specialist (CNS)
    3. Nurse practitioner (NP)

II. Emergency nursing skills and competencies
- A. Performance of a primary survey and initiation of critical interventions
    1. Airway assessment and management (cervical spine immobilization in the injured patient)
    2. Breathing/ventilation assessment and management
    3. Circulation assessment and management
    4. Neurological assessment and management
    5. Exposure management
        a. Temperature
        b. Evidence collection
    6. Vital sign assessment and management
- B. Perform a secondary survey
    1. Obtain a patient history
        a. Chief complaint
        b. Mechanism of injury
        c. Medical history
        d. AMPLE history
    2. Review of the systems using inspection, palpation, auscultation, and percussion as indicated
        a. Neurological
        b. Cardiovascular
        c. Pulmonary
        d. Gastrointestinal
        e. Musculoskeletal
        f. Integumentary
        g. Genitourinary
        h. Psychosocial
        i. Family
    3. Diagnostic
        a. Laboratory values
        b. ECG

c. Gastric lavage

d. Whole blood glucose monitoring

4. Equipment management

a. Airway equipment

b. Ventilation equipment

c. Circulation equipment

d. C-spine immobilization

e. Basic life support (BLS) equipment

f. Advanced life support (ALS) equipment

g. Age-specific equipment (e.g., pediatric)

h. Illness- or injury-specific equipment (e.g., casts, splints, cervical traction)

III. Educational resources

A. Trauma nursing core course (TNCC)[1]

B. Emergency nursing pediatric course (ENPC)[2]

C. Emergency nursing core curriculum[3]

D. Standards of emergency nursing practice[4]

E. Emergency Nurses Association orientation program

F. Emergency nursing procedures[5]

IV. Flight and transport nursing education

A. Knowledge in

1. Basic life support (BLS)

2. Advanced cardiac life support (ALS)

3. Neonatal advanced life support (NALS)

4. Pediatric advanced life support (PALS)

5. Trauma (transport nurse advanced life support)

6. Safety (aircraft, scene, personnel)

7. Survival skills and competencies

8. Medical

9. Infectious diseases

10. Obstetrical

11. Altitude and flight physiology

12. Transport equipment

B. Communication

C. Public relations

D. Legal and ethical issues

E. Outreach education

F. Collaborative care

G. Prehospital care environment

V. Flight and transport nursing skills and competencies

A. Tracheal intubation

1. Endotracheal

2. Nasotracheal

B. Cricothyrotomy

C. Transtracheal jet ventilation

D. Laryngeotracheal mask intubation

E. Needle decompression

F. Chest tube insertion

G. Pericardiocentesis

H. Central line insertion

I. Venous cutdown

J. Escharotomy

K. Vaginal speculum examination

L. Fetal monitoring

M. Ventilator management

N. External pacer application

O. Intraaortic balloon pump

P. Blood and blood products administration

Q. Medication management and administration

R. Extrication management and safety

S. Triage

T. Disaster response

U. Weapons of mass destruction and effect: nuclear, biological, and chemical

VI. Educational resources

A. Transport nurse advanced trauma course (TNATC)[6]

B. Basic trauma life support (BTLS)

C. Neonatal resuscitation certification program

D. Prehospital trauma life support (PHTLS)

E. Trauma nurse specialist (TNS)

F. Mobile intensive care nurse (MICN)

G. Standards of flight nursing practice

H. Standards for ground transport

I. Flight nursing core curriculm[7]

The practice of emergency and transport nursing requires that nurses possess knowledge in all areas of patient care that they may encounter. Emergency and flight/transport nurses provide care for neonatal, pediatric, adult, and geriatric, medical, surgical, trauma, oncology, infectious diseases, and psychological emergencies. The patients may be suffering from minor to life-threatening emergencies. The question then becomes, How does one prepare for everything?

One of the most vital sources of education is experience. It is difficult to procure the knowledge that experience can teach. The more one is exposed to different types of patient care situations, the more comfortable and educated one becomes. The ability to become competent in one's practice is enhanced with experience and continuing education.

The nursing process is the model on which nursing care is based. Using the concepts of assessment, diagnosis, outcome identification, planning, implementation, and evaluation, the emergency and flight/transport nurse can plan care for individuals and groups of patients. Nurses care for the "whole" patient, including the family and environment in which the patient interacts. This process is what makes nurses different from the other health care professionals with whom we work, such as medical and prehospital care providers.

Emergency and transport nursing practice requires a team or collaborative approach to patient care. Depending on the nurses' skill levels and their job description, they may be responsible for additional advanced patient care interventions, such as endotracheal intubation or chest decompression.

Both emergency and transport nurses function in various roles in their practice, including direct patient care, research, education, management, consultation, advocacy, and administration. These roles alone require additional education and preparation in order to function with care and competence.

Emergency and transport nurses need to demonstrate that they are competent practitioners. Competence involves an integration of knowledge and technical skills, while applying the principles of the nursing practice. Competency is also a measure of one's professional growth.[8] Confusion arises as to what describes a competent emergency or transport nurse. Nursing practice varies from state to state, and emergency and flight nursing practice is definitely influenced by the types of patients for whom they provide care. For example, some emergency departments now routinely care for patients with invasive lines and intracranial pressure monitors, while some flight nurses perform transtracheal jet ventilation and insert central lines.

Transport nursing involves care in the field and in the transport vehicles, such as helicopter, fixed-wing aircraft, and ground ambulances. This requires additional training and education to ensure both patient and crew safety. Johnson, Childress, and Herron[9] found that 44, or 88% of the states in the United States have no nursing-oriented credentialing process for registered nurses who practice in the prehospital care environment. Some states require that nurses obtain additional certifications, such as EMT or EMT-P, before they can function in the prehospital environment.[9]

Another important role for the emergency transport nurse involves providing education for patients and the communities that we serve. The Joint Commission on Accreditation of Healthcare Organizations (JCAHO) and the American Hospital Association's Patients Bill of Rights address the need for patients and their families to be provided with information about their health care problems and how to manage them. Developing and providing educational programs for patient, family, and healthcare providers—including prehospital care providers—is an important responsibility of the practice of emergency and transport nursing.[10,11,12]

Both the Emergency Nurses Standard of Care and the Standards of Flight Nursing Practice (in the future

these will expand to include both ground and air transport) provide some guidelines for preparation and continuing education. The following outline contains a catalog of skills, courses, and reference books that may be helpful for educational preparation. As with life, it will continually change and grow, and, as practicing emergency and flight nurses, we must be open to the changes that are an integral part of our practice.

## REFERENCES

1. Jacobs BB: *Trauma nursing core course,* Park Ridge, Ill, 1995, Emergency Nurses Association.
2. Haley K, Baker P, & Eckles N: *Emergency nursing pediatric course,* Park Ridge, Ill, 1999, Emergency Nurses Association.
3. Jordan KS: *Emergency nursing core curriculum,* Philadelphia, 2000, WB Saunders.
4. Donatelli NS et al, editors: *Standards of emergency nursing practice,* ed. 3, St Louis, 1995, Mosby.
5. Proehl J: *Emergency nursing procedures,* ed 3, Philadelphia, 1999, WB Saunders.
6. DeJarnette R, et al: *Flight nurse advanced trauma nurse course manual,* Thorofare, NJ, 1994, National Flight Nurses Association.
7. Krupa D: *Flight nursing core curriculum,* Park Ridge, 1997, National Flight Nurses Association.
8. Ready R: Clinical competency testing for emergency nursing, *J Emerg Nurs* 20: 24-31, 1994.
9. Johnson R, Childress S, Herron H: Regulation of prehospital nursing practice: A national survey, *J Emerg Nurs* 19: 437-440, 1993.
10. Duffy M, Snyder K: Can ED patients read your patient education materials? *J Emerg Nurs* 25:294-297, 1999.
11. Hepp H: *Flight nursing standards of practice,* St Louis, 1995, Mosby.
12. McCafferty M: Teaching tools for heart failure, *J Emerg Nurs* 22: 451-453, 1996.

## ADDITIONAL READINGS

Alspach JG: *Core curriculum for critical care nursing,* ed. 5, Philadelphia, 1998, WB Saunders.
Cardona V, et al: *Trauma nursing: From resuscitation through rehabilitation,* Philadelphia, 1994, WB Saunders.
Kelley S: *Pediatric emergency nursing,* Norwalk, 1994, Appleton & Lange.
Kim MJ, McFarland G, McClane A: *Pocket guide to nursing diagnoses,* St Louis, 1993, Mosby.
Kitt S, et al: *Emergency nursing: A physiologic and clinical perspective,* Philadelphia, 1995, WB Saunders.
Semonin-Holleran R: *Flight nursing principles and practice,* St Louis, 1996, Mosby.
Neff J, Kidd P: *Trauma nursing: Art and science,* St Louis, 1993, Mosby.
Semonin Holleran R: *Prehospital nursing: a collaborative approach,* St Louis, 1994, Mosby.
Frazier E: *Standards for accreditation for medical transport systems,* ed 4, Anderson, SC, 1999, Commission on Accreditation of Medical Transport Systems.

# Chapter 2

# Patient Assessment and Priority Setting: Triage

## REVIEW OUTLINE

I. Definition of triage
  A. History of triage
    1. Military
    2. Civilian
  B. Types of triage
    1. Nursing
    2. Physician
    3. Paramedic, emergency medical technician (EMT)
    4. Disaster, multiple-casualty incident (MCI)
    5. Telephone triage
      a. Protocol based
      b. Nursing-judgment based
      c. Levels of expertise
II. Components of triage
  A. ABCs (airway, breathing, circulation)
  B. Chief complaint
  C. History
  D. Classification
  E. Documentation
  F. Pediatric triage[1,2]
    1. Based on growth and development
    2. Need to collect history from both caregiver and child
    3. Based on assessment of the ABCs, recognizing the differences between the pediatric patient and the adult patient
    4. Use of tables that provide "normal" pediatric values, such as blood pressure, pulse, respirations, and weight
    5. Pediatric assessment triangle
      a. Appearance
      b. Breathing
      c. Circulation to skin
    6. General inspection of the child, looking for things such as rashes or signs of abuse or neglect

7. CIAMPEDS[2]
  a. Chief complaint
  b. Immunizations
  c. Isolation
  d. Allergies
  e. Medications
  f. Medical history
  g. Parents' impressions of the child's condition
  h. Events surrounding the illness or injury
  i. Diet
  j. Diapers
  k. Symptoms associated with the illness or injury
III. Rapid patient assessment
  A. Basic cardiac life support (BCLS)
  B. Advanced cardiac life support (ACLS)
  C. Pediatric advanced life support (PALS)
  D. Emergency nursing pediatric course
  E. Trauma nursing core curriculum (TNCC)
  F. Basic trauma life support (BTLS)
  G. Advanced trauma life support (ATLS)
IV. Chief complaint
  A. P = provocation
  B. Q = quality
  C. R = region and radiation
  D. S = severity of the problem
  E. T = time
V. History
  A. History related to the chief complaint
  B. Medical history
  C. Allergies
  D. Cultural beliefs
  E. Family interaction
VI. Diversity assessment model[3]
  A. Assumptions: Taking for granted the ethnic background of the patient or family

B. Beliefs and behaviors of the patient, families, caregivers

C. Communication: how does the patient communicate

D. Diversity: the way in which people differ, i.e., age, race, ethnicity, gender, sexual orientation, spirituality, and so on

E. Education: learning about the patient's differences

VII. Vital signs

A. Blood pressure

B. Pulse

C. Respirations

   1. Pulse oximetry

D. Temperature

VIII. Physical assessment

A. Subjective data (See previous outline of History, and so on)

B. Objective data

   1. Inspection

   2. Palpation

   3. Auscultation

   4. Percussion

   5. Olfaction (odors)

C. Secondary assessment (review of the systems)

   1. Head

   2. ENT

   3. Chest

   4. Abdomen

   5. Pelvis/perineum

   6. Extremities

   7. Integument (skin)

D. Age-specific assessment

   1. Pediatric

   2. Geriatric

IX. Classification

A. Emergent, urgent, nonurgent

B. Immediate, expected, delayed care

C. Acute, nonacute

D. Emergency severity index[4]

   1. Scores range from 1 (resuscitation) to 5 (nonurgent) used along with an algorithm that includes chief complaint, vital signs, and narrative

X. Documentation

A. SOAP charting (subjective, objective, assessment, plan)

B. Chief complaint

C. History

D. Brief physical assessment

E. Family

F. Allergies

G. Tetanus status

H. Patients at risk for becoming violent

   1. Young males

   2. Gang members

   3. Intoxicated patients

   4. Patients with altered mental status

   5. Patients with psychiatric history

   6. Patients with history of violence

   7. Patients and family under stress

XI. Prehospital triage[5]

A. Primary information survey[5]

   1. Description of event

   2. Location and environment

B. Scene survey

C. Kinematics of injury

D. Levels of care

   1. Level I (academic hospital)

   2. Level II (community hospital)

   3. Level III (rural hospital)

E. Factors in patient assessment in prehospital triage

   1. Clinical status of the patient

   2. Nature and probable severity of the injury

   3. Scoring systems

      a. Glasgow coma scale

      b. Revised trauma score

      c. Baxt's trauma triage rule

   4. Type and availability of transportation

   5. Level of availability and accessibility of hospital care

XII. Nursing diagnoses

A. Airway clearance, ineffective

B. Breathing pattern, ineffective

C. Fluid volume deficit, high risk for

D. Injury, high risk for

E. Knowledge deficit

F. Pain (acute, chronic)

G. Rape-trauma syndrome

H. Spiritual distress (distress of the human spirit)

I. Tissue perfusion, altered

---

The word *triage* has its origin from the French, meaning "to pick, sort, select, or choose." The current use of triage in the emergency department is "to sort out" those in need of emergency services first.

The concept of medical triage evolved during battle, when Napoleon's surgeon developed a system that "sorted out" the wounded on the battlefield. The most critically injured were transported first. Florence Nightingale, using her now-famous lamp, went out during the night after battles during the Crimean War to "sort out" the remaining soldiers and offer them care.[3]

At the end of the nineteenth century, the English introduced the use of casualty and clearing stations where injuries were identified and first aid initiated. Based on their injuries, patients were then sent to an appropriate place for further treatment.[2,4]

During World War II and the Korean War, primary triage of the injured occurred on the battlefield, with secondary triage occurring at the battalion station, and the final destination being a MASH unit.[2,6]

The introduction of helicopter transport of the injured from the battlefield helped to increase the speed that victims were triaged and transported for care. Many casualties could be removed at the same time. Triage was done before and after air evacuation.[7,8]

Civilian triage within hospitals formally began in the 1960s. Physicians initially did triage, but nurses quickly assumed primary triage responsibilities.[3,4,5]

The goals of triage include early patient assessment, brief overall assessment, determination of urgency need, documentation of findings during patient assessment, control of patient flow through the emergency department, assignment of patients to the appropriate care area, initiation of diagnostic measures, initiation of therapeutic interventions, infection control, promotion of good public relations, and health education for patients and families.[1] The goals and their implementation vary from emergency department to emergency department.

In the prehospital or field environment, the goals of triage are not much different. The nurse needs to be able to rapidly assess, identify, and intervene as indicated by the patient's condition. When multiple patients are involved, the flight nurse and other team members will need to be able to recognize who is the emergent patient or patients and provide or assign the appropriate resources so that the patient is stabilized and quickly transported.

Of primary concern in both the prehospital and emergency department environment before triage can occur is safety. Surveying the scene and determining safety, whether it is at the site of the accident or at a referring facility, are the first steps in the triage process. Identifying a potentially unsafe situation or potentially violent patient is imperative to the safety of the nurse as well as emergency department staff and visitors.

Triaging in the emergency department and in the prehospital care environment is based on both art and science. Experience, as well as the science of nursing and medicine, helps the emergency and flight nurse make assessment decisions. The Journal of Emergency Nursing contains a section entitled "Triage Decisions," which provides case studies about specific patient problems that may be seen in the emergency department. These can provide an excellent review for the nurse studying for the Certification in Emergency Nursing

(CEN) examination and the Certification in Flight Nursing (CFRN) examination. *Prehospital and Disaster Medicine, Journal of Air Medical Transport,* and *AirMed* offer case studies that help sharpen one's triage skills by learning from others' experiences.[8]

## REVIEW QUESTIONS

*Three patients present to the triage nurse at one time. The first patient is a 48-year-old man complaining of left-sided chest pain radiating down his left arm. He is awake, diaphoretic, and pale. The second patient is a 3-year-old boy who is drooling and pale and can only breathe sitting straight up on his mother's lap. The third patient has sustained a laceration on his right hand. He currently has a dressing in place, and bright red blood is noted on the dressing. His vital signs are B/P 100/70 and P 100.*

1. Which patient should be taken into the emergency department first?
   - 0  A. The patient with the chest pain
   - 0  B. The child who is drooling
   - 0  C. The patient with the laceration
   - 0  D. Any patient who is bleeding

2. The triage nurse suspects that the child may have epiglottitis. What care should be provided in the triage area?
   - 0  A. Immediately remove the child from his mother and take him back to the treatment areas
   - 0  B. Take an oral temperature to determine if he has a fever and may require a dose of acetaminophen in the triage area
   - 0  C. Leave the child in his most comfortable position and take him as quickly as possible back to the patient care area
   - 0  D. Immediately start an intraosseous infusion to administer methylprednisone and a normal saline bolus

3. The triage nurse should base the initial care of this child on which of the following nursing diagnoses?
   - 0  A. Self-care deficit, feeding, related to the patient not being able to swallow any liquids for several days
   - 0  B. Infection, high risk for, related to his exposure to the influenza virus and possibility of having epiglottitis
   - 0  C. Airway clearance, ineffective, related to the patient's inability to keep his airway clear
   - 0  D. Family processes, altered, related to the patient's inability to interact with his mother because he is ill

4. Focused triage documentation for a patient with potential airway problems (as in this case) should include documentation of:
   - 0  A. Insurance coverage and family physician
   - 0  B. The IV site and catheter size
   - 0  C. Chest and lateral neck radiography results
   - 0  D. The patient's respiratory rate and effort

*An 18-year-old man comes to the triage area complaining of upper body weakness, as well as numbness and tingling in both hands. The patient states that he was involved in a fight the previous night and that his head was shoved between his legs. The patient is alert and oriented. Vital signs are B/P 110/70, P 64, R 18, and Temp 99° F. His pupils are equal and reactive. He is unable to keep his arms extended for longer than 5 seconds, and he cannot make a fist.*

5. The triage classification for this patient would be:
   - 0  A. Delayed care
   - 0  B. Emergent
   - 0  C. Urgent
   - 0  D. Nonurgent

6. The initial care provided by the triage nurse should include application of:
   - 0  A. Heat to the patient's neck
   - 0  B. Ice to the patient's neck
   - 0  C. A cervical collar for immobilization
   - 0  D. Elastic bandage wraps to the patient's hands

7. Of the following, which nursing diagnosis would be most appropriate for the care of this patient?
   - 0  A. Injury, high risk for, related to his spinal cord injury
   - 0  B. Fluid volume deficit, high risk for, related to his spinal cord injury
   - 0  C. Hyperthermia, related to his spinal cord injury
   - 0  D. Infection, high risk for, related to his spinal cord injury

8. Focused triage documentation for this patient (or any patient complaining of neurological trauma) should include documentation of:
   - 0  A. Adventitious breath sounds
   - 0  B. Peripheral and central pulses
   - 0  C. Paradoxical pulses
   - 0  D. Level of consciousness (GCS)

*A granddaughter brings her 83-year-old grandfather to the triage nurse. She states that he has taken 25 tablets of*

*Elavil, 50 mg. His wife recently died, and he is suffering from prostate cancer. The patient states that he has a "living will" and has the right to die. He is refusing to allow the triage nurse to assess him.*

9. Which of the following would be an appropriate action for the triage nurse to take?
   - 0  A. Allow the patient to leave
   - 0  B. Ask the granddaughter to leave
   - 0  C. Explain to the patient why he must stay
   - 0  D. Have the patient arrested

10. All of the following would be emergent conditions except:
   - 0  A. Obvious fractures without vascular compromise
   - 0  B. Hemorrhage from a wound
   - 0  C. Cardiopulmonary arrest
   - 0  D. Respiratory distress

11. Which of the following heart rates would alert the triage nurse to a problem in an infant?
   - 0  A. 120 beats per minute
   - 0  B. 160 beats per minute
   - 0  C. 130 beats per minute
   - 0  D. 220 beats per minute

12. The goals of triage include all of the following except:
   - 0  A. Control of patient flow through the emergency department
   - 0  B. Assignment of patients to appropriate care areas within the emergency department
   - 0  C. Performing and documenting a secondary survey on all patients who come to triage
   - 0  D. Determination of the urgency of the patient's condition

*The flight team has been called to the scene of a head-on motor vehicle crash. There are four victims involved. Victim 1 is a 2-year-old boy who has suffered a moderate head injury. His GCS is 12, but he is maintaining his airway. Victim 2 is an 18-year-old woman (probably the mother of the child). She has a GCS of 15, multiple orthopedic injuries, and severe abdominal pain. Her B/P is 90/40, P is 140, and R 32. Victim 3 is a 72-year-old man who is under full CPR. Finally, Victim 4 is a 70-year-old woman who has a GCS of 15. She is complaining of severe chest pain and shortness of breath. Her vital signs are B/P 80/50, P 120, and R 10. All victims were unrestrained. The helicopter can only transport one patient at a time. The closest facility is 40 miles from the scene of the accident.*

13. Which victim should be transported first?
    0  A. Victim 3
    0  B. Victim 1
    0  C. Victim 2
    0  D. Victim 4

14. Which victim should be transported second?
    0  A. Victim 3
    0  B. Victim 1
    0  C. Victim 2
    0  D. Victim 4

15. Which patient should not be transported by helicopter?
    0  A. Victim 3
    0  B. Victim 1
    0  C. Victim 2
    0  D. Victim 4

16. Respirations that are becoming faster and deeper, followed by a period of apnea, is described as:
    0  A. Kussmaul's breathing
    0  B. Eupnea
    0  C. Apneustic
    0  D. Cheyne-Stokes

17. Which of the following mnemonics may be used to determine and describe a patient's level of consciousness?
    0  A. PQRST
    0  B. AVPU
    0  C. TIPPS
    0  D. AEIOU

18. An example of objective patient data is:
    0  A. History of diabetes mellitus
    0  B. Complaint of pain in the left foot
    0  C. Brief neurological exam
    0  D. Precipitating event/onset of symptoms

19. Telephone triage:
    0  A. Involves decision making under conditions of certainty of what is wrong with the patient upon information gathered by talking with the patient
    0  B. Provides unlimited sensory input from the patient's verbal descriptions of their signs and symptoms
    0  C. Has demonstrated that it is an effective patient management tool and patients appear to be satisfied with it
    0  D. Can be performed by any nurse who has practiced in the emergency department for a year

20. Components of an effective telephone triage protocol include all of the following *except*:
    0  A. Clearly described and defined protocols addressing specific patient populations and the areas served
    0  B. A policy that states that nurses may never use their judgment in decision making about a patient's condition
    0  C. Experienced, educated nurses with education in telephone assessment and communication skills
    0  D. A continuous quality improvement program that evaluates telephone triage decisions and patient outcomes

## ANSWERS

1. **B. Assessment.** Based on rapid patient assessment using both basic and advanced life support principles (airway, breathing, circulation, neurological deficit, exposure [ABCDE], and history), the patient having airway difficulties should be taken into the emergency department first. A child who is drooling and only able to breathe comfortably sitting straight up may have epiglottitis and is at great risk of complete obstruction of his airway.[1-3]

2. **C. Intervention.** Since the child is currently able to comfortably maintain his airway, the triage nurse should leave the child in the position in which he is most comfortable. By removing him from his mother or performing any unnecessary procedures, the nurse may cause the child to become agitated and obstruct his airway.[1-3]

3. **C. Analysis.** Since the patient is having airway difficulties, airway clearance, ineffective, should be the initial nursing diagnosis on which the emergency nurse bases care. Defining characteristics of this nursing diagnosis include abnormal breath sounds, cyanosis, tachypnea, and dyspnea.

4. **D. Evaluation.** The patient's respiratory rate is an important piece of information for the patient who is having respiratory difficulties and should be documented on the triage record. One of the responsibilities of the triage nurse is to sort patients and determine the need for emergency services. The patient's vital signs provide the emergency nurse with observed information about the patient's cardiopulmonary status.[2]

5. **B. Assessment.** Based on rapid patient assessment using ABCDE, this patient would be an emergent patient. He has signs and symptoms of a neurological deficit that could place him at risk for additional complications related to injury of the cervical spine.[5,7]

6. **C. Intervention.** One of the goals of triage is the initiation of therapeutic interventions. Because this patient may have suffered a cervical spine injury, the initial care of this patient should include immobilization of the cervical spine.[1,3]

7. **A. Analysis.** The initial assessment of the patient demonstrates that he is currently in no acute distress, but, because of his mechanism of injury and symptoms, is at great risk for additional injury. Defining characteristics of this nursing diagnosis are divided into host factors such as sensory or motor deficits, tissue hypoxia, and cognitive impairment, agent factors such as chemical and mechanical energy, and environmental factors such as unsafe design, unsafe mode of transportation, and presence of pollutants.

8. **D. Evaluation.** Documentation of a neurological examination includes the level of consciousness, pupillary response, motor response, sensory response, and vital signs.

9. **C. Intervention.** The triage nurse should first try to explain to the patient that a living will does not allow the patient to deliberately harm himself. Rather, the living will allows the patient to decide whether or not medical or nursing care should be given if the patient is dying from natural causes. The emergency department is obligated to treat the patient.[8,9]

10. **A. Assessment.** One method of triage classification is the use of specific patient designations: emergent, urgent, and nonurgent. Emergent patients include those with cardiopulmonary arrest, chest pain indicative of a myocardial infarction, respiratory distress, severe trauma, and attempted suicide. Urgent patients include those with obvious fractures with vascular compromise, abdominal pain of less than 36 hours' duration, sudden headaches, vomiting, and jaundice. Nonurgent patients include those with sprains, minor burns, and closed fractures.[5,7]

11. **D. Assessment.** The normal infant's heart rate will range from 120 to 160 (newborn to 1 year of age). A heart rate greater than 200 is an indication of some type of problem.[1,2]

12. **C. Intervention.** Performing and documenting a secondary survey on all patients who come to triage is an unrealistic goal. The primary goal of triage is to recognize the ill or injured patient who requires treatment in a timely manner. Triage areas are generally not set up to perform an adequate secondary assessment.[5,7]

13. **D. Assessment.** Based on ABCs, the elderly patient having shortness of breath and a decreased respiratory rate should be transported first. The child has a lower GCS, but he is maintaining his airway.

14. **B. Assessment.** Even though the child is maintaining his airway, he has the potential to deteriorate because he has a moderate head injury and a GCS of 12. Based on the length of time and distance to a receiving facility, the child may be at greater risk of additional injury.[7]

15. **A. Assessment.** Patients who suffer a traumatic arrest have less than a 1% chance of survival, which would justify the flight team's decision not to transport the patient under full CPR.[8]

16. **D. Assessment.** Cheyne-Stokes respirations gradually become faster and deeper, then slower, followed by periods of apnea. Apneustic breathing is prolonged, gasping inspiration followed by short expiration. Eupnea is a description of normal respiratory rate and rhythm.[11]

17. **B. Assessment.** Many mnemonics exist that may be used in patient assessment. One that can be used to determine and describe a patient's level of consciousness is AVPU.
   a. A-alert
   b. V-responds to voice
   c. P-responds to painful stimuli
   d. U-unresponsive
   PQRST is a mnemonic that can be used to obtain information about patient history, and TIPPS and AEIOU provide descriptions of causes that may alter a patient's level of consciousness.[12]

18. **C. Assessment.** Objective data includes airway, breathing, circulation and a brief neurological exam.[12]

19. **C. Intervention.** Telephone triage has demonstrated that it can be an effective patient management tool, and patients have expressed satisfaction with the process, especially when it has kept them from unnecessary trips to the ED. However, patient assessment is limited, and only experienced, skilled nurses who receive specific training related to telephone triage should perform it.[13,14]

20. **B. Intervention.** Telephone triage policies, procedures, and protocols must allow for the exercise of nursing judgment when making decisions about the disposition of the patient. Protocols should only serve guidelines and should never be inflexible.[13,14]

## REFERENCES

1. Bracken J: Triage. In Newberry L, editor: *Sheehy's emergency nursing principles and practice,* ed 4, St Louis, 1998, Mosby.
2. Haley K, Eckles N, Baker P: *Emergency nursing core course,* Park Ridge, Ill, 1999, Emergency Nurses Association.

3. Emergency Nurses Association: *Approaching diversity: An interactive journey.* Park Ridge, IL, 1998, ENA.

4. Gilboy N, Travers D, Wuerz R: Re-evaluating triage in the new millennium: a comprehensive look at the need for standardization and quality. *J Emerg Nurs* 25(6):468-473, 1999.

5. Champion H: Prehospital triage. In *Trauma care systems,* Rockville, MD, 1986, Aspen Publications.

6. DeJarnette R et al: *Flight nurse advanced trauma course,* Thorofare, NJ, 1994, National Flight Nurses Association.

7. Rund DA, Rausch TS: *Triage,* St Louis, 1981, Mosby.

8. Semonin Holleran R: *Prehospital nursing: A collaborative approach,* St Louis, 1994, Mosby.

9. Ramler CL, Mohammed N: Triage. In Kitt S et al, editors: *Emergency nursing: a physiologic and clinical approach,* Philadelphia, 1995, WB Saunders.

10. Southard P: Legal and legislative considerations in emergency practice. In Kitt S et al, editors: *Emergency nursing: a physiologic and clinical approach,* Philadelphia, 1995, WB Saunders.

11. Sedlak K: Patient assessment. In Newberry L, editor: *Sheehy's emergency nursing principles and practice,* ed 4, 113-127. St Louis, 1998, Mosby.

12. Twedell D: Nursing process: Assessment and priority setting. In Jordan K, editor: *Emergency nursing core curriculum,* ed 5, Philadelphia, 2000, WB Saunders.

13. Rutenberg CD: What do we really know about telephone triage? *J Emerg Nurs* 26(1):76-78, 2000.

14. Emergency Nurses Association: *Telephone triage advice.* Des Plaines, IL, 1998, Emergency Nurses Association.

# Chapter 3

# Abdominal Emergencies

## REVIEW OUTLINE

I. Anatomy and physiology
  A. Right upper quadrant
    1. Liver
    2. Gallbladder
    3. Pylorus
    4. Duodenum
    5. Head of the pancreas
    6. Portion of the right kidney and adrenal gland
    7. Hepatic flexure of the colon
    8. Section of the ascending and transverse colon
  B. Left upper quadrant
    1. Left lobe of the liver
    2. Stomach
    3. Spleen
    4. Body of the pancreas
    5. Portion of the left kidney and adrenal gland
    6. Splenic flexure of the colon
    7. Sections of the transverse and descending colons
  C. Right lower quadrant
    1. Appendix
    2. Cecum
    3. Lower pole of right kidney
    4. Right ureter
    5. Right ovary
    6. Right spermatic cord
  D. Left lower quadrant
    1. Sigmoid colon
    2. Section of the descending colon
    3. Lower pole of the left kidney
    4. Left ureter
    5. Left ovary
    6. Left spermatic cord
  E. Abdominal vessels
    1. Mesentery
    2. Descending abdominal aorta
    3. Inferior vena cava
    4. Iliac artery
    5. Renal artery
  F. Physiology
    1. Digestion
    2. Absorption
    3. Elimination
    4. Bile production and excretion
    5. Liver functions
    6. Insulin production and use
    7. Red and white blood cell production and destruction

II. Abdominal assessment
  A. History
    1. Pain
      a. Location
      b. Quality
      c. Severity
      d. Radiation
      e. Temporal
      f. Provocation/relief
    2. Nausea/vomiting
      a. Onset
      b. Frequency
      c. Duration
      d. Amount
      e. Color, consistency
    3. Other associated symptoms
      a. Bleeding or bruising
      b. Change in bowel habit
      c. Change in appetite
      d. Recent weight change
      e. Fever, chills
    4. Mechanism of injury
      a. Blunt
      b. Penetrating
      c. Perversion
    5. Pertinent medical history
      a. Current or chronic diseases
      b. Past surgeries
      c. Current medications
        (1) Prescribed

(2) Over-the-counter

(3) Illicit

d. Allergies

e. Alcohol use

f. Recent travel (domestic, international)

B. Physical examination

1. General

a. Positioning

b. Facial expression

2. Vital signs: postural vital signs

3. Inspection

a. Skin

(1) Color

(2) Lesions

(3) Edema

(4) Superficial vascularity

(5) Open areas

b. Contour

(1) Symmetry

(2) Abdominal girth measurement

(3) Protuberance ("Six Fs" [fat, flatus, fetus, feces, fluid, fatal growth])

c. Movement

(1) Abdominal breathing

(2) Visible peristalsis

(3) Visible aortic pulsations (normal)

d. Signs of abdominal trauma/illness

(1) Cullen's sign

(2) Grey Turner's sign

(3) Coopernail's sign

4. Auscultation

a. Bowel sounds

(1) Location

(2) Present

(3) Absent

b. Bruits

c. Venous hum

d. Friction rub

5. Palpation

a. Light

b. Deep

c. Tenderness

d. Guarding

e. Rigidity

f. Rebound tenderness

g. Masses

h. McBurney's point

i. Rovsig's sign

j. Murphey's sign

6. Percussion

a. Dullness or resonance

b. Liver size

c. Borders of any masses

d. Fundus of urinary bladder

e. Costovertebral angle (CVA) tenderness

f. Ballance's sign

C. Diagnostic studies and procedures

1. Complete blood count (CBC) with differential

2. Electrolytes, blood urea nitrogen (BUN), blood glucose, creatinine

3. Amylase/lipase

4. Beta human chorionic gonadotropin (BHCG), blood, urine

5. Liver function tests: aspartate aminotransaminase (AST); alanine aminotransferase (ALT), lactate dehydrogenase (LDH), alkaline phosphatase

6. Coagulation studies

7. Type and screen or crossmatch

8. Blood for *Heliobacter pylori*

9. Sickle cell screen

10. Urinalysis

11. Urine culture

12. Stool for ova/parasites/occult blood/WBC/mucus, protein enzyme-linked immunosorbent assay (ELISA) of stool

13. Test (guiac) for presence of blood in feces, emesis, gastric drainage

14. Upright chest film

15. Upright, left lateral decubitus, flat abdominal x-ray films

16. Contrast studies

17. Scanning (CT with contrast, MRI)

18. Ultrasound

19. Gastroscopy, endoscopy, sigmoidoscopy

20. Peritoneal lavage

21. Local wound exploration

III. Related nursing diagnoses

A. Altered nutrition: less than body requirements

B. Constipation

C. Colonic constipation

D. Diarrhea

E. Infection: potential for

F. Altered gastrointestinal tissue perfusion

G. Fluid volume deficit

H. Tissue perfusion: altered (gastrointestinal, renal)

I. High risk for fluid volume deficit

J. Impaired physical mobility

K. Altered health maintenance

L. Knowledge deficit

M. Pain

N. Chronic pain

IV. Collaborative care of the patient with an abdominal emergency
- A. Ongoing abdominal assessments
- B. Oxygen therapy
- C. Monitoring
  1. Vital signs
  2. Cardiac monitoring
  3. Intake and output
- D. Intravenous fluids
- E. Blood administration
- F. Gastric decompression
- G. Identification and control of bleeding
  1. Cool saline lavage (controversial)
  2. Balloon tamponade
- H. Autotransfusion
  1. Mechanical autotransfer
  2. Pneumatic antishock garment (controversial)
- I. Peritoneal lavage
- J. Urinary catheter
- K. Pharmacological intervention
  1. Analgesics
  2. Antibiotics
  3. Antiemetics
  4. Antispasmodics, anticholinergics
  5. Histamine receptor antagonists
  6. Antacids
  7. Vasopressors
- L. Emotional/psychological support
- M. Patient/family teaching

V. Specific abdominal emergencies
- A. Inflammatory conditions
  1. Gastritis
  2. Gastroenteritis
  3. Appendicitis
  4. Pancreatitis
  5. Cholecystitis
  6. Diverticulitis
  7. Hepatitis
  8. Irritable bowel syndrome
- B. Intestinal obstruction
- C. Intussusception
- D. Esophageal varices
- E. Gastric or duodenal ulcers
- F. Gastroesophageal reflux disorder
- G. Abdominal aortic aneurysm
- H. Mesenteric ischemia
- I. Abdominal trauma
  1. Penetrating
     a. Gunshot wounds
     b. Stab wounds
     c. Shrapnel wounds
  2. Blunt
     a. Organ contusion
     b. Organ laceration
     c. Organ rupture
  3. Insertion of foreign bodies

A bdominal pain or discomfort is one of the most common complaints expressed by patients who come to the emergency department for care.[1] Abdominal pain may be the manifestation of an acute process or a chronic, longstanding problem. Pain may arise from one of many systems located in the abdomen. The gastrointestinal, genitourinary, and reproductive systems occupy most of the organ space in the abdominal cavity. In addition, the vascular and musculoskeletal systems may be involved, especially when bleeding or inflammation is present. Likewise, trauma to the abdomen may involve multiple systems. The abdominal cavity is large and located anteriorly, making it more susceptible to both blunt and penetrating injury. As the diaphragm rises with expiration, the abdominal cavity size increases, and injury to its contents may occur with a lower chest injury. Blunt trauma results in a force being diffused throughout the abdomen. Penetrating injury, caused by any object that penetrates the abdominal wall, usually a bullet, knife, or some type of missile, injures anything in its path.[2] When solid organs of the abdomen, such as the liver, spleen, and kidneys, are injured, significant bleeding results. When hollow organs, such as the stomach and intestines, are damaged, their contents spill, causing massive irritation and infection.

Abdominal pain may be classified according to type. These include visceral, parietal, referred, abdominal pain caused by metabolic disease, neurogenic, and psychogenic pain. Visceral pain, so named because the stretching of a hollow viscus causes it, is characterized by diffuse, crampy pain varying in intensity. Many inflammatory conditions, such as appendicitis, cholecystitis, pancreatitis, and intestinal obstruction, present with visceral pain. The second type, somatic or parietal pain, is a result of bacterial or chemical irritation of nerve fibers. This type of pain is sharp and localized. The patient suffering from somatic pain characteristically assumes the fetal position, either on the side or supine with knees flexed, attempting to prevent any movement that will result in increased pain. The third type of abdominal pain, referred pain, is felt some distance from the source.[1,3] A classic example of referred pain is seen in renal colic, when the pain is located in the groin and external genitalia. Metabolic diseases such as porphyria and lead poisoning cause abdominal pain because they irritate the alimentary tract. Neurogenic abdominal pain results from an irritation of the nerves in the abdomen. The source of the pain can be from the spinal cord or from diseases such as diabetes. Finally, patients may suffer from abdominal pain when there is no organic dysfunction. Life stresses can contribute to intestinal spasms and hypersecretion of stomach acids.[4] Research has also demonstrated that abdominal pain related to diseases such as peptic ulcer disease may actually be caused by an infection rather than excessive acid secretion. *H. pylori* has been implicated in over 80% of peptic ulcer disease.[4]

Diarrhea, a common symptom associated with abdominal pain and discomfort has emerged as a potentially serious health care problem. Diarrhea from person-to-person contact (rotavirus) and from food-borne transmission causes many patients to visit the emergency department each year. Diarrhea can result from antibiotic use, travel, sexual transmission, and day care. Depending on the age of the patient and the type of diarrhea, severe and even lethal complications can occur.[5]

Initial nursing care of the patient with an abdominal emergency is based on subjective and objective assessments. When evaluating the patient, the emergency nurse needs to keep in mind what may be the source of the patient's pain by the location (e.g., the right upper quadrant). A general overview of the patient, including the position he or she assumes, facial expression, and skin color, temperature, and moisture, may give an indication as to the type and severity of pain. Vital signs give important baseline information.

A subjective assessment or history using the PQRST mnemonic (provocation, quality, radiation, severity, timing) is a useful tool in evaluating the patient with an abdominal complaint. It is useful to have the patient point with one finger to where the pain or discomfort is. If the problem cannot be localized, it offers some additional assessment information about the nature of the patient's complaint. Associated signs and symptoms such as nausea, vomiting, fever, or chills will assist in determining which system or systems need further evaluation.

Recognizing abdominal trauma is vital to patient management but is sometimes difficult. The mechanism of injury must be carefully assessed to determine abdominal involvement. In multiple trauma (i.e., trauma involving two or more body systems), abdominal injury is assumed until it has been ruled out. The goal or emergency care in abdominal trauma is to determine whether the patient requires surgery and not to isolate specific injuries.

General management of the patient with an abdominal emergency is determined by evaluation of the ABCs (airway, breathing, circulation) and the initial assessment. Intravenous access for laboratory studies, fluids, and medications is indicated. Other laboratory specimens, such as urine and peritoneal lavage fluid, may be needed. The use of the abdominal CT with contrast and ultrasound has become a foundation for the evaluation of abdominal trauma. Fewer patients are being treated in the operating room and are instead being managed by close observation and initiation of critical interventions as indicated by the patient's injury and condition.[6]

Gastric decompression and bladder catheterization are frequent interventions. Pain management through nursing comfort measures until, and in addition to, pharmacological intervention is important. Infection prevention and/or treatment are indicated. Finally, preparation for admission or discharge involves patient and family teaching and, at discharge, follow-up instructions.[3]

## REVIEW QUESTIONS

1. The correct sequence for performing a physical assessment of the abdomen is:
   - O A. Inspection, palpation, auscultation, percussion
   - O B. Inspection, auscultation, palpation, percussion
   - O C. Inspection, percussion, palpation, auscultation
   - O D. Palpation, auscultation, inspection, percussion

2. When palpating a painful abdomen, the emergency nurse should do which of the following?
   - O A. Palpate nonpainful areas first, then painful areas
   - O B. Begin with deep palpation first, then move to lighter palpation
   - O C. Cover the patient's face when palpating the abdomen to decrease embarrassment
   - O D. Never palpate the abdomen without the physician's permission

3. When assessing the abdomen, the emergency nurse remembers that:
   - O A. Deep palpation should never be used
   - O B. Deep palpation should be performed if splenomegaly is present
   - O C. Normally, one should not be able to palpate the spleen
   - O D. Normally, one should not be able to palpate the liver

4. When listening for bowel sounds, the emergency nurse should remember that:
   - 0  A. Adequate assessment of bowel sounds takes 5 minutes
   - 0  B. Absent bowel sounds always indicate a bowel obstruction
   - 0  C. Audible bowel sounds automatically rule out any GI obstruction
   - 0  D. It is normal to hear bowel sounds in the thoracic cavity

5. If rebound tenderness is found when assessing the abdomen, the emergency nurse knows that:
   - 0  A. It is frequently a sign of a malignancy
   - 0  B. It is normal to have abdominal rebound tenderness
   - 0  C. Rebound tenderness is a sign of peritoneal irritation
   - 0  D. Rebound tenderness indicates a positive beta human chorionic gonadotropin (BHCG)

6. When inspecting a patient's abdomen, the nurse notices an area of ecchymosis around the umbilicus. This is known as:
   - 0  A. Cullen's sign
   - 0  B. Grey Turner's sign
   - 0  C. Chandelier's sign
   - 0  D. McBurney's sign

7. The diagnostic evaluation of a woman of childbearing age with abdominal pain must include:
   - 0  A. Postural vital signs
   - 0  B. Amylase and lipase levels
   - 0  C. BHCG level
   - 0  D. Pap smear

8. All abdominal pain, no matter how minor, is considered to be an emergency:
   - 0  A. In the elderly
   - 0  B. In women of childbearing age
   - 0  C. Until it is relieved
   - 0  D. Until it is diagnosed

## Gastritis

9. Factors that may provoke the symptoms of gastritis include all of the following except:
   - 0  A. Smoking tobacco
   - 0  B. Taking aspirin (ASA) for pain management
   - 0  C. A parent with gastritis
   - 0  D. Meditation and exercise

10. The most common cause of superficial gastritis is:
   - 0  A. Excessive hard alcohol ingestion
   - 0  B. Infection with *H. pylori*
   - 0  C. Severe physiologic stress
   - 0  D. Ingestion of nonsteroidal antiinflammatory drugs (NSAIDs) for arthritis pain

11. The primary treatment for superficial gastritis is:
   - 0  A. Taking antacids such as Maalox every 2 hours
   - 0  B. Taking only antisecretory drugs such as cimetidine or ranitidine
   - 0  C. Changing one's eating habits to eliminate all spices
   - 0  D. Taking a combination of antimicrobial agents and antisecretory drugs

## Bowel Obstruction

12. The four hallmark signs of a bowel obstruction are:
   - 0  A. Absent bowel sounds, nausea, vomiting, and cramping
   - 0  B. Abdominal pain, abdominal distention, vomiting, and constipation
   - 0  C. Hyperactive bowel sounds, distention, fever, and vomiting stool
   - 0  D. Anorexia, normal bowel sounds, vomiting, and cramping

13. All of the following interventions are therapeutic for a patient with a bowel obstruction except:
   - 0  A. Nothing by mouth
   - 0  B. Gastric tube to low suction
   - 0  C. Enemas until bowel is clear
   - 0  D. Intravenous (IV) fluids for rehydration

## Gastroenteritis

14. Acute gastroenteritis is considered more serious in what patient population?
   - 0  A. Athletes
   - 0  B. Infants
   - 0  C. Middle-aged men
   - 0  D. Postpartum women

15. With the persistent vomiting and diarrhea that accompanies acute gastroenteritis, the patient is a candidate for which nursing diagnosis?
   - 0  A. Injury, potential for
   - 0  B. Ineffective airway clearance
   - 0  C. Fluid volume deficit
   - 0  D. Impaired skin integrity

16. Discharge teaching instructions to a patient who has been treated for gastroenteritis should include all of the following except:
    - ○ A. Do not eat or drink anything for 72 hours
    - ○ B. Wash hands, dishes, and eating utensils thoroughly before eating
    - ○ C. Drink an electrolyte replacement solution (e.g., Gatorade, Pedialyte) for the next 24 hours, then advance to regular diet as tolerated
    - ○ D. Throw out any foods that you think may be contaminated or spoiled

17. The most common cause of diarrhea in young children is:
    - ○ A. *Salmonella*
    - ○ B. *Cryptosporidium*
    - ○ C. Adenovirus
    - ○ D. Rotavirus

18. A 3-year-old is brought to the emergency department by his caregiver because of continued abdominal pain and watery diarrhea. When obtaining a history related to his present illness, an important risk factor to identify would be:
    - ○ A. Current diet the child has been on
    - ○ B. Recent use of antibiotics
    - ○ C. Time spent at a day care center
    - ○ D. All of the above

19. A clinical sign that would indicate that the child is suffering severe dehydration is:
    - ○ A. The presence of sunken eyeballs
    - ○ B. The absence of tears
    - ○ C. An increased heart rate
    - ○ D. A slightly increased respiratory rate

20. The child who is mildly dehydrated should initially be treated with:
    - ○ A. A fluid bolus of 20 ml/kg of $D_5W$ over 20 minutes
    - ○ B. A balanced electrolyte solution by mouth
    - ○ C. A fluid bolus of 20 ml/kg of crystalloid solution
    - ○ D. No fluids until the source of the dehydration is identified

## Intussusception

*A young mother brings in her 18-month-old child to the emergency department. She states that he began crying a lot and holding his left lower abdominal area about 4 hours ago. Since then he has vomited twice and after that he had one small stool that looked like "red jelly." She also states she "felt a lump in his stomach where he hurts."*

21. Based on the above information and these symptoms, you suspect:
    - ○ A. Child maltreatment
    - ○ B. Foreign body aspiration
    - ○ C. Intussusception
    - ○ D. Mesenteric injury

22. The emergency physician orders a barium enema. The emergency nurse knows that:
    - ○ A. A barium enema is contraindicated in children no matter what the clinical findings
    - ○ B. A barium enema is diagnostic for intussusception and may even reduce it and eliminate the need for surgery
    - ○ C. Soapsuds enemas until clear will be required before this test can be initiated
    - ○ D. A barium enema will cause intestinal perforation and contribute to the child developing peritonitis

## Appendicitis

*An 18-year-old man is brought to the emergency department with a 12-hour history of abdominal pain. Initially vague and generalized, the pain is now concentrated in his right lower quadrant. Vital signs are B/P 108/60, P 112, R 24, Temp 100.8° F. A diagnosis of acute appendicitis is suspected.*

23. All of the following would be considered a normal finding in acute appendicitis except:
    - ○ A. A pulsatile abdominal mass
    - ○ B. Rebound tenderness
    - ○ C. Nausea with possible vomiting
    - ○ D. Low-grade temperature elevation

24. Which symptoms would best indicate that the appendix might have ruptured?
    - ○ A. Projectile vomiting
    - ○ B. Temperature spikes to 104° F
    - ○ C. Watery, mucoid diarrhea
    - ○ D. Bright red vomitus

25. Five minutes after this patient arrives in the emergency department, which initial nursing action would be inappropriate?
    - ○ A. Explaining upcoming tests and procedures
    - ○ B. Obtaining laboratory specimens
    - ○ C. Continued ongoing assessments
    - ○ D. Giving parenteral analgesics

26. The possibility for unrecognized perforation of the appendix increases:
   - 0 A. In the elderly patient
   - 0 B. In the adolescent patient
   - 0 C. In the middle-age patient
   - 0 D. In the school-age patient

## Pancreatitis

*A 42-year-old man arrives in the emergency department by squad with a 1-day history of epigastric pain radiating through to the mid-back area with nausea and vomiting twice. A diagnosis of pancreatitis is suspected.*

27. Which statement about pancreatitis is true?
   - 0 A. It does not affect the respiratory status of the patient
   - 0 B. It is generally not very painful
   - 0 C. It can be caused by biliary disease
   - 0 D. It only occurs in alcoholics

28. The treatment of pancreatitis would include all of the following except:
   - 0 A. IV fluids for rehydration
   - 0 B. Gastric tube to decrease abdominal distention and vomiting
   - 0 C. Parenteral doses of morphine or codeine for pain
   - 0 D. Parenteral antiemetics to decrease nausea and vomiting

29. A patient with acute pancreatitis is at risk for all of the following potential nursing diagnoses except:
   - 0 A. Fluid volume deficit
   - 0 B. Infection, potential for
   - 0 C. Gas exchange, impaired
   - 0 D. Cardiac output, increased

30. The diagnosis of acute pancreatitis is best confirmed by:
   - 0 A. An elevated white blood cell count
   - 0 B. A markedly elevated amylase level
   - 0 C. Air fluid levels on abdominal x-ray films
   - 0 D. A guaiac-negative emesis and stool test

## Cholecystitis

31. The most common cause of cholecystitis is:
   - 0 A. Cholelithiasis
   - 0 B. Gastritis
   - 0 C. Alcohol consumption
   - 0 D. Smoking

32. When caring for a patient with cholecystitis, what statement made by the patient would be the most important to communicate to the doctor?
   - 0 A. "I vomited twice before coming in tonight."
   - 0 B. "I ate chili dogs and French fries tonight for supper."
   - 0 C. "I hurt in my right side."
   - 0 D. "I've been wanting to see a doctor about this for weeks."

33. Cholecystitis usually affects:
   - 0 A. Thin, fair-skinned males
   - 0 B. Middle-age, fair-skinned females
   - 0 C. Premature, non-breastfed infants
   - 0 D. Middle-age women who have never been pregnant

## Diverticulitis

34. All of the following statements about diverticulitis are true except:
   - 0 A. It is thought to be due to high-fat diets and stress
   - 0 B. The symptoms of an acute attack can mimic appendicitis
   - 0 C. Antibiotics are usually recommended
   - 0 D. Gastric suction should always be used

## Esophageal Varices

*A 52-year-old man is transferred to the emergency department from the local county jail after vomiting a large amount of bright red blood. History includes a long history of alcoholism and hepatitis. He is lethargic and restless. Marked ascites is present. He denies any acute pain. B/P 100/66, P 110, R 32, Temp 100.0° F. He gags and vomits 500 ml bright red blood upon arrival to the emergency department. A diagnosis of bleeding esophageal varices is suspected.*

35. Based on his presentation, the most urgent nursing diagnosis would be:
   - 0 A. Infection, potential for
   - 0 B. Nutrition, altered (potential for)
   - 0 C. Airway clearance, ineffective
   - 0 D. Impaired physical mobility

36. Esophageal varices:
   - 0 A. May rupture spontaneously, causing rapid exsanguination and death
   - 0 B. Are enlarged arterial channels dilated by portal hypertension
   - 0 C. Decrease as portal hypertension increases with medical treatment
   - 0 D. Are not caused by alcoholic cirrhosis in the United States

**37.** Gastric decompression and lavage for this patient would be best accomplished with the use of:

0   A. Salem sump gastric tube

0   B. Levine gastric tube

0   C. Sengstaken-Blakemore gastric tube

0   D. Gastrostomy tube

**38.** Additional interventions that would be appropriate for a patient with bleeding esophageal varices include all of the following except:

0   A. Initiation of two large-bore IV lines

0   B. Dopamine (Intropin) IV maintenance drip

0   C. Close monitoring of vital signs

0   D. Vasopressin (Pitressin) IV maintenance drip

## Irritable Bowel Syndrome

**39.** Clinical symptoms of irritable bowel syndrome include:

0   A. Acute abdominal pain located around the umbilicus

0   B. Regular disturbance of defecation with only diarrhea

0   C. Nausea with projectile vomiting

0   D. Recurrent, episodic, cramplike abdominal pain

**40.** Irritable bowel syndrome is diagnosed by:

0   A. Laboratory values that demonstrate bowel inflammation

0   B. A careful history and physical examination

0   C. An emergent abdominal CT with contrast

0   D. Placing the patient on laxatives for constipation

**41.** One of the significant differences between Crohn's disease and ulcerative colitis is:

0   A. Diffuse abdominal pain

0   B. Frequent episodes of diarrhea

0   C. Considerable weight gain

0   D. Rectal bleeding

**42.** The most common cause of diarrhea is:

0   A. Ingestion of toxins

0   B. Infections

0   C. Food intolerance

0   D. Psychological stress

**43.** A common side effect of diphenoxylate and atropine (Lomotil) is:

0   A. Hypothermia

0   B. Bradycardia

0   C. Dry mouth

0   D. Renal failure

## Abdominal Trauma

**44.** Factors known to contribute to the development of abdominal trauma include:

0   A. Improperly worn seatbelts

0   B. A bent or broken steering wheel

0   C. Rapid acceleration/deceleration injuries

0   D. All of the above

**45.** A patient sustaining liver trauma may be especially prone to developing:

0   A. Coagulopathies

0   B. Hypervolemia

0   C. Fatty emboli

0   D. Peritonitis

**46.** Which of the following mechanisms of injury would predispose a patient to splenic trauma?

0   A. Penetrating trauma to the right upper quadrant

0   B. Blunt trauma to the left upper quadrant

0   C. Blunt trauma to the pelvis

0   D. Penetrating trauma to the left femur

**47.** Referred pain in the left shoulder area is referred to as a:

0   A. Cullen's sign

0   B. Grey Turner's sign

0   C. Chvostek's sign

0   D. Kehr's sign

**48.** The emergency nurse knows that with a ruptured spleen:

0   A. The patient will always present in shock

0   B. There may be a delayed rupture and no symptoms

0   C. Bleeding cannot occur within the splenic capsule

0   D. It cannot occur from deep abdominal palpation

**49.** One of the most common methods used to evaluate the stable patient with abdominal trauma is:

0   A. Abdominal CT with contrast

0   B. Diagnostic peritoneal lavage

0   C. Flat plate of the abdomen

0   D. Exploratory laporatomy

**50.** Postsplenectomy patients are especially prone to and need to be vaccinated against:

0   A. Swine influenza

0   B. Tetanus

0   C. Guillain-Barré syndrome

0   D. Pneumoccocal pneumonia

51. Blunt abdominal trauma is considered to be more deadly than penetrating abdominal trauma because:
    0   A.  Blunt abdominal trauma is more common in men than women
    0   B.  Blunt abdominal trauma is hidden and more difficult to diagnose than penetrating abdominal trauma
    0   C.  Penetrating abdominal trauma is more common in the elderly than young adults
    0   D.  Penetrating abdominal trauma involves a diagnostic peritoneal lavage and blunt abdominal trauma does not

52. In caring for a patient with penetrating abdominal trauma resulting in a partial evisceration of the small intestine, the best nursing action would be to:
    0   A.  Make a gentle attempt to force the organ back into the abdomen
    0   B.  Irrigate the organs with warmed normal saline solution
    0   C.  Cover the organs with moist normal saline dressings
    0   D.  Encourage the patient to cough and breathe deeply

53. Diaphragmatic injury should be suspected when:
    0   A.  The gastric tube is in the right chest on radiograph
    0   B.  Bowel sounds are auscultated in the chest cavity
    0   C.  Blood is obtained upon insertion of a left-sided chest tube
    0   D.  Hematuria is obtained with insertion of a urinary catheter

## Abdominal Aortic Aneurysm

*Mr. West, a 70-year-old man, arrives by squad into the emergency department complaining of intense lower back and lower abdominal pain of 1-hour duration. No nausea or vomiting. His wife states he fainted while sitting on the commode at home. Medical history is positive for mild hypertension. The patient is rapidly being evaluated for a dissecting abdominal aortic aneurysm. B/P 100/52, P 120, R 30, Temp 96.4° F.*

54. In the diagnosis of a dissecting abdominal aortic aneurysm, which emergency diagnostic test would be of most value?
    0   A.  Diagnostic peritoneal lavage
    0   B.  CT scan of abdomen
    0   C.  Abdominal ultrasound
    0   D.  Magnetic resonance imaging (MRI)

55. The most applicable nursing diagnosis for this patient would be:
    0   A.  Tissue perfusion, altered
    0   B.  Infection, potential for
    0   C.  Airway clearance, ineffective
    0   D.  Injury, potential for

56. The pain associated with a dissecting abdominal aortic aneurysm is frequently described as:
    0   A.  Stabbing
    0   B.  Dull ache
    0   C.  Sharp, tearing
    0   D.  Crushing

57. Mr. West wants to see his wife, who is out in the waiting room. The best response would be to say:
    0   A.  "You are too sick to have any visitors."
    0   B.  "You can see her after you have surgery."
    0   C.  "Ask the doctor if you can have visitors."
    0   D.  "I'll bring her in now."

58. Which of the following drugs would be used to manage hypertension in the patient with an abdominal aortic aneurysm?
    0   A.  Dopamine
    0   B.  Dobutamine
    0   C.  Metoprolol
    0   D.  Nitroprusside

## Mesenteric Ischemia

59. Major contributing factors that increase the development of mesenteric ischemia include:
    0   A.  Cardiac disease
    0   B.  Sepsis
    0   C.  Coagulation disorders
    0   D.  All of the above

60. The following are symptoms of mesenteric ischemia except:
    0   A.  Generalized, vague abdominal pain
    0   B.  Abdominal distention and no bowel sounds
    0   C.  Presence of free air on abdominal x-ray films
    0   D.  No formed bowel movements and foul-smelling diarrhea

## ANSWERS

1. **B. Assessment.** The correct sequence for a physical assessment of the abdomen is inspection, auscultation, palpation, and percussion. The abdomen should be auscultated prior to any hands-on assess-

ment. Touching the abdomen may distort bowel sounds as well as cause pain or discomfort that would impede any further attempts at an examination.[7]

2. **A. Assessment.** In palpating a painful abdomen, the nurse should do all of the following: palpate nonpainful areas first, then painful areas last; begin with light palpation, then move to deeper palpation last; and always observe the patient's face and other behaviors while palpating.[7]

3. **C. Assessment.** The spleen would have to swell to nearly three times its size to be palpated. In this case, deep palpation should never be used when splenomegaly is suspected due to the possibility of rupturing the organ. However, deep palpation is a routine part of the physical assessment of the abdomen.[7]

4. **A. Assessment.** The presence or absence of bowel sounds does not necessarily rule in or rule out a gastrointestinal disorder. Although they are still an important part of the physical assessment of the abdomen, their diagnostic value is questionable.[7]

5. **C. Assessment.** Rebound tenderness, pain that occurs when pressure is applied to the area and then released, develops when irritated tissues and peritoneal fluid surround an inflamed appendix. It is commonly seen in patients who have peritonitis and/or appendicitis.[3]

6. **A. Assessment.** Cullen's sign, a periumbilical ecchymosis, is indicative of blood in the peritoneum and is considered a potentially serious sign. Grey Turner's sign is ecchymosis over the flank area resulting from retroperitoneal bleeding. Chandelier's sign, extreme pain (and jumping) when the cervix is touched during a pelvic exam, is indicative of an acute pelvic infection, especially pelvic inflammatory disease (PID). McBurney's sign is tenderness at McBurney's point (the right lower quadrant, 2 inches from the right anterior superior spine of the ileum), which is suggestive of acute appendicitis.[3]

7. **C. Assessment.** In the emergency department, all women of childbearing age are assumed to be pregnant until proved otherwise by a documented negative serum beta human chorionic gonadotropin (BHCG). Many expert clinicians have been "burned" when they forget this basic emergency care rule.[2]

8. **D. Assessment.** All abdominal pain is an emergency until it is diagnosed. It is easy for experienced emergency nurses to be unimpressed with abdominal pain patients. Do not get caught in this trap. Abdominal pain has many potentially life-threatening origins and it should always be thoroughly evaluated.[8]

9. **D. Assessment.** Meditation and exercise are methods that are used to decrease patient stress and decrease the risk of developing gastritis.[9]

10. **B. Assessment.** The most common cause of peptic ulcer disease is *Helicobacter pylori*.[4]

11. **D. Intervention.** The treatment of superficial gastritis is based upon a combination of treatments. If it has been determined that *H. pylori* is the primary cause of the disease process, antimicrobial therapy is initiated, along with an $H_2$ receptor antagonist such as ranitidine. An effectiveness of about 90% was found with a combination of ranitidine, metronidazole, and amoxicillin.[4]

12. **B. Assessment.** The four hallmark signs of a bowel obstruction are (1) abdominal pain, (2) abdominal distention, (3) vomiting, and (4) marked constipation. Again, bowel sounds assessment is not completely reliable.[10]

13. **C. Intervention.** Generally enemas are contraindicated for a patient who has a bowel obstruction. They may cause more harm than good. Remember, the constipation is not necessarily the cause of the obstruction. Keeping the patient NPO, inserting a gasric tube to low suction, and administering IV fluids for rehydration are the basic necessities for a patient with bowel obstruction distress.[10]

14. **B. Assessment.** Infants are less able to tolerate any change in their body fluid status than any other patient population. They are closely followed by the elderly. Infants and small children will dehydrate rapidly, in a matter of hours.[11]

15. **C. Analysis.** Fluid volume deficit is the applicable nursing diagnosis due to the potential for dehydration that accompanies acute gastroenteritis. Potential for injury, ineffective airway clearance, and impaired skin integrity would not apply.

16. **A. Intervention.** A patient with gastroenteritis should drink plenty of fluids, especially an electrolyte replacement solution, then advance to a regular diet. Good handwashing and washing of dishes are crucial, as is disposing of any foods thought to be contaminated.

17. **D. Assessment.** The most common cause of diarrhea in young children is rotavirus, which accounts for 80% of diarrhea infections.[11]

18. **D. Assessment.** Potential causes of diarrhea in children include raw foods, recent use of antibiotics, which may cause *Clostridium difficile*, and time spent at a day care center, which can contribute to exposure to rotavirus, *giardiasis*, and *shigella*.[11]

19. **B. Assessment.** A clinical sign of severe diarrhea is the absence of tearing. It is true that the child's

heart rate will increase, but that is a significant sign of moderate dehydration as well.[11]

20. **B. Intervention.** The initial treatment of mild dehydration should be accomplished through oral hydration with a balanced electrolyte solution as long as the child can tolerate oral fluids.[11]

21. **C. Assessment.** This child has virtually every symptom of intussusception, a telescoping of the lumen of the bowel that occurs mainly in infants and children. It most commonly develops at or near the ileocecal valve or at the point of attachment of a colon tumor, polyp, or Meckel's diverticulum. Death can occur within 2 to 4 days because of the compromised blood supply to the bowel and mesentery and the resulting sepsis and gangrene.[12]

22. **B. Intervention.** A barium enema is diagnostic of intussusception and may even reduce it, thus eliminating the need for surgery. A soapsuds enema would not be helpful at this point.[12]

23. **A. Assessment.** A pulsatile mass is suggestive of an abdominal aortic aneurysm, not appendicitis. Symptoms of appendicitis commonly occur in children and young adults and include anorexia, nausea, vomiting, right lower- quadrant pain, rebound tenderness, low-grade fever, and an elevated white blood cell count with shift.[9]

24. **B. Assessment.** A temperature spike may be seen a few hours after the appendix has ruptured. Surprisingly, there may also be an initial relief of pain with an appendix rupture, then a few hours later, fever and worsening abdominal pain.[9]

25. **D. Intervention.** It is sometimes unwise to relieve abdominal pain until it is diagnosed because the symptoms can be masked by the analgesics. Recently, some clinicians disagreed with this rule and instead recommended medicating the patient early on and then giving a narcotic antagonist if pain assessment is required. Explaining upcoming tests and procedures, obtaining laboratory specimens, and continuing to assess the abdomen are all appropriate actions.[9]

26. **A. Analysis.** Pain perception and pain patterns change with age. It is not uncommon to have a completely different presence of appendicitis in the elderly or for them not to present until the appendix has perforated and they are suffering from peritonitis.[8]

27. **C. Assessment.** The most common cause of pancreatitis is alcoholism and it can occur years after the patient is sober. Other causes of pancreatitis include abdominal surgery or trauma, local infections, drugs at normal or toxic levels (especially glucocorticoids, thiazide diuretics, sulfonamides,

antihypertensives, opiates, estrogens, antibiotics, and acetaminophen), mechanical obstruction of the biliary tract, hyperlipidemia, and hypercalcemia. Patients with a positive family history, previous bacterial infection (especially mumps or scarlet fever), or a connective tissue disease such as Crohn's disease are at increased risk for pancreatitis.[13]

28. **C. Intervention.** Morphine and codeine are contraindicated in pancreatitis as these drugs can cause a constriction of the sphincter of Oddi. Meperidine (Demerol) or another potent analgesic should be used instead. IV fluids for rehydration, a gastric tube to decrease abdominal distention and relieve vomiting, and drugs such as anticholinergics and antiemetics, are all appropriate interventions for pancreatitis.[9,13]

29. **D. Analysis.** Increased cardiac output does not generally occur with pancreatitis. Fluid volume deficit and potential for infection are definite problems associated with pancreatitis. The patient also has a great potential for impaired gas exchange due to several factors. Because pancreatitis is an extremely painful condition, the patients tend to steadily hypoventilate, thereby affecting their oxygen saturation levels. The concurrent loss of fluids and electrolytes may also alter the delicate acid-base balance.[13]

30. **B. Assessment.** A markedly elevated amylase (and even lipase) level is diagnostic for acute pancreatitis. The white blood cell count can elevate from numerous other factors, not just pancreatitis. Air-fluid levels are indicative of an abdominal perforation, and emergency surgery is required for that. Pancreatitis may or may not cause blood in the vomitus or stool, so negative guiac tests are not reliable.[9,13]

31. **A. Assessment.** The number one cause of cholecystitis is cholelithiasis (gallstones). Other factors that can lead to the development of cholecystitis include typhoid fever, tumors, systemic staphylococcus or streptococcus infections, obesity or heavy fatty food diet, pregnancy, oral contraceptives, diabetes, celiac disease, cirrhosis of the liver, and pancreatitis.[9]

32. **B. Assessment.** An attack of cholecystitis is typically preceded by consumption of a large, fatty, spicy meal, especially before going to bed. It is not uncommon to have vomiting with the right upper quadrant or epigastric area pain.[9]

33. **B. Analysis.** Middle-age, fair-skinned females are at greatest risk for developing cholecystitis. Pregnancy and obesity may also contribute to the development of cholecystitis.[9]

34. **D. Assessment.** Fortunately many exacerbations of diverticulitis do not require gastric suction. The symptoms can mimic appendicitis and are thought to be due to high-fat diets and stress. Antibiotics are recommended.[9]

35. **C. Analysis.** Because of the high volume of blood in the esophagus and oropharynx, the patient is prone to ineffective airway clearance. Although the other nursing diagnoses apply, the airway involvement receives the highest priority.

36. **A. Assessment.** Esophageal varices are very serious and may rupture spontaneously, causing rapid exsanguination and death. When portal hypertension develops, small veins at the gastroesophageal junction are forced to receive large amounts of shunted blood, which causes distention and hypertrophy of these vessels. The abrupt bleeding may be caused by acid pepsin erosion, mechanical trauma (gastric tube placement), increased abdominal pressure, or coughing, retching, or vomiting. The bleeding is made worse by the fragility of the vessels and the poor blood-clotting abilities that accompany liver disorders.[9,14]

37. **C. Intervention.** A Blakemore nasogastric tube has a balloon along the length of the tube that is inflated and used to tamponade the bleeding esophageal vessels. There are other trade names for this tube, such as Miller-Abbott, Minnesota, and Sengstaken-Blakemore.[9,14]

38. **B. Intervention.** Dopamine (Intropin) would generally be contraindicated for a patient who has bleeding esophageal varices. This peripheral vasoconstrictor would probably lead to increased esophageal bleeding. Vasopressin (Pitressin) is the drug of choice.[9]

39. **D. Assessment.** Clinical symptoms of irritable bowel syndrome (IBS) include chronic or recurrent abdominal pain, generally in the lower abdomen. The pain is cramplike and episodic. Other symptoms associated with IBS include an irregular disturbance in bowel movements, ranging from diarrhea to constipation, and nausea without vomiting.[15]

40. **B. Analysis.** A careful history and a good physical examination provide the data to make the diagnosis of IBS. Limited testing should be directed at ruling out diseases such as ulcerative colitis or colon cancer.[15]

41. **D. Analysis.** Rectal bleeding is a clinical finding of ulcerative colitis. Both disease processes manifest diffuse abdominal pain and weight loss.[16]

42. **B. Assessment.** Acute diarrhea occurs in the majority of all adults. There are multiple causes including food intolerance, psychological stresses, ingestion of toxins, and adverse reactions to medications. Most cases, however, are thought to be caused by an infectious process, which can originate from bacteria, parasites, and viruses.[5]

43. **C. Analysis.** Because of the atropine in Lomotil, a dry mouth is one of the most common symptoms. A delayed toxic response to Lomotil can involved bloating, constipation, and the development of a paralytic ileus or toxic megacolon.[18]

44. **D. Assessment.** Factors known to contribute to the development of abdominal trauma include improperly worn seatbelts, a broken or bent steering wheel, rapid acceleration/deceleration injuries, contact-sports injuries, falls, stabbings, shootings, and other intentional injuries.[1,2]

45. **A. Assessment.** Among numerous other physiological responsibilities, the liver plays a major role in synthesizing blood products and clotting factors. Any injuries to this organ may result in major coagulation problems.[1,2]

46. **B. Assessment.** The spleen is likely to be injured in acceleration/deceleration accidents, trauma associated with left rib fractures, and *any blunt abdominal trauma*. Sled-riding accidents and handlebar injuries frequently cause splenic trauma.[2]

47. **D. Assessment.** Kehr's sign is seen in patients who have a ruptured spleen and sometimes other forms of intraabdominal bleeding. This referred pain is felt in the left shoulder and may worsen when the patient is laid flat or placed in Trendelenburg position.[3]

48. **B. Assessment.** A ruptured spleen is not always obvious in the early phases of the treatment, and up to 20% of patients with splenic injuries may have a delayed rupture or delayed onset of symptoms.[2]

49. **A. Assessment.** Abdominal CT with contrast has become one of the most common methods of evaluating the patient with abdominal injury—particularly blunt trauma. However, if the patient is unstable, diagnostic peritoneal lavage should be performed to rule out abdominal hemorrhage.[6]

50. **D. Intervention.** Patients who have had their spleens removed have a tendency to develop pneumococcal infections. Because of this tendency, every effort is made to salvage the spleen whenever possible. If the spleen must be removed, the patient should receive pneumococcal polysaccharide vaccine (Pneumovax). This procedure is especially important in children, who are particularly susceptible to the pneumococcal virus.[1,2]

51. **B. Assessment.** Patients with blunt abdominal trauma tend to have a higher mortality rate than

those with penetrating abdominal trauma. This is due to the fact that nearly all patients with penetrating abdominal trauma undergo immediate surgery for their obvious injuries. Patients with blunt abdominal trauma are frequently observed rather than aggressively evaluated and treated, generally because their injuries are not as obvious as a bullet wound or stabbing. Unfortunately, when they are finally treated, catastrophic events may have already occurred. This entire scenario gives true meaning to the rule "the most obvious is not always the most severe."[6]

52. **C. Intervention.** Eviscerated organs should always be covered with dressings soaked with normal saline. This keeps the tissue viable for later surgery. The organs should never be forced back into the abdominal cavity. The patient should be encouraged to lay still and not cough or vomit, as this may lead to further evisceration.[2]

53. **B. Assessment.** The presence of bowel sounds in the chest cavity is an indication of a ruptured diaphragm. If the bowel has entered the chest cavity, insertion of chest tube may actually drain fecal material.[2]

54. **B. Assessment.** A stat CT scan of the abdomen would be the most important diagnostic test to be done. A complete blood count (CBC) and an electrocardiogram (ECG) are helpful but not crucial to the diagnosis of an abdominal aortic aneurysm. An MRI would not be practical at this point due to the time factor and patient condition.[9]

55. **A. Analysis.** The obvious hypotension and tachycardia are indicative of hypovolemic shock and subsequent altered tissue perfusion, all commonly associated with ruptured abdominal aortic aneurysm. The potentials for infection and injury, as well as airway clearance problems, are not applicable.

56. **C. Assessment.** Pain associated with a dissecting abdominal aortic aneurysm is frequently described as sharp and tearing and is commonly located in the lower back, lower abdomen, and possibly the upper thigh areas. It is constant and is not relieved with changes in position.[9]

57. **D. Intervention.** Because of the high mortality rate associated with a dissecting aortic aneurysm, it would be advisable to have this patient be with his wife as soon as possible. Despite the urgency of the situation, priority should be given to his emotional needs as well. Depending on the wife's response and behavior, she should be allowed to be with the patient as long as possible.[9]

58. **D. Intervention.** Nitroprusside is commonly used to manage the hypertension that may occur with an abdominal aortic aneurysm. It is fast acting and easily controllable.[9,18]

59. **D. Assessment.** Cardiac disease, especially congestive heart failure and atrial fibrillation, place a patient at risk for developing mesenteric ischemia. Additional cardiac conditions include myocardial infarction and valvular heart disease. Other predisposing conditions are advanced age, hypovolemia, hypercoaguable states, rheumatoid arthritis, polyarteritis nodosa, sickle cell disease, and systemic lupus erythematosus. Certain medications, such as digitalis, oral contraceptives, and psychotropic medications have also been associated with mesenteric ischemia.[9]

60. **C. Assessment.** The presence of free air on abdominal x-ray films is associated with an acute abdomen and/or possible organ perforation. It requires a surgical exploration. The symptoms of mesenteric ischemia include colicky, intermittent abdominal pain out of proportion to the physical findings associated with generalized vague abdominal tenderness, voluntary guarding, and rebound tenderness. Bowel sounds may be hyperactive initially but then become decreased to absent as an ileus develops. The abdomen usually becomes distended late in the course of acute intestinal ischemia. Distention may be the only sign in a patient with ischemia not experiencing pain. Anorexia, nausea, and absent or diarrhea bowel movements may accompany the pain.[9]

## REFERENCES

1. Noventy-Dinsdale J: Gastrointestinal emergencies. In Kitt S et al, editors: *Emergency nursing: a physiologic and clinical perspective,* Philadelphia, 1995, WB Saunders.
2. Freeman LM, Newberry L: Gastrointestinal trauma. In Newberry L, editor: *Sheehy's emergency nursing: principles and practice,* St Louis, 1998, Mosby.
3. Wright J: Seven abdominal assessment signs every emergency nurse should know. *J Emerg Nurs* 23:446-450, 1997.
4. Navuluri R, Yue S: Understanding peptic ulcer disease pharmacotherapeutics, *Nurs Pract* 21:128-132, 1999.
5. Powell D: Approach to the patient with diarrhea. In Goldman L, Bennett JC, editors: *Cecil textbook of medicine,* Philadelphia, 2000, WB Saunders.
6. Elliott D, Militello P: Pitfalls in the diagnosis of abdominal trauma. In Maull K, Rodriguez, Wiles C, editors: *Complications in trauma and critical care,* Philadelphia, 1996, WB Saunders.
7. Cauthorne-Burnette T, Estes MEZ: *Clinical companion for health assessment and physical examination,* Albany, NY, 1998, Delmar Publishers.
8. Pisarra VH: Recognizing the various presentations of appendicitis, *Nurs Pract* 24:42-53, 1999.
9. Huey TR: Gastrointestinal emergencies. In Newberry L, editor, *Sheehy's emergency nursing: principles and practice,* St Louis, 1998, Mosby.

10. Jess LW: Acute abdominal pain: revealing the source, *Nursing 93* 23(9):34-42, 1993.

11. Haley K, Baker P, Eckles N: *Emergency nursing pediatric course,* Park Ridge, 1999, Emergency Nurses Association.

12. Waisman Y: Intussception. In Barkin R, editor: *Pediatric emergency medicine,* St Louis, 1997, Mosby.

13. Brown A: Acute pancreatitis: pathophysiology, nursing diagnosis, and collaborative problems, *Focus on Critical Care* 18(2):121-130, 1991.

14. Friedman S: Alcoholic liver disease, cirrhosis, and its major sequelae. In Goldman L and Bennett JC, editors: *Cecil textbook of medicine,* Philadelphia, 2000, WB Saunders.

15. Talley NJ: Functional gastrointestinal disorders; irritable bowel syndrome; non-ulcer dyspepsia; and non-cardiac pain. In Goldman L and Bennett JC, editors: Philadelphia, 2000, WB Saunders.

16. Rayhorn N: Inflammatory bowel disease, *Nursing 99* 29:57-61, 1999.

17. Kaplan MA, Prior MJ, Ash RS, et al: Loperamide-simethicone vs loperamide alone, simethicone alone, and placebo in the treatment of acute diarrhea with gas-related abdominal discomfort, *Arch Fam Med* 8:243-248, 1999.

18. McKenry LM, Salerno E: *Pharmacology in nursing,* St Louis, 1998, Mosby.

# Chapter 4

# Cardiovascular Emergencies

**REVIEW OUTLINE**

I. Anatomy
  A. Heart
    1. Right ventricle
    2. Left ventricle
    3. Right atrium
    4. Left atrium
    5. Valves
    6. Cardiac muscle
  B. Cardiac vasculature
    1. Superior vena cava
    2. Aortic arch
    3. Coronary arteries
    4. Inferior vena cava
    5. Pulmonary arteries
    6. Pulmonary veins
II. Physiology
  A. Preload
  B. Afterload
  C. Starling's law
III. Electrical conduction
  A. Cardiac cells
  B. Sinoatrial (SA) node
  C. Atrioventricular (AV) node
  D. Bundle of His
  E. Right bundle
  F. Left bundle
  G. Purkinje fiber
  H. P wave
  I. Q wave
  J. R wave
  K. ST segment
  L. T wave
IV. Cardiovascular assessment
  A. History
    1. Chest pain differentiation (PQRST)
      a. Provocation and palliation
      b. Quality and intensity
      c. Region and radiation
      d. Severity
      e. Temporal: When did it start? How long has the pain been there? Is there any time it is not there?

2. Medical history
3. Risk factors for cardiac disease
    a. Hypertension
    b. Pulmonary disease
    c. Previous cardiovascular disease
    d. Smoking
    e. Family history
    f. Diabetes
    g. Renal disease
    h. Obesity/higher than average body mass
    i. Postmenopausal women
    j. Personality traits
    k. Elevated serum cholesterol level
    l. Adverse dietary pattern
    m. Lack of exercise
4. Associated signs and symptoms
    a. Syncope
    b. Weakness
    c. Nausea and vomiting
    d. Dizziness
    e. Orthopnea
    f. Dependent edema
    g. Fatigue
    h. Paroxysmal nocturnal dyspnea
    i. Palpitations
    j. Irregular heart beat
5. Identification of possible contraindications to fibrinolytic therapy
    a. History of recent major surgery
    b. History of cerebral vascular disease or event
    c. Intracranial neoplasm
    d. Recent trauma
    e. Recent gastrointestinal or genitourinary bleeding
    f. Puncture of a noncompressible vessel such as the insertion of a central catheter
    g. Uncontrolled hypertension
    h. Pregnancy
    i. Menstruation (relative contraindication)

j. Known bleeding diathesis

k. Acute pericarditis

B. Physical examination

1. Obvious signs and symptoms of trauma

    a. Penetrating trauma: gunshot wound, knife wound, penetrating objects

    b. Blunt trauma: bruising and abrasions of the chest wall—anterior and posterior

    c. Obvious deformity

    d. Paradoxical movement

    e. Respiratory distress

2. Level of consciousness

3. Patient's skin color and temperature

    a. Pallor

    b. Cyanosis

    c. Diaphoresis

4. Jugular vein distention

5. Hepatomegaly

6. Clubbing of digits

7. Rate and rhythm of respirations

8. Palpation of peripheral pulses

9. Auscultation of breath sounds

    a. Comparison from side to side

    b. Presence or absence of breath sounds

    c. Rales

    d. Rhonchi

    e. Wheezes

    f. Pleural friction rub

10. Auscultation of heart sounds

    a. $S_1$

    b. $S_2$

    c. $S_3$

    d. $S_4$

    e. Friction rub

    f. Murmurs

    g. Bruits

11. Assessment of edema

    a. Location

    b. Pitting or nonpitting

12. Dysrhythmia recognition

13. Blood pressure evaluation

    a. Hypotension

    b. Hypertension

    c. Variances in pulse pressure

    d. Pulsus alterans

    e. Pulsus paradoxus

    f. Comparison of blood pressure from side to side

C. Age-related changes[1-3]

1. Pediatric patient

    a. Infant's heart is large in relation to its size, lies horizontally, and takes up a large portion of the thoracic cavity

    b. Around age 7, the heart is closer to adult size

    c. Apical pulse more easily palpable in children

    d. $S_3$ is more common in children

    e. Children and young adults may have a benign systolic murmur

    f. Congenital cardiac anomaly in children

        (1) Tetralogy of Fallot

        (2) Cardiac enlargement

        (3) Mitral stenosis

        (4) Aortic regurgitation

        (5) Ventricular septal defect

        (6) Patent ductus arteriosus

    g. Blood pressure, pulse, and respirations vary depending on age of the child

2. Geriatric patient

    a. Stiffening of aorta and large arteries with age

    b. Increase in blood pressure with age

    c. Peripheral arteries lengthen and harden

    d. Some elderly develop postural hypotension

    e. Development of an aortic systolic murmur

    f. Development of a systolic murmur of mitral regurgitation

    g. Cardiac dysrhythmia common

    h. Perception of chest pain is less

D. Diagnostic studies or procedures

1. Electrocardiogram (ECG), 12 and 15 leads

2. Echocardiogram

3. Chest radiographic studies

4. Serum enzyme studies

    a. Myoglobin levels

    b. Cardiac troponins

5. Cardiac catheterization

6. Pericardiocentesis

7. Needle thoracostomy

8. Chest tube insertion

9. Open thoracotomy

10. Doppler studies

11. Arteriogram

V. Collaborative care

A. Activity intolerance

B. Airway clearance, ineffective

C. Breathing pattern, ineffective

D. Cardiac output, decreased

E. Fatigue

F. Fear

G. Fluid volume deficit, high risk for

H. Fluid volume excess

I. Gas exchange, impaired

J. Grieving, anticipatory

K. Injury, high risk for

L. Knowledge deficit

M. Pain

N. Spiritual distress (distress of the human spirit)

O. Tissue perfusion, altered

P. Trauma, high risk for

VI. Collaborative care of the patient with a cardiovascular emergency

   A. A, B, C, D, E (airway, breathing, circulation, deficit [neurological], exposure)

     1. BCLS (basic cardiac life support)

     2. ACLS (advanced cardiac life support)

     3. PALS (pediatric advanced life support)

     4. ENPC (emergency nursing pediatric course)

     5. TNCC (trauma nursing core course)

     6. ATNC (advanced trauma nursing core course)

     7. TNATC (transport nurse advanced trauma course)

     8. BTLS (basic trauma life support)

     9. ATLS (advanced trauma life support)

   B. Oxygen therapy

   C. Cardiac monitoring

   D. Pulse oximetry

   E. External pacemaker

   F. Transvenous pacemaker

   G. Chest tube insertion

   H. Open thoracotomy

   I. Drug therapy

     1. Vasoactive drugs

     2. Antidysrhythmics

     3. Antibiotics

     4. Analgesics

     5. Inotropic agents

     6. Fibrinolytic agents

       a. Endogenous

         (i) t-PA

         (ii) u-PA

       b. Therapeutics

         (i) streptokinase

         (ii) urokinase

         (iii) alteplase

         (iv) reteplase

     7. Glycoprotein inhibitors IIb/IIIa receptor antagonists

     8. Digitalis antibodies

     9. Antihypertensive agents

     10. Calcium channel blockers

     11. Anticoagulants

       a. UFH (unfractionated heparin)

       b. LMWH (low molecular weight heparin) beta blockers

     12. Beta-blockers

     13. ACE inhibitors

     14. Angiotensin II antagonists

   J. Defibrillation and cardioversion

   K. Pericardiocentesis

   L. Frequent assessment

   M. Arterial line insertion

   N. Pulmonary artery catheters

   O. Intraaortic balloon pump

   P. Cardiopulmonary bypass

   Q. Doppler assessment

   R. Automatic implantable cardioverter defibrillator (AICD)

VII. Specific cardiovascular emergencies

   A. Congestive heart failure, acute pulmonary edema

   B. Dysrhythmia

     1. Ventricular fibrillation

     2. Ventricular tachycardia

     3. Asystole

     4. Heart block

     5. Premature ventricular contractions (PVCs)

     6. Supraventricular tachycardia

   C. Malignant hypertension

   D. Digitalis intoxication

   E. Venous thrombosis

   F. Arterial occlusion

   G. Myocardial infarction (Q wave, non–Q wave)

   H. Angina/unstable angina

   I. Aortic aneurysm

   J. Cardiac trauma

     1. Penetrating

       a. Gunshot wounds

       b. Stab wounds

     2. Blunt

       a. Myocardial contusion

       b. Pericardial tamponade

*I*t has been found that cardiovascular diseases account for more deaths in the United States than the other causes of death combined.[4,5] The majority of these patients seek treatment in the emergency department, which presents a particular challenge to emergency nursing practice. All the changes that continue to occur in the management of cardiovascular emergencies—especially chest pain and myocardial infarction—require that emergency nurses keep abreast of the current research and treatment to ensure that patients receive the best care.

Research has demonstrated that a patient suffering chest pain should be treated the same as a trauma patient—rapid assessment and timely treatment. In other words, time and skill are of the essence in preventing additional injury to the patient's myocardium.[6,7] Today, cardiac teams, Rapid Treatment and Diagnostic Centers (RDTC), and Chest Pain Centers have demonstrated that "door-to-treatment" times can be reduced and the patient placed in the appropriate care area. The management of a patient with chest pain requires knowledge about multiple medications, their effects, and what additional interventions may be necessary when initial intervention fails.[6,7]

Cardiovascular emergencies can have either a medical or a traumatic origin. Occasionally a patient may sustain a cardiovascular emergency of both a medical and a traumatic nature, such as in the case of the elderly patient who has an acute myocardial event that precipitates a motor vehicle crash.

The care of the patient who is experiencing a cardiovascular emergency begins with the assessment and stabilization of the patient's airway, breathing, and circulation (ABCs). The emergency nurse needs to possess knowledge about the anatomy and physiology of the cardiovascular system. These topics are included in the Review Outline at the beginning of the chapter. Advanced cardiac life support (ACLS), pediatric advanced life support (PALS), and the emergency nursing pediatric course (ENPC) offer guidelines for the care of both the adult and the pediatric patient who is experiencing a cardiovascular emergency.

Since the cardiovascular system affects all other body systems, inspection of the patient who is suffering from a cardiovascular emergency will encompass airway patency, breathing patterns, and perfusion. Palpation should include evaluation of both the central and the peripheral pulses. Auscultation of heart sounds, cardiac rhythm, and breath sounds should be included.

Identifying the origins of the patient's chest pain, or chest pain differentiation, presents a demanding challenge to the assessment skills of the emergency department nurse. One method that can be used to differentiate a patient's chest pain is based on four different factors: the patient's description of the pain (crushing, burning, tearing, sudden onset, location); factors that relieve the pain (stopping activity, sitting up, analgesics, relief with nitroglycerin, no relief); associated symptoms (friction rub, shortness of breath, nausea, vomiting, diaphoresis); and ECG findings (no changes, elevated ST segments, transient ST and T wave changes).[8]

Diagnostic data related to cardiovascular emergencies include an ECG, echocardiogram, chest x-ray film, serum cardiac enzyme levels, electrolytes (particularly potassium and calcium), and Doppler studies. The use of cardiac enzymes used to be limited due to the amount of time it took to confirm their presence and significance. Bedside testing has made the use of defining cardiac injury with enzymes more feasible. Cardiac troponin T and I have been identified as sensitive and specific indicators of an acute myocardial infarction. They have also been found to be sensitive indicators of non-Q wave injury and unstable angina.[9]

Specific collaborative procedures for the patient who is suffering from a cardiovascular emergency include the insertion of chest tubes,[3,5] pericardiocentesis, open thoracotomy, portable extracorporeal circulation,[10] and thrombolytic therapy.[4-8] The emergency nurse needs to review the indications, the nurse's role, and the nursing interventions required to provide emergency nursing care to patients who are undergoing these procedures.

Over the past 10 years, the management of cardiovascular emergencies has expanded in the prehospital environment to include the use of automatic external defibrillators. These are not only being carried by emergency service but also are being used by flight attendants, factory workers, and many others who have received the appropriate training. The reaction to cardiovascular emergencies continues to be focused on a community response. Emergency nurses play an integral role in this response as teachers and providers of care.

The care of the patient who is suffering from a cardiovascular emergency begins with an understanding of the anatomy and physiology of the cardiovascular system. The emergency nurse needs to be able to differentiate the sources of chest pain. Recognition and treatment of potentially lethal dysrhythmia is a very important component of the care provided to the emergency cardiovascular patient. Finally, possessing current knowledge about the care of the patient with acute myocardial infarction—particularly fibrinolytic therapy—and recognizing and providing treatment for the patient who may have experienced blunt or penetrating cardiac trauma contribute to the emergency nurse's ability to provide optimal care to the emergency cardiovascular patient.[11,12]

## REVIEW QUESTIONS
### Myocardial Infarction

*A 48-year-old man comes to the emergency department complaining of midsternal chest pain. He is awake, alert, pale, and diaphoretic. His vital signs are B/P 100/72, P 100 and irregular, R 22, and Temp 98.6° F.*

1. The pain pattern of myocardial infarction frequently is described as:
   0   A. Tearing, radiating to the back
   0   B. Sudden, sharp, increasing with a change in position
   0   C. Sudden, crushing, radiating to the jaw and neck
   0   D. Sudden, sharp over the lung fields, increasing with inspiration

2. Fibrinolytic therapy is being considered for this patient. All of the following should be considered as initial indicators for fibrinolytic therapy *except:*
   0   A. Serum cardiac enzyme levels
   0   B. A 12-lead ECG with significant ST elevation
   0   C. A history of cardiovascular disease and diabetes
   0   D. Onset of chest pain greater than 6 hours

3. ST elevation on a 12-lead ECG indicates:
   0   A. Infarction
   0   B. Ischemia
   0   C. Dysrhythmia
   0   D. Injury

4. The emergency nurse obtains a 12-lead ECG. There is ST elevation greater than 2 cm in leads $V_2$, $V_3$, and $V_4$. The patient is having an acute:
   0   A. Anterior wall infarction
   0   B. Inferior wall infarction
   0   C. Posterior wall infarction
   0   D. Lateral wall infarction

5. Tissue plasminogen activator (t-PA) is ordered for this patient. In preparation for administration of this therapy, the emergency nurse may:
   0   A. Place an external pacemaker on the patient in anticipation of a dysrhythmia

   0   B. Draw all the initial blood studies before administering the drug
   0   C. Administer platelets to the patient to prevent the possibility of bleeding
   0   D. Start a dopamine or dobutamine drip to prevent hypotension

6. The patient is to be transported to the cardiac catheterization unit. In preparation for transport, the emergency nurse should:
   0   A. Change all the patient's IV fluids to normal saline
   0   B. Place blood tubing on one of the IV lines
   0   C. Bring along a defibrillator and ACLS drugs
   0   D. Place a pulse oximeter on the patient

7. After the t-PA has been infused, the emergency nurse should:
   0   A. Purge the IV tubing to get all of the drug
   0   B. Draw a CBC and an arterial blood gas
   0   C. Insert a Foley catheter to monitor for hematuria
   0   D. Draw a PT and a PTT to monitor clotting time

8. A common dysrhythmia associated with reperfusion is:
   0   A. Ventricular fibrillation
   0   B. Complete heart block
   0   C. Accelerated idioventricular rhythm
   0   D. Asystole

9. The most common complication of fibrinolytic therapy is:
   0   A. Dysrhythmia
   0   B. Bleeding
   0   C. Thrombosis
   0   D. Hypocalcemia

10. Which group of patients is at greater risk of having a stroke after treatment with fibrinolytic therapy?
   0   A. Elderly patients with a history of headaches
   0   B. Women being treated with fibrinolytics for MI
   0   C. Men who have had previous infarctions
   0   D. Men who have a history of headaches

11. Because of the possibility of an intracerebral hemorrhage occurring as the result of fibrinolytic administration, the emergency nurse should evaluate the patient for:
    - O  A. The presence of petechiae
    - O  B. Changes in level of consciousness
    - O  C. Blood in the urine
    - O  D. Fever and chills

12. The emergency nurse performs a baseline neurological assessment as part of the initial care of a patient who is to receive thrombolytic therapy for an acute anterior myocardial infarction. The patient is given retavase, and a weight-based heparin drip is initiated. During infusion of these drugs, the nurse notes that the patient has a sudden deterioration in mental status and weakness on his left side. What actions should the emergency nurse initiate?
    - O  A. Notify the emergency physician and obtain an emergency CT scan
    - O  B. Discontinue the heparin drip and notify the emergency physician
    - O  C. Continue the patient's infusions and reevaluate the patient in 15 minutes
    - O  D. Immediately obtain PT, PTT, and a platelet count from the patient

13. Medications that may be given to reverse the effects of streptokinase and heparin are:
    - O  A. D$_{50}$, naloxone, and oxygen
    - O  B. Fresh frozen plasma and platelets
    - O  C. Diphenhydramine and normal saline
    - O  D. Protamine zinc and aminocaproic acid

14. The most appropriate nursing diagnosis for the patient receiving fibrinolytic therapy is:
    - O  A. Airway clearance, ineffective
    - O  B. Fluid volume deficit, high risk for
    - O  C. Injury, high risk for
    - O  D. Gas exchange, impaired

15. T-PA:
    - O  A. Is clot specific
    - O  B. Causes a lytic state
    - O  C. Is not clot specific
    - O  D. Has a prolonged effect on the coagulation system

*A 53-year-old man comes to the emergency department complaining of chest pain for the past 12 hours. He states that it is crushing and goes down his left arm.*

16. Control of chest pain is important in the patient having a myocardial infarction because:
    - O  A. It may interfere with the patient's level of consciousness
    - O  B. It will increase the patient's anxiety and fear
    - O  C. Pain releases catecholamines and may increase myocardial damage
    - O  D. Pain may cause nausea and vomiting

17. The patient states, "I do not know what this heart attack is going to do to my life." The most appropriate nursing diagnosis on which the emergency nurse should base care is:
    - O  A. Fear related to the implications of the patient's illness
    - O  B. Body image disturbance related to the acute myocardial infarction
    - O  C. Thought processes, altered, related to chest pain
    - O  D. Spiritual distress (distress of the human spirit) related to pain

18. After providing the patient with information about his condition, the emergency nurse should use which of the following to evaluate the effectiveness of the intervention?
    - O  A. The patient's pulse and blood pressure increases
    - O  B. The patient is able to talk about his fears
    - O  C. The patient states that he wants to be alone
    - O  D. The patient says that he does not want to see his family

*A 60-year-old patient is diagnosed as having an acute inferior wall myocardial infarction and a right ventricular infarction. He is awake and alert. The patient develops profound hypotension while in the emergency department. His vital signs are B/P 80/50, P 60, and R 32.*

19. The initial management of this patient should include:
    - O  A. Administration of furosemide (Lasix) to prevent congestive heart failure
    - O  B. Administration of a 200 ml normal saline fluid bolus
    - O  C. Insertion of a transvenous pacemaker to improve the patient's hypotension
    - O  D. Endotracheal intubation to prevent hypoxia and cardiac dysrhythmia

20. A right ventricular infarction is diagnosed by:
    O  A. A chest x-ray film to rule out cardiomyopathy
    O  B. Placement of right-sided precordial leads
    O  C. Serum cardiac enzymes
    O  D. Congestive heart failure (CHF)

21. Diagnosis of an acute myocardial infarction in the emergency department is based on which of the following clinical criteria?
    O  A. Emergent cardiac catheterization
    O  B. Elevation of an ST segment greater than 2 cm in one lead
    O  C. The patient's history and a 12-lead ECG
    O  D. Pathological Q waves in two leads on the ECG

22. Mr. J has been diagnosed with an acute inferolateral myocardial infarction. A nitroglycerin drip has been started to help manage the patient's chest pain, which he states is 8/10. Benefits of intravenous nitroglycerin include:
    O  A. An increase in myocardial oxygen demand
    O  B. A decrease in collateral flow to the myocardium
    O  C. A reduction of coronary artery spasm
    O  D. An increase in mean arterial pressure

23. Large, inappropriate dosages of nitroglycerin may:
    O  A. Cause a reflex hypertension
    O  B. Cause a reflex tachycardia
    O  C. Cause a reflex bradycardia
    O  D. Cause an increase in coronary perfusion pressure

24. Heparin administration is more effective when weight-based because:
    O  A. Bleeding is less likely to occur with a smaller dose
    O  B. Absorption of heparin varies from patient to patient
    O  C. Diseases such as diabetes may affect heparin
    O  D. Bradycardia may result with inadequate doses of heparin

25. The diagnosis of an acute myocardial infarction includes all of the following *except:*
    O  A. ST-segment changes or new Q waves
    O  B. Abnormally elevated serum cardiac enzyme levels
    O  C. No ST-segment changes or new Q waves

    O  D. Abnormally elevated serum myoglobin levels

26. Which of the following enzyme changes indicate myocardial reperfusion?
    O  A. Creatinine kinase (CK)
    O  B. CK-MB subforms: MB1 and MB2
    O  C. Cardiac troponin T
    O  D. Lactate dehydrongenase (LDH)

27. Preload is measured in the right side of the heart by:
    O  A. Pulmonary wedge pressure (PWP)
    O  B. Central venous pressure (CVP)
    O  C. Left arterial pressure (LAP)
    O  D. Diastolic blood pressure (DAP)

28. Systemic vascular resistance is increased by:
    O  A. Chronic obstructive pulmonary disease
    O  B. Administration of nitroprusside intravenously
    O  C. Primary pulmonary hypertension
    O  D. Sympathetic nervous system compensation

29. A 68-year-old female presents to the emergency department with 4 hours of crushing chest pain, diaphoresis, and vomiting. She is diagnosed with an acute inferior myocardial infarction. She is treated with fibrinolytic therapy. Her heart rate remains at 100 without any ectopy. The emergency department physician orders metoprolol 15 mg to be administered over 15 minutes. The desired effect of metoprolol is:
    O  A. To increase the patient's heart rate
    O  B. To decrease the patient's heart rate
    O  C. To increase the heart's oxygen consumption
    O  D. To increase cardiac metabolic demand

30. A 37-year-old obese male presented to the emergency department complaining of midsternal crushing chest pain. He has a history of diabetes controlled by diet and smoking for the past 20 years. An ECG demonstrates some anterior wall ischemia. The patient is diagnosed with acute coronary syndrome. Abciximab (ReoPro) has been ordered. The physiological effect of abciximab (ReoPro) is:
    O  A. Lysing clots that have formed in the coronary arteries

B. Blocking fibrinogen's ability to cause platelet aggregation

C. Blocking thromboxane $A_2$ to stop platelet aggregation

D. Enhancing platelet aggregation in the coronary artery

31. The antiplatelet effect of glycoprotein IIb/IIIa receptor inhibitors can be reversed by:
    A. Administration of platelets
    B. Administration of protamine zinc
    C. Administration of packed red blood cells
    D. Administration of clopidogrel

32. A costly complication of myocardial infarction is:
    A. Excessive medication administration in the emergency department
    B. A 50% chance of suffering a CVA when fibrinolytics are administered
    C. Decrease in research related to the management of myocardial infarction
    D. The development of congestive heart failure

33. An advantage of bolus administration of rPA is:
    A. There is a decreased risk of bleeding when administering the drug as a bolus when compared with continuous infusion
    B. Less chance of a medication error because dosages do not have to be adjusted to weight of the patient
    C. The longer half-life of rPA makes it easy to reverse the effects of a bolus-administered medication
    D. There is no advantage to administering fibrinolytic agents by bolus or as a continuous infusion

34. Resuscitation can be withheld in which of the following circumstances?
    A. In emergency departments where policies permit resuscitation to be withheld without consulting the patient or his or her family
    B. In emergency departments where "slow" resuscitation is allowed to be initiated until the patient or family is consulted
    C. For patients who have clear advanced directives directing healthcare providers not to begin resuscitation in the event of a cardiac arrest

D. For patients whose body temperature is less than 90° F and have a heart rate of 20 beats per minute

35. Aspirin is a primary treatment for the patient with acute coronary syndrome because it targets:
    A. Fibrin
    B. Platelets
    C. Fibrinogen
    D. Red blood cells

## Advanced Cardiac Life Support

*A family pulls up to the emergency department entrance and asks for help. They state that their 35-year-old daughter would not wake up. The patient is removed from the car and brought into the resuscitation room.*

36. When the patient is placed on the monitor, the following rhythm is found. What is it?

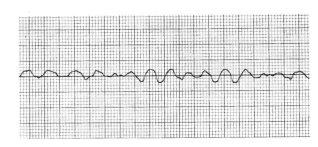

    A. Sinus rhythm
    B. Ventricular tachycardia
    C. Ventricular fibrillation
    D. Asystole

37. The patient has been defibrillated twice, but remains in the same rhythm. What should the emergency team do next?
    A. Defibrillate at 360 W/sec
    B. Continue CPR until an IV line is established
    C. Intubate and hyperventilate the patient
    D. Give the patient 10 mg of epinephrine

38. The patient's monitor shows a rhythm, but a pulse cannot be palpated. What interventions should the emergency nurse consider?
    A. Stopping CPR and transferring the patient to the ICU
    B. Giving two ampules of sodium bicarbonate
    C. Giving calcium chloride through a central line
    D. Giving the patient a fluid bolus of normal saline

**39.** A 52-year-old man comes to the emergency department complaining of chest pain. When placed on the monitor, he is found to be in an irregular rhythm. What rhythm is he in?

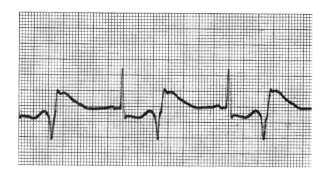

- 0    A. Ventricular tachycardia
- 0    B. Ventricular bigeminy
- 0    C. Asystole
- 0    D. Complete heart block

**40.** This patient's rhythm is treated with:
- 0    A. Atropine, 0.5 mg IV push
- 0    B. Lidocaine, 1 mg/kg IV push
- 0    C. Sodium bicarbonate, 1mEq/kg IV push
- 0    D. Bretylium 5 mg/kg IV push

**41.** The patient's dysrhythmia continues and he is now in the following rhythm:

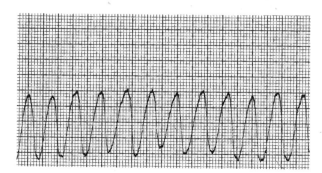

- 0    A. Ventricular tachycardia
- 0    B. Ventricular fibrillation
- 0    C. Atrial fibrillation with a rapid ventricular response
- 0    D. Sinus rhythm with frequent PVCs

**42.** The patient continues to have a pulse, but is not responding to a repeated lidocaine bolus and a lidocaine infusion at 4 mg. The emergency physician orders an amiodarone bolus and infusion. The initial bolus is:
- 0    A. Rapid infusion of 50 mg/20 minutes
- 0    B. Slow infusion of 150 mg/30 minutes

- 0    C. Rapid infusion of 300 mg/10 minutes
- 0    D. Rapid infusion of 150 mg/10 minutes

**43.** The most common side effect of amiodarone is:
- 0    A. Hypertension
- 0    B. Tachycardia
- 0    C. Hypotension
- 0    D. Hepatic failure

**44.** The patient continues to intermittently respond to the amiodarone. A diagnosis of torsades de pointes is being considered. What other medication can effectively abolish torsades?
- 0    A. Aminophylline 5 mg/kg infusion
- 0    B. Morphine 1 to 3 mg IV
- 0    C. Digoxin .25 mg IV
- 0    D. Magnesium sulfate 1 to 2 g IV

**45.** An 82-year-old man is brought to the emergency department after having collapsed while mowing the lawn. When his family found him, he was apneic and pulseless, and CPR was initiated. When the patient arrives in the emergency department, the monitor shows the following rhythm. What is it?

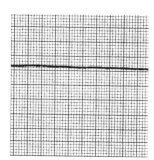

- 0    A. Asystole
- 0    B. Ventricular tachycardia
- 0    C. Sinus rhythm
- 0    D. Electrical mechanical dissociation

**46.** The patient is intubated, but an IV line has not yet been established. All of the following drugs can be placed down the endotracheal tube except:
- 0    A. Lidocaine
- 0    B. Atropine
- 0    C. Naloxone
- 0    D. Sodium bicarbonate

47. The emergency physician orders that the initial dose of epinephrine should be given down the endotracheal tube. The patient weighs 110 kg. How much medication should the emergency nurse administer down the tube?
    - O  A. 1 mg of epinephrine, followed by 10 ml flush of normal saline
    - O  B. 2.5 mg of epinephrine, followed by 10 ml flush of normal saline
    - O  C. 0.5 mg of epinephrine, followed by 15 ml flush of normal saline
    - O  D. 3 mg of epinephrine, followed by quick sufflation with the ambu bag

48. A 78-year-old woman is brought to the emergency department after having passed out at home. She has no history of any cardiac disease and has not seen a doctor for over 20 years. When the patient is placed on the monitor, the following rhythm is found. What is it?

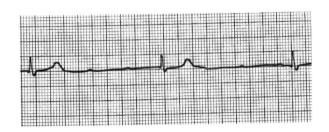

    - O  A. Asystole
    - O  B. First-degree heart block
    - O  C. Third-degree heart block
    - O  D. Sinus rhythm

49. A patient has a blood pressure of 80/50, with an HR 30 and RR 12. She is complaining that she feels "dizzy." An external pacemaker is placed and pacing is initiated. A common complication of external pacing in the awake patient is:
    - O  A. Failure to capture through the patient's skin because of decreased elasticity
    - O  B. Failure of pacing pads to stick to the patient's chest wall because of age
    - O  C. Pain from muscle spasms induced by the external pacemaker
    - O  D. Shortness of breath because the patient has to lie flat during pacing

50. External pacemaker mechanical capture is demonstrated by:
    - O  A. Palpable femoral pulse
    - O  B. Decreased level of consciousness
    - O  C. Decreased blood pressure
    - O  D. Pacer spikes on the monitor

51. Interventions to improve external pacemaker mechanical capture include:
    - O  A. Decreasing the MA until a pulse can be palpated
    - O  B. Increasing the cardiac rate setting of the external pacemaker
    - O  C. Checking the battery power of the external pacemaker
    - O  D. Adding an additional set of pads in a different position on the chest

52. An 18-year-old woman comes to the emergency department complaining of a "funny" feeling in her chest and shortness of breath. The patient's B/P is 80/60, P is 200, and Valsalva maneuvers do not decrease or change the patient's rhythm. Which of the following drugs may be ordered to treat this dysrhythmia?

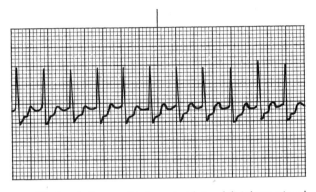

From Kitt S et al: *Emergency Nursing: a physiologic and clinical perspective*, ed 2, Philadelphia, 1995, WB Saunders.

    - O  A. Epinephrine, 1 mg/kg IV push
    - O  B. Atropine, 1 mg IV push
    - O  C. Adenosine, 6 mg IV push
    - O  D. Procainamide, 50 mg IV push

53. After 2 minutes, the patient's rhythm has not changed and her blood pressure has decreased to 70 by palpation. The next treatment she would be given is:
    - O  A. 10 mg verapamil IVP
    - O  B. 0.5 mg digitalis slow IVP
    - O  C. Lidocaine 50 mg IVP
    - O  D. Adenosine 12 mg IVP

54. Emergency nursing care of the patient receiving adenosine, based on a common side effect of this drug, would include which of the following nursing diagnoses?
    - O  A. Injury, high risk for, related to the generalized seizures adenosine may cause
    - O  B. Hyperthermia related to the thermoregulatory side effects of adenosine

C. Self-care deficit related to the dizziness that is a side effect of adenosine

D. Fear related to the sudden change in cardiac rhythm that precedes conversion

55. A 55-year-old woman is brought to the emergency department after complaining of "weakness." The BLS squad reported that her heart rate was around 75 and very irregular. Upon arrival in the emergency department, the patient is placed on the monitor and found to be in this rhythm. In what rhythm is the patient?

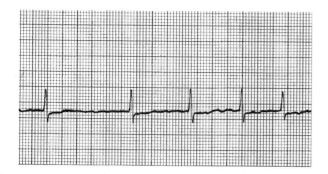

A. Atrial fibrillation

B. Atrial flutter

C. Normal sinus rhythm

D. Nodal tachycardia

56. The patient has no history of any medical problems, and her ECG shows no evidence of previous injury. She states she exercises every day and thought that her irregular heart rate may have been related to physical exertion. During her evaluation, her heart rate increases to 180 beats per minute, and she complains of chest pain. This rhythm leaves the patient at risk for:

A. Developing complete heart block (CHB)

B. Developing congestive heart failure

C. Having a transient ischemic attack (TIA)

D. Developing ventricular fibrillation

57. The patient's blood pressure is 84/52, heart rate 180 and irregular, and RR 18. Because of her unstable rhythm, cardioversion is indicated. The emergency nurse sets the defibrillator to:

A. 200 J defibrillation mode

B. 25 J synchronous mode

C. 360 J defibrillation mode

D. 100 J synchronous mode

58. The patient is sedated and successfully cardioverted to a rate of 110. The emergency physician has decided to treat this patient's dysrhythmia by giving her a dose of diltiazem. Her body weight is 65 kg. Which of the following doses would the emergency nurse administer to this patient?

A. 50 mg diltiazem IVP

B. 14.5 mg diltiazem IVP

C. 10 mg diltiazem IVP

D. 20 mg diltiazem IVP

59. Treatment of diltiazem toxicity would include all of the following drugs except:

A. Calcium chloride IV

B. Verapamil IV

C. Bretylium IV

D. Labetalol IV

60. A 3-month-old infant is brought to the emergency department because of respiratory distress. The infant's pulse is over 260 beats per minute. The mother states that the child has not been ill and that this incident started suddenly. The infant is lethargic and cyanotic. The emergency physician has decided to cardiovert the infant. The emergency nurse would calculate the joules to be used to cardiovert the baby using the following:

A. 2 J/kg

B. 0.5 J/kg

C. 3 J/kg

D. 25 J/kg

61. Because of possible cardiovascular collapse, which of the following drugs should not be given to infants who are in a supraventricular rhythm?

A. Epinephrine

B. Adenosine

C. Verapamil

D. Amiodarone

62. The mother of a 4-week-old infant brings the infant to the emergency department. She states that the child has been "turning blue" when she cries. Today, she "turned blue" when she was sucking on her bottle. The baby is tachypneic (RR 60); HR 150, diaphoretic, and becomes cyanotic when she cries. The mother has not had any follow-up care since

she was discharged home 24 hours after her daughter's birth. A loud heart murmur is auscultated. Tetralogy of Fallot is suspected. The initial treatment of this infant should include:

- 0   A.   Administration of diltiazem IV to decrease her heart rate
- 0   B.   Administration of propanolol IV to relieve right ventricular outflow spasms
- 0   C.   Immediate sedation, neuromuscular blocking, and intubation
- 0   D.   Referral to the outpatient pediatric clinic for a 12-lead ECG

63. How should the paddles be placed for the patient who has an implanted cardioverter defibrillator and who needs to be defibrillated?
- 0   A.   The patient should not be defibrillated
- 0   B.   The paddles should be placed on the apex and sternum
- 0   C.   The paddles should be placed anteriorly and posteriorly
- 0   D.   The patient's chest should be opened for internal defibrillation

64. A 50-year-old man with a history of a heart transplant presents to the emergency department in complete heart block. His BP is 78/52; HR 42; RR 16. He is lethargic, but can be aroused. An external pacemaker has been placed, but is not effectively pacing the patient. Which medication would provide chronotropic support and increase his heart rate until a transvenous pacemaker can be inserted?
- 0   A.   Isoproterenol 2 µg/min
- 0   B.   Dobutamine 10 µg/min
- 0   C.   Diltiazem 2 mg/min
- 0   D.   Norepinepherine 1 µg/min

## Hypertension

*The family of a 47-year-old African American male brings him to the emergency department. He is complaining of a headache, blurred vision, and chest pain. He has no known medical problems and is not taking any medication. He states his brother has been treated for high blood pressure and a myocardial infarction. His vital signs are B/P 220/142 (right arm), P 100, and R 22. The emergency nurse takes his blood pressure in his left arm and finds it to be 218/138.*

65. A hypertensive emergency is occurring when the patient's diastolic blood pressure is greater than:
- 0   A.   90 mm Hg
- 0   B.   100 mm Hg
- 0   C.   120 mm Hg
- 0   D.   130 mm Hg

66. Signs and symptoms of complications related to hypertension include:
- 0   A.   A diastolic blood pressure of 80 mm Hg
- 0   B.   Right ventricular hypertrophy
- 0   C.   Impaired renal function
- 0   D.   Normal potassium levels

67. The emergency physician orders labetalol, 20 mg IV push, for the patient. A possible side effect of this drug is:
- 0   A.   Orthostatic hypotension
- 0   B.   Tachycardia
- 0   C.   Excessive salivation
- 0   D.   Headache

68. The labetalol has not effectively lowered the patient's blood pressure. His chest pain continues, but a 12-lead ECG shows no acute changes with evidence of left-ventricular hypertrophy. A nitroprusside drip is initiated at .2 µg/kg. The most accurate blood pressure readings would be obtained by:
- 0   A.   Placing a noninvasive blood pressure cuff on the patient's left arm
- 0   B.   Placing a noninvasive blood pressure cuff on the patient's right arm
- 0   C.   Inserting an arterial line for continuous blood pressure monitoring
- 0   D.   Placing the patient on a continuous 12-lead ECG monitor

69. A toxic effect of the long-term use of intravenous nitroprusside is:
- 0   A.   Hypocalcemia leading to muscle weakness
- 0   B.   Hyperkalemia leading to peaked T waves
- 0   C.   Thiocyanate and cyanide toxicity
- 0   D.   Bradycardia leading to asystole

70. A patient with newly diagnosed hypertension is prescribed hydrochlorothiazide (Hydrodiuril), 50 mg bid, by the emergency physician. The patient states, "I have never taken any medication for my blood pressure before." The emergency nurse should base discharge instructions on which of the following nursing diagnoses?
- 0   A.   Knowledge deficit related to the use of a new drug for a newly diagnosed disease process
- 0   B.   Body image disturbance related to physical changes that occur with hypertension

0  C. Thought processes, altered, related to the cerebral changes brought about by chronic hypertension

0  D. Family processes, altered, related to the need for a family member to take a new medication

71. The emergency nurse provides information to the patient about his disease process and refers him for follow-up care. Which of the following measures could the emergency nurse use to evaluate the effectiveness of this intervention?

0  A. The patient returns to the emergency department for follow-up care

0  B. The patient keeps his appointment at the hypertension clinic

0  C. The patient does not take his medicine and returns in a hypertensive crisis

0  D. The patient leaves his referral information at the emergency department

**Congestive Heart Failure**

*The rescue squad brings a 62-year-old woman to the emergency department. She was awakened by severe shortness of breath and chest pain. On arrival in the emergency department, she is awake, short of breath, diaphoretic, and pale. Her vital signs are B/P 160/100, P 120, RR 32. Crackles are auscultated in both lung fields two thirds of the way up. She has a history of hypertension, renal failure, and an inferior myocardial infarction.*

72. Which of the following disease processes most often contributes to congestive heart failure in the adult patient?

0  A. Cardiomyopathy

0  B. Congenital cardiac disease

0  C. Myocardial infarction

0  D. Atrial fibrillation

73. A nitroglycerin infusion is started at 20 $\mu$g/min. The clinical effect of nitroglycerin is to:

0  A. Increase preload

0  B. Increase afterload

0  C. Decrease preload

0  D. Increase afterload

74. Morphine, 2 mg, is administered by IV push by the emergency nurse. Morphine is an effective

drug for the patient with congestive heart failure because it:

0  A. Produces respiratory arrest

0  B. Produces myocardial depression

0  C. Increases the patient's heart rate

0  D. Reduces venous return

75. The patient is given 40 mg of furosemide (Lasix) for diuresis. One intervention the emergency nurse could perform to decrease patient exertion would be to:

0  A. Insert a urinary catheter

0  B. Place the patient in Trendelenburg position

0  C. Give the patient oxygen by nasal cannula

0  D. Place a pulse oximeter on the patient

76. The patient's blood gas results are as follows: pH, 7.37; $P_{CO_2}$, 25; $P_{O_2}$, 60; and $HCO_3$, 18. Using the data collected from these blood gas results, which of the following nursing diagnoses would the emergency nurse use to base care?

0  A. Fluid volume deficit related to diuresis with furosemide

0  B. Gas exchange, impaired, related to the patient's congestive heart failure

0  C. Activity intolerance related to the low $P_{O_2}$

0  D. Tissue integrity, impaired, related to the patient's acute congestive heart failure

77. The patient's oxygen source is changed to a 100% nonrebreather mask. In addition to arterial blood gases (ABGs), what other data could the emergency nurse use to evaluate the patient's condition?

0  A. Level of consciousness

0  B. Hemoglobin and hematocrit

0  C. Urinary output

0  D. Palpation of peripheral pulses

78. Recent research has demonstrated better management of left ventricular systolic dysfunction when patients with CHF are treated with a combination of:

0  A. ACE inhibitors and beta-blockers

0  B. Beta-blockers and calcium channel blockers

0  C. ACE inhibitors and angiotensin II antagonists

0  D. Digitalis and loop diuretics

## Thrombophlebitis and Arteriovascular Disease

79. Risk factors that would contribute to the development of thrombophlebitis include all of the following *except:*
    - 0   A. Wearing antiembolic stockings
    - 0   B. Taking oral contraceptives
    - 0   C. Sepsis from a urinary tract infection
    - 0   D. Prolonged bed rest

80. Signs and symptoms of venous thrombosis include:
    - 0   A. No palpable peripheral pulses
    - 0   B. Lack of pain in the affected extremity
    - 0   C. Absence of Homans' sign
    - 0   D. An extremity that is red, hot, and swollen

81. A 25-year-old patient with a previous history of deep vein thrombosis once again has an abnormal duplex ultrasonography. The patient is to be treated at home with enoxaparin (Lovenox) subcutaneously and warfarin orally. The advantages of low molecular weight heparin (enoxaparin) over unfractionated heparin include:
    - 0   A. Enoxaparin has a shorter half-life than heparin
    - 0   B. Enoxaparin has a predictable anticoagulant response
    - 0   C. Enoxaparin has lower bioavailability than heparin
    - 0   D. Enoxaparin can only be administered orally

82. The patient is taught how to administer the enoxaparin subcutaneously. She performs the return demonstration well. What other instructions should the patient be able to demonstrate a full understanding of before discharge from the emergency department?
    - 0   A. Because the patient is on anticoagulant therapy, she may resume her normal physical activities
    - 0   B. If excessive bruising develops around the injection site, she should just ignore it because that is a common side effect of anticoagulation medications
    - 0   C. Her blood should be drawn daily to monitor her prothrombin time for the first few days at home
    - 0   D. If she has any blood in her stool, this should not be reported until it has occurred for several days

83. The advantage of using the international normalized ratio (INR) to monitor warfarin therapy instead of a prothrombin time includes:
    - 0   A. It can only be used to monitor anticoagulant therapy for patients taking warfarin for the treatment of pulmonary embolus
    - 0   B. The INR is reliable anywhere the patient may require treatment, allowing the patient more flexibility
    - 0   C. It is governed by the sensitivity of the reagents used to measure the effectiveness of the amount of warfarin the patient is taking
    - 0   D. There is no advantage to using INR over prothrombin time to monitor the effectiveness of anticoagulant therapy

*An 82-year-old man is brought to the emergency department because of severe pain in his left leg. He has a history of atrial fibrillation and hypertension. He states that the pain began suddenly when he got out of bed prior to arrival in the emergency department.*

84. The physical examination of a patient with an acute arterial occlusion would reveal:
    - 0   A. Palpable peripheral pulses
    - 0   B. A red, warm extremity
    - 0   C. A pale, cold extremity
    - 0   D. Presence of Homans' sign

85. The emergency nurse should prepare the patient with an acute arterial occlusion for:
    - 0   A. Surgery for embolectomy to decrease the risk of extremity loss
    - 0   B. Anticoagulant therapy low molecular weight heparin at home
    - 0   C. Application of ice to, and elevation of, the affected extremity to relieve pain
    - 0   D. Application of antiembolic hose to decrease the risk of pulmonary embolus

86. The appropriate nursing diagnosis on which the emergency nurse should base the care of this patient is:
    - 0   A. Gas exchange, impaired, related to an acute arterial occlusion
    - 0   B. Tissue perfusion, altered (peripheral), related to an acute arterial occlusion

C. Fluid volume deficit related to an acute arterial occlusion

D. Disuse syndrome, potential for, related to an acute arterial occlusion of a lower extremity

## Digitalis Toxicity

*A 4-year-old child has ingested an unknown amount of his grandmother's digitalis. The family is unsure when the child took the pills. He is currently awake, nauseated, and vomiting.*

87. The most common dysrhythmia seen in patients with digitalis toxicity who do not have cardiac disease is:
    - A. Ventricular bigeminy
    - B. Ventricular tachycardia
    - C. Sinus bradycardia
    - D. AV junctional tachycardia

88. The child's monitor shows a sinus bradycardia. He progresses to a third-degree block with a blood pressure of 70/40. Which drug should the emergency team administer?
    - A. Lidocaine, 1 mg/kg IV push
    - B. Isoproterenol drip of 4 mg in 250 $D_5W$
    - C. Atropine, 0.5 mg IV push
    - D. Epinephrine, 0.1 mg/kg

89. Digibind is to be administered to this child. All of the following are indications for the use of digoxin-specific antibody fragments except:
    - A. Cardiac arrest from digitalis toxicity
    - B. Bradyarrhythmias unresponsive to atropine
    - C. Severe hyperkalemia
    - D. Conversion to sinus rhythm after atropine

90. Plants that contain cardiac glycosides include all of the following except:
    - A. Foxglove plant
    - B. Lily of the valley
    - C. Ramp
    - D. Hellebore

## Cardiac Trauma

*A 24-year-old man is brought to the emergency department following an accident in which he was struck by a car while riding his bicycle. The patient was thrown from the bike, landing on his chest. He was wearing a helmet. On arrival in the emergency department, the patient is awake, moving all his extremities, and complaining of midsternal chest pain. His vital signs are B/P 100/79, P 132, R 28.*

91. The most common sign or symptom associated with myocardial contusion is:
    - A. Sinus tachycardia
    - B. Pericardial effusion
    - C. Chest pain referred to the shoulder
    - D. Hemothorax

92. The initial evaluation of the patient with a suspected myocardial contusion in the emergency department should include:
    - A. A MUGA scan
    - B. Clotting studies
    - C. A 12-lead ECG
    - D. Serial hemoglobin and hematocrit

93. Beck's triad includes:
    - A. Increased blood pressure, distended neck veins, and muffled heart sounds
    - B. Decreased blood pressure, distended neck veins, and muffled heart sounds
    - C. Decreased blood pressure, flat neck veins, and audible heart sounds
    - D. Increased blood pressure, flat neck veins, and muffled heart sounds

94. The most sensitive enzyme that determines myocardial damage is:
    - A. Creatine kinase (CK)
    - B. CK-MB subforms: MB 1 and MB 2
    - C. Lactic dehydrongenase (LDH)
    - D. Cardiac troponin I

95. A 7-year-old boy is brought to the emergency department in full arrest. He was playing baseball and was struck in the chest with a baseball. He immediately collapsed, and bystander CPR was initiated. He was transported in a private car to the emergency department. When placed on the monitor, he is found to be in ventricular fibrillation. Despite aggressive resuscitation, including an open thoracotomy, the child expired. The most likely cause of his arrest is:
    - A. Pulmonary contusion from the ball that struck him in the chest
    - B. Cardiac concussion from a blunt blow to the chest
    - C. Cerebral embolus from being struck with the ball
    - D. Congenital cardiac problem brought on by playing baseball

**96.** A 24-year-old man has been brought to the emergency department with a stab wound in his midsternum. Initially awake, he has become unresponsive. He has a palpable pulse. The emergency nurse should prepare the patient for:

   0   A.  Insertion of a trauma catheter

   0   B.  Insertion of bilateral chest tubes

   0   C.  Emergency thoracotomy

   0   D.  Insertion of a CVP line

**97.** A 19-year-old woman is brought to the emergency department after having been involved in a head-on collision with a truck. She was entrapped for over an hour and has obvious signs of severe chest trauma. All of the following would indicate an aortic injury except:

   0   A.  Chest wall bruising

   0   B.  A first rib fracture

   0   C.  The trachea in the midline

   0   D.  Paraplegia

**98.** An 85-year-old woman presents to the emergency department with a complaint of severe abdominal pain. Her vital signs are B/P 110/40, P 100, R 24. Upon physical examination, a palpable pulsating mass is found in her lower abdomen. The patient will need to be transferred to another facility for further treatment. What medications may be used to manage the patient's pain?

   0   A.  Esmolol to decrease the patient's blood pressure, which will decrease the pressure on the arterial wall and relieve her pain

   0   B.  Morphine sulfate for analgesia and a benzodiazepine to manage her anxiety related to being transferred

   0   C.  Norepinephrine to increase her blood pressure and decrease the risk of shock, which may cause further vasoconstriction and pain

   0   D.  No pain medication should ever be given to a patient with an aortic aneurysm

**99.** Cardiac arrest due to electrolyte abnormalities results from:

   0   A.  Hypercalcemia

   0   B.  Hypernatremia

   0   C.  Hyperkalemia

   0   D.  Hyperphosphatemia

**100.** A 20-year-old man was working on some electrical connections in his house. His friends who called 911 found him unresponsive. The initial management of this patient would include:

   0   A.  Securing the patient's airway through endotracheal intubation

   0   B.  Starting chest compressions after checking a pulse

   0   C.  Defibrillating the patient before placing on the monitor

   0   D.  Turning off the electrical power before rescue attempts are started

## ANSWERS

1. **C. Assessment.** The pain pattern described by the patient having a myocardial infarction is usually sudden in onset, crushing, and substernal; the pain may radiate to the patient's neck, jaw, and back.[5]

2. **A. Assessment.** Serum cardiac enzyme levels can provide information about the evolution and resolution of injury to the myocardium. The information these tests can provide, however, is generally not available in the emergency department, and waiting for it could delay important treatment, such as thrombolytic therapy.[5,6]

3. **D. Assessment.** ST segment elevation indicates injury; T wave inversion indicates ischemia; and pathological Q waves indicate infarction.[5]

4. **A. Assessment.** ST elevation in leads $V_2$, $V_3$, and $V_4$ is indicative of an anterior infarction.[2,5]

   ST elevation in II, III, and aVF is indicative of an inferior infarction. ST elevation in leads I, $Av_1$, $V_5$, and $V_6$ is indicative of a lateral infarction. Leads showing wave changes in $V_1$ and $V_2$, a tall, broad initial R wave, ST segment depression, and a tall upright T wave would indicate a posterior infarction.[4,5]

5. **B. Intervention.** Drawing all the blood studies before drug administration will decrease the potential for additional sites that may bleed during the administration of fibrinolytics.[4]

6. **C. Intervention.** Because of the potential for reperfusion dysrhythmia during the administration of fibrinolytics, the emergency nurse needs to be prepared by bringing along a defibrillator and ACLS drugs.[5]

7. **A. Intervention.** To ensure that all of the medicine has been infused, it is recommended that the tubing be purged after the infusion.[5]

8. **C. Evaluation.** Accelerated idioventricular rhythm is frequently associated with reperfusion. The usual rate is 60 to 100 beats per minute.[13]

9. **B. Assessment.** The most common complication of thrombolytic therapy is bleeding. Intracranial hemorrhage is the most dangerous complication of thrombolytic therapy.[4]

10. **B. Assessment.** Women who have had a myocardial infarction and were treated with fibrinolytics have a greater incidence of having a stroke.[12]

11. **B. Evaluation.** Since intracranial hemorrhage is one of the most serious complications of thrombolytic therapy, it is important that the emergency nurse assess the patient for changes in level of consciousness, nausea and vomiting, headache, and confusion.[12]

12. **B. Intervention.** If during the course of infusion of fibrinolytics that patient should exhibit signs and symptoms of intracerebral hemorrhage, the emergency nurse should immediately stop the infusions and notify the emergency physician.[4,12]

13. **D. Intervention.** Medications used to reverse the effects of fibrinolytic therapy with streptokinase and heparin include protamine sulfate and aminocaproic acid. Protamine sulfate is the antidote for heparin overdose. It works by binding with heparin to form an inactive complex that cannot cause anticoagulation. Aminocaproic acid prevents the recurrence of subarachnoid hemorrhage and produces amegakaryoctic thrombocytopenia to decrease the need for platelet transfusion.[14]

14. **C. Analysis.** Because the patient is receiving a drug that has several serious potential side effects, the emergency nurse's care needs to be directed at preventing any injury that could result. Examples of this prevention are drawing blood from the IV site, minimizing the number of IV sites, minimizing the number of punctures, and performing invasive procedures such as Foley catheter insertion before the administration of the drug.[15]

15. **A. Assessment.** T-PA is clot specific. It is a direct activator of plasminogen. Urokinase and streptokinase cause lytic states.[14]

16. **C. Intervention.** Pain stimulates the release of catecholamines, which can lead to additional oxygen demands on an already compromised myocardium.[14]

17. **A. Analysis.** The defining characteristics of this nursing diagnosis include increased tension, verbalization of fear, decreased self-assurance, and sympathetic stimulation. A related factor that would contribute to the use of this nursing diagnosis on which to base emergency nursing care is the fact that the patient is separated from his support system in a potentially life-threatening situation.[15]

18. **B. Evaluation.** One of the expected outcomes for emergency nursing interventions related to this diagnosis would be that the patient is able to verbalize his feelings about the source of his fear and how he is able to deal with it.[15]

19. **B. Intervention.** Right ventricular infarction occurs in about 40% of patients who suffer inferior wall myocardial infarctions. Treatment for the hypotension that occurs with right ventricular infarction is the administration of fluids.[4,5]

20. **B. Assessment.** Right ventricular infarcts are diagnosed by the placement of right-sided precordial leads.[4,5]

21. **C. Assessment.** The diagnosis of an acute myocardial infarction (MI) is based on three factors: history, clinical examination, and a 12-lead ECG. The history and clinical evaluation help the emergency nurse identify risk factors for heart disease, such as smoking and hypertension. A 12-lead ECG may show ischemia, injury, or infarction. Enzyme analysis (not generally available in the emergency department) will show the extent of damage that has occurred.[4,5]

22. **C. Intervention.** The benefits of nitroglycerin in the treatment of myocardial infarction include a reduction in myocardial oxygen consumption, an increase in flow to ischemic myocardium, and a decrease in coronary artery spasm.[14]

23. **B. Intervention.** Nitroglycerin administered in large, inappropriate doses may cause reflex tachycardia, which will increase myocardial oxygen consumption.[14]

24. **B. Intervention.** The absorption of heparin has been found to vary from patient to patient. Weight-based heparin helps to ensure that the patient is receiving an effective dose.[16]

25. **D. Analysis.** The WHO definition of the diagnosis of an acute MI includes (1) ST-segment changes and new Q waves; (2) chest pain characteristics; and (3) abnormally elevated serum cardiac enzyme levels. However, some patients experience acute myocardial infarctions with no ECG changes or chest pain. Myoglobin may also be elevated by strenuous exercise, renal failure, IM injections, or heavy use of alcohol. The patient's age and sex also may influence myoglobin levels.[9]

26. **C. Analysis.** Cardiac troponin complex is a basic component of the myocardium. These levels begin to increase 3 hours after myocardial ischemia and remain elevated for 5 to 7 days. A sharp increase in cardiac troponin T indicates reperfusion because of the "washout" of cytoplasmic cardiac troponin T after reperfusion.[9]

27. **B. Assessment.** Preload is measured in the right side of the heart by the right arterial pressure or the central venous pressure. This reflects the blood being returned from the systemic circulation.[17]

28. **D. Assessment.** Systemic vascular resistance is increased by compensatory constriction of peripheral blood vessels caused by epinephrine.[17]

29. **B. Intervention.** Metoprolol is a beta blocker, and its effects provide a protective mechanism for an injured myocardium by decreasing the heart rate, oxygen consumption, and metabolic demand.[18]

30. **B. Intervention.** Abciximab (ReoPro) is a glycoprotein IIb/IIIa receptor inhibitor. This drug inhibits platelet aggregation by binding with the site where fibrinogen binds when platelets are activated. This stops platelet aggregation and thrombus formation. Research has demonstrated that glycoprotein IIb/IIIa receptor inhibitors, along with aspirin and weight-based heparin, have been found to be effective in preventing thrombosis.[19,20]

31. **A. Intervention.** Administration of platelets will inhibit the antiplatelet effect of glycoprotein IIb/IIIa receptor inhibitors. Protamine zinc is the antidote for heparin, and clopidogrel is an oral antiplatelet drug.[19]

32. **D. Evaluation.** A growing and costly epidemic in the United States is the prevalence of congestive heart failure after acute myocardial infarction. Approximately 20% of patients who suffer an MI will develop CHF within 6 years of their MI. The cost of caring for patients with CHF is estimated to be more than $35 billion. This points to the important role emergency nurses can play in early recognition of potential myocardial injury and the need to teach preventive strategies such as diet, exercise, and blood pressure management to at risk patients who come to the emergency department for care.[21]

33. **B. Intervention.** Bolus administration of fibrinolytics offers some advantages over continuous infusion, including ease of administration and less risk of a medication error because the dosage does not have to be adjusted for patient weight. However, the longer half-life of these medications makes it more difficult to reverse the effects of bleeding complications.[22]

34. **C. Intervention.** Resuscitation may be withheld in the following circumstances:
   - Patients who have a clear advanced directive asking healthcare workers not to begin resuscitation in the event of a cardiac arrest.

   - Patients with signs of irreversible death such as rigor mortis or decapitation.[23]

35. **B. Assessment.** Aspirin targets the platelet and fibrinolytic therapy targets the fibrin component of the clot.[22]

36. **C. Assessment.** Ventricular fibrillation.

37. **A. Intervention.** The emergency team should confirm the rhythm and then defibrillate the patient with 360 W/sec. The ACLS algorithm for ventricular fibrillation/pulseless ventricular tachycardia (VF/VT) states that the patient should be defibrillated up to three times for persistent VF/VT at 200 J, 200-300 J, and 360 J.[13]

38. **D. Intervention.** When electrical activity is detected but no pulse is palpated, the patient is in pulseless electrical activity (PEA). When the patient is in PEA, the emergency nurse needs to consider the possibility of hypovolemia, cardiac tamponade, tension pneumothorax, acidosis, pulmonary embolism, and hypoxemia, as well as what interventions could be used to correct any of these possible origins of PEA.[13]

39. **B. Assessment.** Ventricular bigeminy.

40. **B. Intervention.** The patient would be treated with lidocaine, 1 mg/kg.[13]

41. **A. Assessment.** Ventricular tachycardia.

42. **D. Intervention.** Amiodarone is administered in three phases:
   - Rapid infusion of 150 mg/10 minutes
   - Early maintenance infusion 1 mg/min for 6 hours
   - Late maintenance infusion 0.5 mg/min[13]

43. **C. Evaluation.** Hypotension is the most common side effect of amiodarone. It is not dose-related.[13]

44. **D. Intervention.** Torsades de pointes should be considered when patients display ventricular tachycardia refractory to treatment by lidocaine and amiodarone. Magnesium sulfate has demonstrated the ability to abolish torsades. It is administered IV for 1 to 2 minutes at a dosage of 1 to 2 g. Up to 4 to 6 g may be administered to treat torsades.[13]

45. **A. Assessment.** Asystole.

46. **D. Intervention.** Lidocaine, atropine, naloxone, and epinephrine can be put down the endotracheal tube. Valium, although not a cardiac drug, can also be given down the endotracheal tube.[13]

47. **B. Intervention.** Drugs administered down the endotracheal tube should be given in 2 to 2.5 times the usual dose and then be followed with a 10 ml flush of normal saline. The initial dose of epinephrine is 1 mg.[13,24]

48. **C. Assessment.** Third-degree heart block.

49. **C. Evaluation.** A common problem with the use of an external pacemaker in the awake patient is pain from the muscle spasms that occur from the pacemaker. Patients may need to be sedated until a transvenous pacemaker can be placed.[13,25]

50. **A. Evaluation.** A palpable pulse demonstrates that there has been mechanical capture. Pacer spikes on the monitor demonstrate electrical capture, but no mechanical capture or functional myocardial contracture.[13,25]

51. **C. Intervention.** The battery may be low and not generating enough power to effectively pace the patient. Adding an additional set of pacer pads would not be helpful, but changing the current pads and repositioning them may increase the chance of capture.[25]

52. **C. Intervention.** Adenosine slows conduction time through the AV node. It is indicated for the treatment of paroxysmal supraventricular tachycardia because it can interrupt the reentry pathway and restore sinus rhythm.[13,26]

53. **D. Intervention.** If there is no change in the patient's rhythm 1 to 2 minutes after administration of the adenosine, the next step is to double the dose of adenosine to 12 mg.[13,26]

54. **D. Analysis.** Adenosine causes conversion dysrhythmia, including sinus bradycardia, heart block, and a brief period of asystole. If the patient is not warned about this side effect, it can be very frightening. In addition, many patients complain of feeling warm and experience flushing, which is another common side effect.[13,26]

55. **A. Assessment.** Atrial fibrillation.

56. **C. Assessment.** Atrial fibrillation leaves the patient at risk for developing clots and emboli. Any of these may result in a transient ischemic attack (TIA) or progress to stroke.[4]

57. **D. Intervention.** Unstable atrial fibrillation should be immediately cardioverted to prevent serious complications such as hypotension, CHF, chest pain, and rhythm deterioration, particularly in the presence of an acute MI. The defibrillator should be set at 100 J, synchronous mode for the initial shock and the Electrical Cardioversion Algorithm followed to manage this patient.[13]

58. **B. Intervention.** The initial intravenous adult dose of diltiazem is calculated using 0.25 mg/kg. If the initial dose is not adequate, the dose may be repeated at 0.35 mg/kg.[13,14]

59. **A. Intervention.** Drugs that are used to treat diltiazem toxicity would depend on the type of physiological reactions the patient was having. If the patient is hypotensive, fluids, vasopressors, and calcium chloride could be used. For symptomatic bradycardia, atropine, calcium, and norepinephrine may be used. Verapamil, which is another calcium-channel blocker, would only potentiate the effects of the diltiazem.[13,14]

60. **B. Intervention.** Synchronized cardioversion is the treatment of choice for a child with unstable tachydysrhythmia. The recommended dose is 0.5 to 1 J/kg.[27]

61. **C. Intervention.** Cardiovascular collapse has been reported in infants when verapamil has been used.[27]

62. **B. Intervention.** Tetralogy of Fallot has four components. These include ventricular septal defect; pulmonary stenosis; right ventricular hypertrophy; and overriding aorta. Unfortunately, many infants are discharged earlier before problems can be identified and may appear as this child did in the emergency department for care. IV propanolol may relieve the spasms of the right ventricular outflow tract and therefore improve oxygenation. The child should receive oxygen and measures initiated to keep her calm to decrease her oxygen consumption.[28]

63. **C. Intervention.** The paddle position for the patient who has an implanted cardioverter defibrillator is the anterior/posterior position.[29]

64. **A. Intervention.** Isoproterenol is recommended for the treatment of bradycardia in the denervated transplanted heart. It has both inotropic and chonotropic properties. The dose needed for chonotropic support in complete heart block begins at 2 $\mu$g/min and should not exceed 10 $\mu$g/min. Because isoproterenol markedly increases myocardial oxygenation, it should be used only temporarily.[4,13,30] It is also important to note here that in the 1999 ILCOR Advisory Statements: Special Resuscitation Situations[23] the treatment for bradyasystolic rhythms in a denervated heart is the use of an adenosine-blocking agent such as aminophylline 250 mg IV bolus if pacing, atropine, or epinephrine fails.

65. **D. Assessment.** A hypertensive crisis is defined as a diastolic blood pressure greater than 130 mm Hg. This constitutes an emergent patient problem.[4,13,30]

66. **C. Assessment.** Complications of hypertension include papilledema, left ventricular hyper-

trophy, congestive heart failure, impaired renal function, and intracranial or subarachnoid hemorrhage.[4,13,30]

67. **A. Evaluation.** Side effects of labetalol include orthostatic hypotension at the beginning of therapy, facial flushing, dry mouth, bradycardia, and fatigue.[14]

68. **C. Intervention.** When a nitroprusside infusion is initiated, an arterial line should be inserted to provide the most accurate assessment of the patient's blood pressure.[4]

69. **C. Analysis.** Toxic side effects of long-term infusions of nitroprusside are thiocyanate and cyanide toxicity.[14]

70. **A. Analysis.** The defining characteristics of this nursing diagnosis include verbalization of inadequate information about one's illness and the patient's requesting information about the disease process. Related factors include lack of exposure to accurate information, lack of motivation to learn, and cultural and language barriers.[15]

71. **B. Evaluation.** The expected outcome for nursing interventions related to this diagnosis would be the patient following through as instructed.[15]

72. **C. Assessment.** Congestive heart failure is a common consequence of acute myocardial infarction. As many as 20% of patients who suffer an MI will develop CHF. Because of the increased incidence of CHF, it is being viewed as a serious epidemic in this country and costs billions of dollars each year in patient care.[4,21]

73. **C. Intervention.** Nitroglycerin is a vasodilator that decreases preload and helps in decreasing myocardial oxygen consumption.[14]

74. **D. Intervention.** Morphine reduces venous return by venodilation. It also reduces the respiratory rate and can decrease the patient's anxiety.[14]

75. **A. Intervention.** Inserting a urinary catheter in the patient who is experiencing diuresis will help decrease patient exertion, as well as provide a method for the emergency nurse to keep an accurate record of output for the patient.

76. **B. Analysis.** Based on the data provided by the blood gases, the patient is hypoxic, probably as a result of impairment of gas exchange. Related factors contributing to this nursing diagnosis include alveolar capillary membrane changes and altered capacity of the blood to carry oxygen.[15]

77. **A. Evaluation.** Defining characteristics of gas exchange, impaired, include confusion, restlessness, hypoxia, and irritability. Evaluation of the patient's level of consciousness would provide information about the effect of 100% oxygen by mask.[15]

78. **C. Intervention.** New recommendations for the management of congestive heart failure include the combination of ACE inhibitors and angiotensin II antagonists. The combination of these drugs have been found to improve left ventricular pump function and increases heart muscle cell response to inotropic stimulus. Some of the names of these drugs are lorsartan (Cozaar) (angiotensin II antagonist) and captopril (Capoten) ACE inhibitor.[14,21,31]

79. **A. Assessment.** Risk factors relating to the development of venous thrombosis include medications such as oral contraceptives, prolonged bed rest, trauma, varicose veins, sepsis, and stasis.[4]

80. **D. Assessment.** Signs and symptoms of venous thrombosis include swelling; a red, warm extremity; the presence of Homans' sign; and pain that may be aggravated by walking.[4,5]

81. **B. Analysis.** The advantages of low-molecular-weight heparin over unfractionated heparin include its predictable anticoagulant response, high bioavailability, and longer half-life, which requires fewer daily dosages. Absorption of heparin varies from patient to patient.[16,32,33]

82. **C. Evaluation.** The patient who is being treated for DVT at home must demonstrate a thorough understanding of how the medications work, their potential side effects, physical activities, and how the medication should be monitored. Any excessive bruising or bleeding must be immediately reported. The patient's blood should be drawn daily to monitor the prothrombin time for the first few days.[32]

83. **B. Analysis.** The international normalized ratio (INR) is reliable anywhere. Prothrombin time results vary from place to place and even sometimes within the same lab, depending on the reagents used. The INR can be used to monitor the effectiveness of warfarin and LMH in the treatment of DVT, pulmonary emboli, prevention of systemic emboli from MI, atrial fibrillation, or the use of mechanical valves.[34]

84. **C. Assessment.** The physical examination of an extremity that has an acute arterial occlusion would show a cool, pale limb, pain, changes in motor and sensory function, lack of pulses distal to the occlusion, and slow capillary filling.[35]

85. **A. Intervention.** The treatment for acute arterial occlusion is surgical removal of the clot, or embolectomy. The quicker the occlusion is relieved, the better the patient will do. However, if surgery is delayed, the patient may be started on a regimen of heparin.[35]

86. **B. Analysis.** The defining characteristics of this nursing diagnosis include decreased or absent arterial pulses, pale extremities, cold extremities, loss of motor/sensory function, and pain.[15]

87. **C. Assessment.** Digitalis toxicity can cause numerous types of cardiac dysrhythmia, including, for the patient who does not have preexisting cardiac disease, such as the pediatric patient, AV conduction disturbances. The patient with cardiovascular disease is more likely to have lethal dysrhythmia.[36]

88. **C. Intervention.** Atropine is the drug of choice. The recommended dose is 0.5 mg to 2.0 mg IV.[36]

89. **D. Intervention.** Digibind, or digoxin-specific antibody fragments, is indicated for the treatment of life-threatening digitalis overdose. Digibind works by increasing the speed of digitalis excretion and reversing tissue affinity for digitalis.[36]

90. **C. Assessment.** Plant toxicity can be a source of many types of problems. Some plants contain toxins that affect the heart in the same manner as cardiac glycosides do. These include the foxglove plant, lily-of-the-valley, and hellebore.[37]

91. **A. Assessment.** The most common sign or symptom of myocardial contusion is sinus tachycardia. Other signs and symptoms of myocardial contusion include severe chest pain, chest wall contusion, hypotension, and dyspnea.[38]

92. **C. Evaluation.** The patient with chest trauma needs to have a 12-lead ECG. Enzymes may be helpful, but the information may not be available in a timely manner.[38,39]

93. **B. Assessment.** Beck's triad includes decreased blood pressure, distended jugular veins, and muffled heart sounds. These signs may be indicative of cardiac tamponade.[38,39]

94. **D. Assessment.** Cardiac troponin I is a sensitive and specific marker of cardiac necrosis. CK-MB do increase with cardiac injury, but they also increase with skeletal muscle damage.[39]

95. **B. Assessment.** Cardiac contusion is a rare occurrence. It results from a blunt blow to the chest such as being struck by a baseball. The dysrhythmia related to cardiac concussion is very hard to convert, and the mortality rate is high.[40]

96. **C. Intervention.** Thoracotomy is indicated for penetrating cardiac trauma, tension pneumothorax, and crush injuries to the chest.[38]

97. **C. Assessment.** Indications of aortic injury include first and second rib fractures, signs of hypovolemic shock, tracheal deviation to the right, chest wall bruising, paraplegia, and sternal fracture.[39]

98. **B. Intervention.** The patient with an aortic aneurysm should have both pain management and blood pressure management when indicated. The patient's blood pressure should be maintained between 100 and 120 mm Hg. Since her vital signs are adequate, her pain should be managed with an analgesic and a sedative to prevent any further detrimental side effects from pain.[4,5]

99. **C. Assessment.** Cardiac arrest from electrolyte abnormalities are not very common except for hyperkalemia. Hypernatremia can be identified by ECG changes (peaked T-waves, bradycardia) and by history (presence of renal failure).[23]

100. **D. Intervention.** The electrical power or the energy source must be stopped before rescue is attempted.[23]

## REFERENCES

1. Engel J: *Pocket guide to pediatric assessment,* St Louis, 1993, Mosby.

2. Bates B: *A guide to physical examination and history taking,* Philadelphia, 1995, Lippincott.

3. Newman P: Trauma in the elderly. In Neff J, Kidd P, editors: *Trauma nursing: The art and science,* St Louis, 1993, Mosby.

4. Barnason S: Cardiovascular emergencies. In Newberry L, editor: *Sheehy's emergency nursing: principles and practice,* St Louis, 1998, Mosby.

5. Howland-Gradman J, Kitt S: Cardiac emergencies. In Kitt S et al, editors: *Emergency nursing: a physiologic and clinical perspective,* Philadelphia, 1995, WB Saunders.

6. Drake D: Cardiac team: an ED quality improvement success story, *J Emerg Nurs* 24:324-328, 1998.

7. Kosnik L: Treatment protocols and pathways: improving the process of care, *Crit Care Nurs* (October suppl): 3-7, 1999.

8. Belle-Isle C: Patients selection and administration of thrombolytic therapy, *J Emerg Nurs* 15:155-164, 1989.

9. Murphy M, Berding CB: Use of measurements of myoglobin and cardiac troponins in the diagnosis of acute myocardial infarction, *Crit Care Nurs* 19(1): 58-66, 1999.

10. Brown C: Portable extracorpeal circulation: A new standard in myocardial infarction care? *J Emerg Nurs* 16:226-228, 1990.

11. Bennett K, Grines C: Current controversies in patient selection for thrombolytic therapy, *J Emerg Nurs* 16:191-194, 1990.

12. Pickett S: Women, thrombolytic therapy, and the gender gap: Recommendations for practice, *J Emerg Nurs* 19:491-497, 1993.

13. American Heart Association: *Advanced cardiac life support,* Dallas, 1997-1999, The American Heart Association.

14. McKenry L, Salerno E: *Pharmacology in nursing,* St Louis, 1998, Mosby.

15. Kim M, McFarland G, McLane A: *Pocket guide to nursing diagnoses,* St Louis, 1993, Mosby.

16. Horvanessian H: New-generation anticoagulants: The low molecular weight heparins, *Ann Emerg Med* 34(6):768-779,1999.

17. Lieberman K: Beyond the basics: Monitoring with a pulmonary artery (Swan-Ganz) catheter, *J Emerg Nurs* 24(3):218-222, 1998.

18. Futterman L, Lemberg L: Heart rate is a simplistic marker of mortality in acute myocardial infarction, *Am J Crit Care* 8: 197-199,1999.

19. MacCallum E, Hanlon S, Byrne K: How glycoprotein inhibitors ease coronary syndromes, *Nursing 99* 29(12): 34-40,1999.

20. Gibler BW, Wilcox RG, Bodie C, et al: Prospective use of glycoprotein IIb/IIIa receptor blockers in the emergency department setting, *Ann Emerg Med* 32(6): 712-722, 1998.

21. Moser D, Frazier S, Worster P, Clarke J: The role of the critical care nurse in preventing heart failure after myocardial infarction, *Crit Care Nurse* (October suppl): 11-15,1999.

22. Dracup K, Cannon C: Combination treatment strategies for management of acute myocardial infarction: new directions with current therapies, *Crit Care Nurse* (suppl): 3-17, 1999.

23. Kloeck W, Working Group Chair. *ILCOR advisory statements: Special resuscitation situations,* Dallas, 1999, American Heart Association.

24. Saver C: Decoding the ACLS algorithms, *J Emerg Nurs* 20:27-36, 1994.

25. Gamarth B, Del Monte L, Richards K: Noninvasive pacing: What you should know, *J Emerg Nurs* 24(3):223-233, 1998.

26. Corcoran J: The new ACLS tachycardia algorithm: Flexible guidelines for an old problem, *J Emerg Nurs* 20:93-101, 1994.

27. Chameides L, Hazinski M: *Pediatric advanced life support,* Dallas, 1997-1999, American Heart Association.

28. DeBoer S: The case of the blue baby: ED management of tetralogy of Fallot, *J Emerg Nurs* 22(1): 73-76, 1996.

29. Schuster DM: Patients with an implanted cardioverter: a new challenge, *J Emerg Nurs* 16:219-225, 1990.

30. Foley J: Pharmacologic management of hypertensive crisis in the ED, *J Emerg Nurs* 20:134-135, 1994.

31. Coodley E: Newer drug therapy for congestive heart failure, *Arch Intern Med* 159:1177-1183, 1999.

32. Colucciello S: Protocols for deep vein thrombosis (DVT): A state-of-the-art review. Part II: Patient management, anticoagulation, and special considerations, *Emerg Med Rep* 20(3):25-32, 1999.

33. Zed PJ, Tisdale JE, Borzak S: Low-molecular-weight heparins in the management of acute coronary syndromes, *Arch Intern Med* 159:1849-1857, 1999.

34. Ortel L: Monitoring warfarin therapy: how the INR keeps your patient safe, *Nursing 99* 29:41-44, 1999.

35. Go S: Extremity pain. In Davis M, Votey S, Greengough P, editors: *Signs and symptoms in emergency medicine,* St Louis, 1999, Mosby.

36. Goodman LS: Digitalis. In Haddad L, Shannon M, Winchester J, editors: *Poisoning and drug overdose,* ed 3, Philadelphia, 1998, WB Saunders.

37. Edgerton PH: Symptoms of digitalis-like toxicity in a family after accidental ingestion of lily of the valley plant, *J Emerg Nurs* 15:220-223, 1989.

38. Hurn P, Hartsock R: Thoracic injuries. In Cardona V et al, editors: *Trauma nursing,* Philadelphia, 1994, WB Saunders.

39. Flynn MB, Bonni S: Blunt chest trauma: case report, *Crit Care Nurs* 19:68-77, 1999.

40. Snyder O: A 17-year-old man with history of trauma and dizziness, *J Emerg Nurs* 24(4):371-373, 1998.

# Chapter 5

# Dental, Ear, Nose, and Throat Emergencies

**REVIEW OUTLINE**

I. Anatomy and physiology
- A. Anatomical structures
  - 1. Oral cavity and contents
  - 2. Deciduous and permanent teeth
  - 3. Pharynx
  - 4. Larynx
  - 5. Salivary glands
  - 6. Thyroid cartilage and gland
  - 7. Cricoid cartilage and membrane
  - 8. Trachea
  - 9. Mastoid process
  - 10. Nose, nasal cavity, and contents
  - 11. Four paranasal sinuses
  - 12. Temporomandibular joint (TMJ)
  - 13. External, middle, and inner ear
  - 14. Cranial nerves
- B. Physiology
  - 1. Process of taste
  - 2. Process of hearing
  - 3. Process of smelling
  - 4. Process of mastication
  - 5. Process of swallowing

II. Assessment
- A. Primary survey
  - 1. A, B, C, D, E (airway, breathing, circulation, deficit [neurological], exposure)
  - 2. Stabilization
- B. Secondary survey
  - 1. History of illness or injury
    - a. Mechanism and time
    - b. AMPLE history
      - (1) Allergies
      - (2) Medications
      - (3) Past medical history
      - (4) Last meal
      - (5) Events or treatment prior to arrival
  - 2. Chief complaint
    - a. Pain: PQRST
      - (1) Provocation
      - (2) Quality
      - (3) Radiation
      - (4) Severity
      - (5) Timing
    - b. Bleeding
    - c. Shortness of breath
    - d. Edema/ecchymosis
    - e. Foreign body
    - f. Asymmetry
    - g. Fever/chills
    - h. Nausea/vomiting
    - i. Dysphasia/dysphagia
    - j. Paresthesia
    - k. Foul odor/taste in mouth
    - l. Loss of hearing
    - m. Tinnitus/vertigo
    - n. Trismus
    - o. Loss of smell
    - p. Deformity/dislocation
  - 3. Physical exam
    - a. General appearance
    - b. Teeth
      - (1) Number and condition of teeth
      - (2) Dental prosthesis
      - (3) Gaps between existing teeth
    - c. Gingival, oral mucosa, lips, oropharynx, tongue, floor of mouth, hard and soft palates, and salivary glands
      - (1) Symmetry
      - (2) Abnormalities
    - d. External ear and canal
      - (1) Position
      - (2) Blood or cerebrospinal fluid (CSF) drainage

e. Tympanic membrane
  (1) Intact
  (2) Abnormalities
f. External nose
  (1) Position, size, symmetry
  (2) Blood or cerebrospinal fluid (CSF) drainage
g. Internal nose
  (1) Septum, turbinates, mucosa
  (2) Abnormalities
h. Neck
  (1) Symmetry of structures
  (2) Abnormalities
i. Palpation
  (1) Symmetry
  (2) Localized point tenderness
  (3) Abnormal mobility
  (4) Crepitus
  (5) Mobility of teeth
  (6) Temporomandibular joint (TMJ) mobility

III. Diagnostic methods for dental, ear, nose, and throat emergencies
  A. Radiology
  B. Laboratory
  C. Visualization
    1. Pharyngeal mirror
    2. Tongue blades
    3. Otoscope
    4. Nasal speculum
    5. Laryngeal mirror
    6. Suction

IV. Related nursing diagnoses
  A. Alteration in comfort: pain
  B. Anxiety
  C. Airway clearance, ineffective
  D. Fluid volume deficit, high risk for
  E. Infection, high risk for
  F. Nutrition, alteration in
  G. Sensory deficit

V. Age-related changes
  A. Pediatric patient
    1. Foreign bodies are common and should be considered in children under 3 years during ear, nose, and throat (ENT) exams.[1]
  B. Geriatric patient
    1. Decrease in hearing due to aging process needs to be considered during assessment.
    2. Most dental and ENT injuries are related to falls, motor vehicle accidents, and assaults.[1]

VI. Dental, ear, nose, and throat emergencies
  A. Odontalgia
  B. Periodontal disease
  C. Dental trauma
  D. Ludwig's angina
  E. Acute otitis media
  F. Ruptured tympanic membrane
  G. Meniere's disease
  H. Rhinitis
  I. Epistaxis
  J. Nasal fracture
  K. Pharyngitis
  L. Tonsillitis
  M. Fractured larynx
  N. Peritonsillar abscess
  O. Foreign bodies

Dental, ear, nose, and throat emergencies are not generally life-threatening emergencies. However, to the patient presenting to the emergency department with a chief complaint involving one of these structures, an emergent situation exists because the patient or their family (especially a crying infant) believes they must have this condition alleviated immediately. It is important for the emergency nurse to realize the patient's perception of an emergent situation and to intervene rapidly. By doing so, they will meet the patient and the family's needs and expectations, as well as engender trust. Patients with dental, ear, nose, and throat emergencies frequently need education and referral to a specialist as part of their emergency care.

Dental, ear, nose, and throat emergencies are emergent when they obstruct the airway, cause hypovolemia, or have the potential to cause permanent sensory loss.

## REVIEW QUESTIONS

### Odontalgia

*Mr. Brown, a 19-year-old man, presents to the emergency department at 3:00 AM complaining of a severe toothache (odontalgia) for 1 week. His vital signs are as follows: B/P 130/80, P 90, and RR 18. His skin is warm and dry and color is pink.*

1. The most serious complication of odontalgia is:
   O  A. Pain when drinking a cold beverage
   O  B. Loss of the tooth from decay and damage
   O  C. Pain when drinking a hot beverage
   O  D. Development of an abscess and facial cellulitis

2. The appropriate nursing diagnosis applicable to Mr. Brown is:
   O  A. Swallowing, impaired
   O  B. Fluid volume deficit, high risk for
   O  C. Alteration in comfort, pain
   O  D. Alteration in thought process

3. The most appropriate nursing action would be to:
   O  A. Administer an analgesic
   O  B. Administer an antibiotic
   O  C. Administer an antiemetic
   O  D. Administer an antiinflammatory

4. Mr. Brown tells you in 45 minutes that the pain medication is not working. You know that the onset of action of the particular medication you administered should have begun by now. You suspect:
   O  A. The patient is exhibiting drug-seeking behavior and should be directed to another emergency department for treatment
   O  B. The cause of the toothache is advanced dental caries, and additional pain medication may be required
   O  C. The patient is desperate for sleep and wants to be sure he can do so when he gets home
   O  D. The patient really is not having pain, but an anxiety reaction to being treated in the emergency department

5. Baby Brown, a 1-year-old, is brought to the emergency department by his parents for a "cold." The parents report that the baby has a clear nasal discharge and is drooling, is irritable, has trouble sleeping, has a normal temperature, and has reddened, swollen gums. You suspect:
   O  A. Epiglottitis
   O  B. Odontalgia
   O  C. Tooth eruption
   O  D. Nasal foreign body

6. A 43-year-old female is triaged to the Fast Track Area with the complaint of painful, swollen, and bleeding gums. She states that her teeth are "coming loose." Systemic risks that contribute to the development of periodontal disease include:
   O  A. Adequately fitting upper and lower dentures
   O  B. Good daily fluid and nutrient intake

   O  C. Cardiovascular disease
   O  D. Pregnancy, cigarette smoking, and neoplasm

7. No evidence of acute infection is identified after evaluation in the emergency department and she is sent home and instructed to rinse her mouth with peroxide mouthwash. She returns 48 hours later with extensive facial swelling and cellulites over the lower part of her jaw. Her tongue is swollen, and she is complaining of difficulty swallowing and shortness of breath. The most probable cause of her symptoms is:
   O  A. Pericoronitis
   O  B. Vincent's disease
   O  C. Ludwig's angina
   O  D. Multiple dental abscesses

8. The emergency nurse should prepare for a potential:
   O  A. Circulatory compromise
   O  B. Airway compromise
   O  C. Neurological compromise
   O  D. Febrile seizure

## Acute Otitis Media

*An 18-month-old infant is brought to the emergency department by her parents for complaints of fever, irritability, vomiting, and diarrhea. The parents relate that the child has a history of frequent ear infections.*

9. Risk factors that contribute to the development of recurrent otitis media in children include:
   O  A. Children older than 4 years of age
   O  B. Consistent care provided in the home
   O  C. Recent use of antimicrobial agents
   O  D. No previous antimicrobial treatment

*Further assessment reveals a child who is awake with hot moist skin and a purulent nasal discharge. Her vital signs are as follows: P 150, R 32, Temp 103.2° F (rectal).*

10. Your priority nursing diagnosis for this child would be:
    O  A. Anxiety
    O  B. Hyperthermia
    O  C. Swallowing, impaired
    O  D. Airway clearance, ineffective

11. The most common bacterial cause of acute otitis media is:
    O  A. *S. pneumoniae*
    O  B. *Haemophilus influenzae*

O  C. Respiratory syncytial virus

O  D. *Streptococcus pneumoniae*

12. The parents are given a prescription for high-dose amoxicillin. Discharge instructions should include:

O  A. If symptoms such as ear pain, fever, and vomiting persist greater than 3 days, the child should be seen again by their pediatrician or return to the ED

O  B. If the child takes all of her medicine, there is no need to return for follow-up care with either the pediatrician or the ED

O  C. Amoxicillin orally will cause vomiting, and the parents should not be concerned if the child cannot take all her medicine

O  D. Amoxicillin may cause a rash, and the parents should not call their pediatrician or return to the emergency department

13. Symptomatic treatment for an acute otitis media for a child who is clinically stable and not toxic may include:

O  A. Administration of liquid aspirin three times a day

O  B. Use of antibiotic eardrops bought from the pharmacy

O  C. Administration of warm oil ear drops

O  D. Cleaning the ears with cotton-tipped applicators three times a day

## Nosebleed (Fracture)

*Ms. Lee, a 27-year-old woman, is admitted per Life Squad with severe epistaxis. She was the unrestrained passenger in the front seat of a car that was struck from behind. Ms. Lee reportedly struck her face on the dashboard. She is awake and oriented. Her vital signs are as follows: B/P 110/70, P 92, and RR 24. She is appropriately immobilized on a backboard with a cervical collar in place. Ms. Lee has an obvious nasal deformity and moderate nasal bleeding.*

14. Your initial nursing assessment should be directed at:

O  A. The patency of the patient's airway

O  B. The effectiveness of her breathing

O  C. Any changes in mental status

O  D. Obtaining a manual blood pressure

15. Ms. Lee's cervical spine is cleared; her cervical collar and backboard are removed. Her nose continues to bleed. Your initial nursing intervention to stop the epistaxis should be:

O  A. Apply direct pressure

O  B. Prepare for cauterization

O  C. Provide a suction device

O  D. Prepare for nasal packing

16. Once the bleeding stops, Ms. Lee's nose should be inspected internally for the presence of:

O  A. Blood clots

O  B. Bone chips

O  C. A septal hematoma

O  D. Purulent discharge

17. Ms. Lee requests a mirror so she can look at her nose. Upon observation, Ms. Lee becomes very upset. An appropriate nursing diagnosis would be:

O  A. Fear of treatment

O  B. Pain related to fracture

O  C. Anxiety related to possible permanent alteration in facial appearance

O  D. High risk for injury related to the patient's behavior

18. Ms. Lee is referred to an ENT specialist for treatment after 48 hours, when the edema has subsided. To prevent further epistaxis during this 48-hour period, Ms. Lee should be instructed:

O  A. To avoid cold food

O  B. To sleep in an upright position

O  C. To open her mouth when sneezing

O  D. To forcefully blow her nose to remove all clots on a routine basis

## Pharyngitis

*Mr. Blue, age 31, presents to the triage desk with complaints of a sore throat for 5 days. Mr. Blue reports he has tried throat lozenges and aspirin for pain but nothing has helped. His voice is muffled. You as the triage nurse know that a great majority of sore throats do not represent a serious illness.*

19. To assist in differentiating an urgent vs. nonurgent condition, the triage nurse should ask Mr. Blue if he has had:

O  A. A sinus headache

O  B. Posterior neck tenderness

O  C. To lie flat in bed

O  D. Difficulty swallowing

*Mr. Blue states he has been having increasing difficulty swallowing. He is immediately taken into the emergency department for care. His vital signs are as follows: B/P 110/70, P 104, R 28, Temp 102° F. While assessing his vital signs you note that Mr. Blue is drooling.*

20. Your initial nursing diagnosis for Mr. Blue would be:
    0   A. Violence, high risk for
    0   B. Infection, high risk for
    0   C. Body image disturbance
    0   D. Airway clearance, ineffective, high risk for

21. Mr. Blue is diagnosed as having a peritonsillar abscess. Your initial nursing intervention for Mr. Blue should be:
    0   A. Have Mr. Blue lie flat on his side
    0   B. Have Mr. Blue lie on his stomach
    0   C. Elevate the head of the bed 60 to 90 degrees
    0   D. Place Mr. Blue in Trendelenburg position

*Mr. Blue is given oxygen, antibiotics, and an analgesic and antipyretic. You realize the importance of monitoring Mr. Blue's respiratory status.*

22. To evaluate the effectiveness of your nursing interventions, you would want to see:
    0   A. Pale, diaphoretic skin
    0   B. A decrease in pulse rate
    0   C. A decrease in blood pressure
    0   D. An increase in respiratory rate

*A 4-year-old is brought to the emergency department by his family with a complaint of a sore throat, cough, and fever. When you observe the child at the triage desk he has assumed an upright position on his mother's lap is very quiet and drooling. His color is pale RR 32, and HR 140R.*

23. Epiglottitis is caused by:
    0   A. An acute viral illness
    0   B. Acute tracheobronchial obstruction
    0   C. Acute bacterial illness
    0   D. The onset of winter

24. Epiglottitis is also characterized by:
    0   A. A muffled voice
    0   B. A barky cough
    0   C. A hoarse voice
    0   D. Normal voice tone

*The child is brought into the department and allowed to sit on his mother's lap.*

25. The appropriate nursing diagnosis would be:
    0   A. Hypothermia related to the ED environment
    0   B. Hopelessness related to the cause of his illness

    0   C. Body image disturbance related to the drooling
    0   D. Airway clearance, ineffective, related to the swollen epiglottis

26. The most effective tool in the prevention of epiglottitis is:
    0   A. Administration of prophylactic antibiotics when other children become sick
    0   B. Receiving recommended childhood immunizations in a timely manner
    0   C. Taking large amounts of vitamin C during the cold and flu season each year
    0   D. Providing a cool mist when the child sleeps at night

27. Antibiotic, antipyretic, and analgesic therapies are all administered. To evaluate the effectiveness of these therapies, you would expect to see:
    0   A. An increase in drooling
    0   B. An increase in capillary refill time
    0   C. A decrease in blood pressure
    0   D. A decrease in respiratory rate

## Trauma

28. Mrs. Bush brings her 5-year-old son to the emergency department. He has a history of falling in the hospital parking lot and knocking his tooth out. She hands you the tooth. In order to "save" the tooth, you immerse it in:
    0   A. Cold milk
    0   B. Iced tap water
    0   C. Normal saline
    0   D. Lactated Ringer's solution

29. For successful reimplantation, the avulsed tooth should be reinserted into the socket within:
    0   A. 15 minutes
    0   B. 30 minutes
    0   C. 60 minutes
    0   D. 120 minutes

30. Mrs. Grill brings her 12-year-old daughter to the emergency department. She has fallen off her bicycle and struck the lateral aspect of her head on the curb. There was no loss of consciousness. The patient complains of ear pain, hearing loss on the affected side, nausea, and has blood coming from the affected ear. She is diagnosed with a ruptured tympanic membrane. Mrs. Grill asks if the hearing loss will be permanent. Your response is:
    0   A. Yes, the hearing loss is usually permanent.

O    B. No, hearing usually returns to normal once the tympanic membrane heals.

O    C. You tell the mother you are unsure and she should ask the doctor.

O    D. You tell the mother that the child probably can hear, but is afraid to admit it because she destroyed her bike when she fell.

**31.** The most common cause of tympanic membrane rupture is:

O    A. Trauma

O    B. Infection

O    C. Self-induced

O    D. Exposure to a loud sound

**32.** A 15-year-old boy is brought to the triage desk by his parents. He is complaining of difficulty swallowing and a hoarse voice. He states that earlier in the day he had been struck in the throat by a baseball bat during a game. You suspect:

O    A. Fractured larynx

O    B. Peritonsillar abscess

O    C. Cervical spine injury

O    D. Upper respiratory tract infection

**33.** Your triage classification of this adolescent is:

O    A. Urgent

O    B. Emergent

O    C. Nonurgent

O    D. Delayed care

**34.** Objective signs of a fractured larynx include:

O    A. Normal respiratory rate

O    B. Neck swelling/edema

O    C. Distended neck veins

O    D. $O_2$ saturation of 100%

**35.** Palpation of the neck when the larynx has been injured would reveal:

O    A. No tenderness in the injured area

O    B. Subcutaneous emphysema

O    C. Normal tracheal position

O    D. Normal and equal breath sounds

## ANSWERS

1. **D. Assessment.** The presence of an abscess and facial cellulites will require more aggressive treatment and the potential for tooth and jaw bone loss as well as putting the patient at risk of developing a systemic infection.[1,2]

2. **C. Analysis.** Fluid volume deficit is a potential for Mr. Brown if his tooth is sensitive to hot or cold, causing him to decrease his fluid intake. However, a review of his vital signs and skin signs demonstrates that he is not dehydrated at this time.[1]

3. **A. Intervention.** Because it is 3:00 AM, the patient's most obvious need is relief of pain. After this primary need is met, associated needs can be addressed.[1]

4. **B. Evaluation.** Irreversible tooth pain is an indication that the patient may require a root canal or tooth extraction.[1,2]

5. **C. Assessment.** Baby Brown has classic signs of tooth eruption. These patients are frequently seen in the emergency department with first-time parents.[1,2]

6. **D. Assessment.** Systemic risk factors that contribute to the development of periodontal disease include pregnancy, diabetes mellitus, human immunodeficiency (HIV) infection, advanced age, male gender, and heredity. Ill-fitting dentures and neoplasm also contribute to the development of periodontal disease. Research has demonstrated that periodontal disease is a risk factor for the development of diabetes mellitus and coronary artery disease.[3]

7. **C. Assessment.** Ludwig's angina is characterized by bilateral swelling of the jaw and neck, marked elevation the tongue, shortness of breath, difficulty swelling. Vincent's disease or acute necrotizing ulcerative gingivitis presents signs and symptoms that include bleeding, edematous gums, poor oral hygiene, and bad breath. Ludwig's angina results from a secondary infection involving the second and third molars.[1]

8. **B. Intervention.** The displacement of the patient's tongue because of the extensive swelling places the patient at risk of airway compromise. Emergency airway equipment, particularly for emergent cricothyrotomy, should be placed at the patient's bedside.[1]

9. **C. Assessment.** Risk factors for the development of recurrent otitis media include recent use of microbial agents, age younger than 2 years of age, and day care attendance.[4]

10. **B. Analysis.** Your initial nursing diagnosis should address the patient's priority problem. For baby White, the initial nursing concern should be her fever, as febrile children have a high potential for seizure.[1]

11. **D. Assessment.** *Streptococcus pneumoniae* causes 40% to 50% of acute otitis media (AOM). Unfortunately, there has been a significant increase in the

emergence of drug-resistant *S. pneumoniae,* which has made treatment of AOM difficult, and an increase in children returning to the ED because of failed treatment.[4,5]

12. **A. Intervention.** If symptoms persist beyond 3 days, the child should be reevaluated by their pediatrician or return to the ED. Inabilities to complete the medical regimen or the development of a rash are indications for return to the pediatrician or the ED.[4]

13. **C. Intervention.** Because of the emergence of antibiotic-resistant bacteria causing AOM, symptomatic treatment alone in a stable, nontoxic patient may prove to be useful in relieving the symptoms of AOM. These include warm oil ear drops, use of normal saline nose drops, holding a hair dryer on low setting over the affected ear, and administration of acetaminophen or ibuprofen for pain relief.[4]

14. **A. Assessment.** For any trauma patient, the initial assessment should address the airway while maintaining cervical spine immobilization. Ms. Lee's mouth should be opened and observed for the presence of blood and/or broken teeth, as foreign bodies can potentially obstruct the airway. Ms. Lee's airway should especially be inspected for blood from her obvious nasal fracture.[1]

15. **A. Intervention.** The patient may indeed require nasal packing and/or cauterization. Initially, however, direct pressure is the first nursing intervention. Suctioning may exacerbate the bleeding.[1]

16. **C. Assessment.** A septal hematoma is a grapelike hematoma sitting on the nasal septum. It is imperative that the hematoma be recognized and drained or septal necrosis may occur.[1]

17. **C. Analysis.** Patients with facial fractures are frequently anxious due to a fear of permanent facial deformities.[1]

18. **C. Intervention.** Other measures Ms. Lee should be instructed on include: avoiding straining (lifting, stooping), avoiding further nasal trauma, such as the insertion of a cotton-tipped applicator, and avoiding forceful nose blowing, hot liquids, and high altitudes.[1]

19. **D. Assessment.** Patients complaining of sore throats should be assessed for stridor, fever, dehydration, and difficulty swallowing or talking. If any of these symptoms are present, the patient should be given an urgent status, as they are indicative of serious illness.[6]

20. **D. Assessment.** Mr. Blue is exhibiting a muffled voice, reports difficulty swallowing, is drooling, and has a fever. These are all symptoms of an infectious process in the throat, which should alert the nurse to the potential for airway obstruction.[6,7]

21. **C. Intervention.** This is the best position to maintain an open airway.

22. **B. Evaluation.** A return of vital signs to within normal range is an indicator of successful treatment. All other choices are indicators for reevaluation and further interventions.[5,6]

23. **C. Assessment.** Epiglottitis is caused by an acute onset of a bacterial illness, generally *Haemophilus influenzae* type B. Other bacteria that may cause it include *Streptococcus pneumoniae* and *Staphylococcus aureus.*[8]

24. **A. Assessment.** A barky cough is characteristic of croup.[8]

25. **D. Analysis.** The patient's drooling is an obvious sign of his inability to handle his own secretions, making airway clearance ineffective.[8]

26. **B. Intervention.** In many communities, epiglottitis has been eradicated because of immunization.[8,9]

27. **D. Evaluation.** A normal respiratory rate in a 4-year-old is less than 32 breaths per minute. A return to normal respiratory rate indicates that therapies are working.[8]

28. **A. Intervention.**[5]

29. **B. Intervention.**[5]

30. **B. Intervention.**[3]

31. **B. Assessment.**[1]

32. **A. Assessment.**[6]

33. **B. Assessment.** The patient should be treated emergently due to his potential for airway obstruction.[10]

34. **B. Assessment.** Loss of the normal prominence of the thyroid cartilage is a classic sign of fractured larynx.[10]

35. **B. Assessment.** The presence of subcutaneous emphysema is indicative of a fractured larynx and may be a precursor for tension pneumothorax.[1,6]

## REFERENCES

1. Coimbra-Emanuele DM: Dental, ear, nose and throat emergencies. In Jordan KS, editor: *Emergency nursing core curriculum,* ed 5, Philadelphia, 2000, WB Saunders.

2. Parshall M: Ear, nose, throat, and facial/dental conditions. In Kidd P, Sturt P, editors: *Mosby's emergency nursing reference,* Philadelphia, 1996, WB Saunders.

3. Cavendish R: Periodontal disease. *Am J Nurs* 99(3):36-37, 1999.

4. Fitzgerald MA: Acute otitis media in an era of drug resistance: implications for NP practice, *Nurs Pract* (suppl): October, 1999.

5. Dowell SF, Butler JC, Giebink S, et al: Acute otitis media: management and surveillance in an era of pneumococcal resistance, *Nurs Pract,* (suppl): October, 1999.

6.  Normandin P, Brown J: A 19-year-old with a cough and hemoptysis, *J Emer Med* 24(4):306-308, 1998.
7.  Greenough G: Sore throat. In Davis M, Votey SR, Greenough PG, editors: *Signs and symptoms in emergency medicine,* St Louis, 1999, Mosby.
8.  Haley K, Eckles N, Baker P, editors: *Emergency nursing pediatric course,* Park Ridge, IL, 1998, Emergency Nurses Association.
9.  Flaherty L, Snyder JA: Public health service centers for disease control and prevention: recommended childhood immunization schedule, *J Emer Nurs* 25(4):302, 199
10. Jacobs BB, Hoyt S: *Trauma nursing core course,* Park Ridge, IL, 2000, Emergency Nurses Association.

## ADDITIONAL READINGS

Kitt S et al: *Emergency nursing: a physiological and clinical perspective,* Philadelphia, 1995, WB Saunders.

Krasner PR: Treatment of tooth avulsion by nurses, *J Emerg Nurs* 16(1):29-35, 1990.

Lower J: Maxillofacial trauma, *Nurs Clin North Am* 21(4):611-628, 1986.

Manson PN, Kelly KJ: Evaluation and management of the patient with facial trauma, *Emerg Med Serv* 18(6):22-30, 1989.

Newberry L, editor: *Sheehy's emergency nursing principles and practice,* ed 4, St Louis, 1998, Mosby.

# Chapter 6

# Environmental Emergencies

## REVIEW OUTLINE

I. General management of the patient who is experiencing an environmental emergency
  A. Assess the safety of the environment
    1. Safety of the rescue crew
    2. Safety of the healthcare providers
      a. Care providers should be appropriately dressed for the particular environmental emergency
    3. Control of the environment (e.g., animal, snake loose in the area)
    4. Additional hazards that may be in the environment
    5. Contact and use of appropriate authorities and experts (e.g., zoo, Environmental Protection Agency)
    6. Preparation of the emergency department for the victim(s)
  B. General patient management
    1. A, B, C, D, E (airway, breathing, circulation, deficit [neurological], exposure): exposure of the patient could be particularly important to identify the cause of the problem and any additional injuries
    2. Vital signs: blood pressure, pulse, respiratory rate, temperature
    3. History
      a. What happened and when did it occur?
      b. In what type of environment was the patient found?
        (1) Enclosed space
        (2) Water temperature
        (3) Length of time in the environment
      c. Symptoms experienced before coming to the ED
        (1) Nausea and vomiting
        (2) Headache
        (3) Dizziness
        (4) Temperature
        (5) Skin lesions
      d. Medical history
        (1) Tetanus status
        (2) Diabetes
        (3) Cardiovascular disease
        (4) Cancer
        (5) Alcoholism
        (6) Obesity
        (7) Spinal cord injury
        (8) Medications
      e. Social situation
      f. Witnesses
      g. Type of burn
        (1) Flame
        (2) Scald
        (3) Chemical
      h. History suggestive of abuse
    4. Physical assessment
      a. Inspection
        (1) Airway (patency, signs of obstruction)
        (2) Respiratory status
        (3) Level of consciousness
        (4) Pupillary function
        (5) Motor function
        (6) Skin appearance
          (i) Hyperemia
          (ii) Blistering
          (iii) Edema
          (iv) Ulceration
          (v) Rash
          (vi) Hives
          (vii) Ticks
          (viii) Fang/bite marks
          (ix) Stingers
        (7) Wounds
          (i) Size
          (ii) Shape
          (iii) Depth
          (iv) Visible skin structures
          (v) Debris (fangs, teeth)

b. Palpation
  (1) Heart rate and rhythm
  (2) Pulses—central and peripheral
  (3) Blood pressure
  (4) Motor and sensory response
  (5) Skin temperature
  (6) Crepitus
  (7) Deformities
  (8) Sensation to injured area
c. Percussion
  (1) Chest
  (2) Abdomen
d. Auscultation
  (1) Breath sounds
  (2) Blood pressure
  (3) Bowel sounds

C. Age-related characteristics
  1. Pediatric
    a. Skin thinner and immature temperature control
    b. Drowning is a leading cause of death in the pediatric patient
    c. Alcohol abuse related to disability and death in the adolescent
    d. Weight of child places children at greater risk of suffering complications from envenomation
    e. Size of child leaves them at greater risk for complications from bite injuries
  2. Geriatric
    a. Changes in senses such as vision and peripheral sensation leave older patient at risk for injury
    b. Thermoregulatory changes leave elderly at risk
    c. Changes in peripheral sensation from aging leave elderly at risk for burn injury
    d. Age changes leave patient at greater risk for complications from envenomation
    e. Age changes leave patient at risk for complications from bite injuries

D. Diagnostic procedures
  1. CBC, PT, PTT
  2. Platelet, fibrin, fibrin split products
  3. Electrolytes
  4. Drug screen
  5. ABGs
  6. Chest radiograph
  7. Cervical spine
  8. CT
  9. ECG

II. Related nursing diagnoses
  A. Airway clearance, ineffective
  B. Breathing patterns, ineffective
  C. Fluid volume deficit
  D. Thermoregulation, ineffective
  E. Knowledge deficit related to specific environmental emergency and prevention
  F. Injury, high risk for
  G. Infection, high risk for
  H. Poisoning, high risk for
  I. Spiritual distress

III. Collaborative care for the patient experiencing an environmental emergency
  A. Determine priorities of care
    1. Control and maintain ABCs (provide cervical spine immobilization as indicated)
    2. Monitor vital signs, particularly temperature
    3. Obtain a history related to the environmental emergency
    4. Prepare the patient for specific interventions related to the environmental emergency
      a. Fluid resuscitation
      b. Wound care
        (1) Dressings
        (2) Fasciotomy
        (3) Escharotomy
      c. Warming procedures
      d. Cooling procedures
    5. Medications
      a. Antibiotics
      b. Tetanus prophylaxis
      c. Medications for anaphylaxis
      d. Antivenin
      e. Rabies prophylaxis
    6. Sedation/pain management
      a. Dextran
      b. Mannitol
      c. Antibiotics
      d. Immunizations
    7. Consult experts as indicated

IV. Specific environmental emergencies
  A. Thermoregulatory emergencies
    1. Heat cramps
    2. Heat exhaustion
    3. Heat stroke
    4. Frostbite
    5. Hypothermia
  B. Near-drowning
  C. Lightning injuries
  D. Electrical injuries
  E. Thermal injuries
    1. Thermal
    2. Chemical
    3. Radiation
  F. Bites and stings
    1. Human bites
    2. Animal bites

3. Snake bites
4. Insect stings
5. Tick bites
6. Spider bites
7. Aquatic organisms

The environment that surrounds us not only provides us with beauty but is a source of potential danger as well. Throughout human evolution, we have learned to adjust to our surroundings; one method of doing this is by controlling our environment. However, there are still forces in the environment that cannot be controlled. In these circumstances, humankind has had to learn to live within the environment or suffer the consequences. To understand the effects of the environment on a patient, one must be familiar with how the body interacts with the environment. Body temperature, or thermoregulation, is maintained by the hypothalamus. The preoptic anterior hypothalamus receives body temperature information from the peripheral and central nervous systems. Several systems interact to help control or adjust the body temperature. These include the pituitary and adrenal glands and the sympathetic nervous system. The sympathetic nervous system manages vasodilatation and vasoconstriction. In addition, the processes of convection, radiation, and evaporation contribute to the regulation of body temperature.[1]

The integumentary system provides sensation, regulation, and protection from the environment. Age, chronic illnesses, and medications can influence the integumentary, cardiovascular, neurological, and pulmonary systems, which may leave patients at risk for suffering an environmental emergency.

There are other living organisms that coexist in the environment that may be sources of injury, including snakes, spiders, and ticks. As humankind ventures into new environments either to live or for pleasure, they also encounter animals that may inflict trauma and require specific treatments, such as rabies prophylaxis. Domestic and humans have also been known to be another source of environmental emergencies.

The initial care of the patient who has suffered an illness or injury from the environment is to remove the patient from the injurious environment when possible and ensure that the environment in which the caregivers (including the emergency nurse) are to work is safe. The caregivers need to be appropriately dressed; additional hazards such as radiation or chemical toxins need to be contained; and the appropriate authorities need to be notified so that the victim receives the best possible care.

The general management of the patient who has suffered an illness or injury from the environment is based on the initial evaluation and stabilization of the ABCs. It is important to expose the patient. Exposure will help the emergency nurse identify the cause of the problem, as well as any additional injuries. Vital signs, particularly the patient's temperature, should be evaluated.

Obtaining a history of what happened will help the emergency nurse recognize the type of environmental illness or injury the patient has suffered. Information should include the type of environmental surroundings in which the patient was found, any significant exposure to toxins, the length of time the patient was exposed, the patient's previous medical history, current medications, and any recent use of alcohol or drugs.

The initial emergency nursing interventions are based on the specific illness or injury suffered by the patient. Intravenous access will need to be obtained and medications administered as needed. A baseline neurological assessment should be obtained to set the foundation for further assessment and to evaluate the effects of specific treatments. Wound care is initiated in the prehospital care environment and continued in the emergency department. Finally, the appropriate authorities and/or experts will need to be notified and/or consulted in order to provide additional information for patient care.[1,2,3]

## REVIEW QUESTIONS
### Heat-Related Emergencies

*An 85-year-old woman is brought to the emergency department. She was found in her apartment with the windows closed and no air conditioning or fans. It is the second week of a summer heat wave, with temperatures over 100° F and 88% humidity. The patient is unconscious, and her vital signs are B/P 90/50, P 120, R 28 with shallow respirations, and temp 106° F.*

1. The major difference between heat exhaustion and heat stroke is:
   - O A. The patient's level of consciousness
   - O B. The patient's blood pressure and pulse
   - O C. The patient's inability to dissipate heat
   - O D. The patient's age and skin integrity

2. One of the primary interventions in the care of the patient who is suffering from heat stroke is:
   - O A. Removing all the patient's clothes, wrapping her in wet cloths, and cooling her with fans
   - O B. Insertion of a rectal temperature probe to monitor the patient's temperature during resuscitation
   - O C. Performing a baseline neurological assessment and documenting the findings

O   D. Giving the patient oral fluids to decrease the body temperature and prevent dehydration

3. Based on this patient's blood pressure and pulse, the following is the most appropriate nursing diagnosis:

O   A. Airway clearance, ineffective related to airway obstruction from airway edema

O   B. Pain related to an increase in the body's temperature; interventions need to decrease the body's temperature

O   C. Fluid volume deficit, related to decreased circulating blood volume from fluid loss

O   D. Breathing pattern, ineffective related to hypoxia from an increase in body temperature

4. The patient is being cooled with wet sheets and large fans. During the cooling process, the emergency nurse should frequently evaluate which physiological system for complications?

O   A. Cardiovascular

O   B. Pulmonary

O   C. Renal

O   D. Neurological

5. Drugs that leave a patient at greater risk for developing a heat-related emergency include:

O   A. Narcotics

O   B. Benzodiazepines

O   C. Phenothiazines

O   D. Calcium channel blockers

6. Monitoring for rhabdomyolyis during resuscitation from heat stroke would include:

O   A. Monitoring for changes in the patient's level of consciousness

O   B. Monitoring the color of the patient's urine and output

O   C. Monitoring the patient's electrolytes for hypokalemia

O   D. Monitoring the patient for rhonchi and rales

**Heat Cramps**

*An 18-year-old man comes to the emergency department complaining of weakness and cramps in his legs. He has been out working with a paving crew. The outside temperature is 90° F, and the humidity is 80%.*

7. The major cause of heat cramps is:

O   A. Fluid retention that causes swelling in the lower extremities and general circulation

O   B. Loss of salt in thermal sweat without adequate replacement in oral fluids

O   C. Hyperventilation tetany that occurs with trying to decrease the body's temperature

O   D. Drinking excessive amounts of a sports drink during outside exercise in a hot environment

8. The preferred treatment for the patient with heat cramps is:

O   A. Inserting two large-bore IV needles and giving a fluid bolus of normal saline

O   B. Elevating the extremities that are ccausing the patient discomfor

O   C. Oral rehydration with a balanced electrolyte solution

O   D. Insertion of a gastric tube and irrigation with cool saline solution

9. The patient is treated for heat cramps. On what nursing diagnosis should the emergency nurse base the patient's discharge planning?

O   A. Fear related to suddenly experiencing a heat-related emergency

O   B. Knowledge deficit related to the causes of heat cramps

O   C. Fluid volume deficit related to the hot environment

O   D. Self-esteem disturbance related to becoming ill on the job

10. One evaluation criterion the emergency nurse could use to assess whether this patient understood his discharge instructions would be the fact that the patient:

O   A. States methods to prevent heat cramps while working

O   B. Returns the next day with heat cramps and continues to work

O   C. Quits his job because it is too hot outside

O   D. Returns in a hypernatremic state to the emergency department

11. Infants and young children are at risk for suffering from a heat-related emergency because:

O   A. They have a decreased metabolic rate while they are young

O   B. They have an increased amount of subcutaneous tissue

O   C. They have a large body surface area in proportion to volume

O   D. They have an increased ability to protect themselves from the environment

## Cold-Related Emergencies

**12.** Superficial frostbite is treated by:
- 0  A. Warming the tissue in warm water
- 0  B. Rubbing the affected area with snow
- 0  C. Covering the affected area with wool
- 0  D. Protecting the patient from infection

**13.** Signs and symptoms of frostbite include all of the following except:
- 0  A. The presence of erythemic tissue
- 0  B. Blistering of the injured tissue
- 0  C. Blackened tissue
- 0  D. Soft and pliable tissue

**14.** Tissue injury results from frostbite because:
- 0  A. Enhanced circulation to the injured extremity as a response to the cold
- 0  B. Indirect injury to the protoplasm of the tissue as a response to the cold
- 0  C. Disruption of the cellular and tissue structures by ice crystal formation
- 0  D. Direct thermal injury to the tissue through rewarming with hot water

## Hypothermia

*A 40-year-old man is brought to the emergency department after having been found lying under a bridge in a sleeping bag. The outside temperature has ranged from 20° to 35° F. No one knows how long the man had been lying there. The patient is alone and no medical history is available. He is responding only to deep pain. Vital signs are B/P 100/70, P 48, R 10, Temp 85° F per rectum.*

**15.** What is the potentially lethal cardiac dysrhythmia associated with hypothermia?
- 0  A. Ventricular fibrillation
- 0  B. Paroxysmal atrial tachycardia
- 0  C. Sinus bradycardia
- 0  D. Multifocal premature ventricular contractions (PVCs)

**16.** What additional laboratory studies would be of value in the initial management of this patient?
- 0  A. Aminophylline level
- 0  B. Phenytoin level
- 0  C. Alcohol level
- 0  D. Minoxidil level

**17.** During the initial rewarming of the hypothermic patient, the most appropriate nursing diagnosis is:
- 0  A. Knowledge deficit related to proper dress during the winter
- 0  B. Pain related to the increase in circulation to the extremities after rewarming

- 0  C. Injury, high risk for related to the effects of rewarming
- 0  D. Infection, high risk for related to being outside in the winter

**18.** Because of the sludging of blood that can occur in the hypothermic patient, fluid resuscitation will need to be initiated to prevent complications such as acute tubular necrosis. What criteria should the emergency nurse use to evaluate the effectiveness of the fluid resuscitation?
- 0  A. Decreased mental status
- 0  B. Increase in body temperature
- 0  C. Decrease in peripheral pulses
- 0  D. Increase in central venous pressure (CVP) and urinary output

**19.** Signs and symptoms of "afterdrop" include:
- 0  A. Cardiac arrhythmia and hypotension
- 0. B. Hypertension and hypoventilation
- 0  C. Shivering and hyperthermia
- 0  D. Sinus rhythm and normothermia

**20.** Active external rewarming involves:
- 0  A. Using warm humidified oxygen by mask
- 0  B. Removing the patient's wet clothing
- 0  C. Performing peritoneal lavage with warm fluids
- 0  D. Using cardiopulmonary bypass

**21.** Active core rewarming involves:
- 0  A. Putting on dry clothes
- 0  B. Turning on a radiant heater
- 0  C. Using "body-to-body" contact
- 0  D. Heated, humidified oxygen

**22.** When using active external rewarming devices, caution must be exercised to prevent:
- 0  A. Additional vasoconstriction in the affected extremities from the application of heat
- 0  B. Decrease in patient's core body temperature from the application of heat
- 0  C. Injury to the patient's skin from heat applications because of peripheral vasoconstriction
- 0  D. The development of hypertension from heat application

## Submersion Injuries

*An 18-month-old boy is brought to the emergency department after having been found at the bottom of a swimming pool. CPR was initiated by his mother and continued by the BLS squad. On arrival in the emergency department, he is intubated and high-dose epinephrine administered. He now has a palpable peripheral pulse. His BP is 82/50; HR 150R; Rectal temperature 95° F. He has no spontaneous respirations.*

23. The history obtained about the near-drowning incident should contain all of the following except the:
    - 0   A. Age of the victim who has drowned
    - 0   B. Length of time the victim was under the water
    - 0   C. Temperature of the water the victim was found in
    - 0   D. The number of people who found the child

24. Initial critical interventions for the near-drowning victim should include:
    - 0   A. Rewarming the patient immediately upon arrival of the rescue squad
    - 0   B. Immobilization of the cervical spine to protect the cervical spine
    - 0   C. Drawing blood gases upon arrival in the emergency department
    - 0   D. Obtaining a radiograph before the child is intubated

25. This child's initial blood gases are pH, 7.25; $PO_2$, 78; $PCO_2$, 30; and $HCO_3$, 25. The most appropriate nursing diagnosis is:
    - 0   A. Gas exchange, impaired related to aspiration
    - 0   B. Fluid volume deficit related to fluid loss
    - 0   C. Cardiac output, decreased related to fluid loss
    - 0   D. Tissue perfusion, altered (cerebral) related to hypoxia

26. The following is a useful tool for continuous cerebral evaluation of the unconscious near-drowning victim in the emergency department:
    - 0   A. Ice water calorics
    - 0   B. Occulocephalic reflex
    - 0   C. Glasgow coma scale
    - 0   D. Deep tendon reflexes

27. All of the following are risk factors for near-drowning to occur except:
    - 0   A. Ability to swim
    - 0   B. Use of alcohol
    - 0   C. Hyperventilation
    - 0   D. Child maltreatment

28. The most effective treatment for near-drowning incidents among pediatric patients is:
    - 0   A. Teaching basic life support to baby-sitters of children under 5 years of age
    - 0   B. Placing the patient on ECHMO to manage the pulmonary injury after aspiration
    - 0   C. Developing and implementing community prevention programs, including education about pool barriers
    - 0   D. Using transtracheal ventilation to manage the cerebral edema after aspiration

29. Favorable prognostic factors in near-drowning incidents include:
    - 0   A. Conscious on arrival in the emergency department
    - 0   B. Submersion greater than 10 minutes
    - 0   C. CPR needed on admission to the emergency department
    - 0   D. Arterial blood gas pH less than 7.0

30. Pulmonary dysfunction may be exacerbated when a patient suffers a submersion injury in:
    - 0   A. Salt water in a fish tank
    - 0   B. Fresh water in a lake
    - 0   C. Bathwater with bubble bath
    - 0   D. Freshwater in a toilet bowel

## Thermal Injuries

*A 17-year-old boy is brought to the emergency department after having been pulled out of a burning building. He is unconscious and has sustained second- and third-degree burns to his face, chest, and arms. The BLS squad has wrapped him in wet sheets and are bagging him with a BVM at 100%.*

31. Signs and symptoms of a potential inhalation injury include:
    - 0   A. First-degree burns to the face
    - 0   B. Second-degree burns to the chest
    - 0   C. Normal respiratory effort
    - 0   D. Upper airway edema

32. Based on this patient's history, what additional laboratory test should be obtained during his initial evaluation?
    - 0   A. Hepatic profile
    - 0   B. Carboxyhemoglobin
    - 0   C. Type and screen
    - 0   D. Cardiac enzymes

33. Burn injury below the glottis is distinguished by:
  0   A. Pharyngeal burns
  0   B. Stridor
  0   C. Hoarseness
  0   D. Expiratory wheezes

34. A partial-thickness burn causes injury to:
  0   A. Muscles and tendons
  0   B. Subcutaneous tissues
  0   C. Regenerative epithelial cells
  0   D. The upper portion of the dermis

35. The burns around this patient's chest are found to be circumferential. Because of this type of injury, the most appropriate nursing diagnosis on which the emergency nurse may base care is:
  0   A. Breathing pattern, ineffective
  0   B. Fluid volume deficit
  0   C. Cardiac output, decreased
  0   D. Family processes, altered

36. Using the fluid resuscitation formula (Parkland formula)—4 ml of Ringer's lactate solution times total body surface area (TBSA) burned times patient's weight in kilograms—how much fluid should this patient receive in the first 8 hours (rounded to the nearest 10 ml)? His body weight is 150 pounds. The amount of body surface burned is 35%.
  0   A. 10,500 ml
  0   B. 5250 ml
  0   C. 8000 ml
  0   D. 5000 ml

37. Because of the potential pulmonary injury this patient has suffered, what would be the best evaluative criterion the emergency nurse could use to monitor this patient?
  0   A. A capillary refill time greater than 2 seconds
  0   B. The patient's ability to cough
  0   C. The patient's ventilatory pattern
  0   D. The patient's tidal volume

38. The patient has received 3000 ml of fluid while awaiting transfer to the burn center. In order to determine if the fluid resuscitation is adequate, the patient's urinary output should be:
  0   A. 25 ml per hour
  0   B. 20 ml per hour
  0   C. 30 ml per hour
  0   D. 10 ml per hour

39. Wound care of a minor burn (partial thickness less than 15% in the adult and less than 10% in the child) would consist of:
  0   A. Putting crushed ice directly on the wound
  0   B. Pouring povidone-iodine solution directly on the wound
  0   C. Washing with a mild soapy solution
  0   D. Rinsing the wound with turpentine and distilled water

40. Complications from petroleum burns include all of the following *except*:
  0   A. Hydrocarbon toxicity
  0   B. Full-thickness burns
  0   C. Ion-bonding
  0   D. Lead toxicity

41. The most common type of thermal burn in children under age 3 is:
  0   A. Scald burn
  0   B. Chemical burn
  0   C. Flame burn
  0   D. Petroleum burn

42. Factors that may alert the emergency nurse that a burn injury in a child may be intentional include:
  0   A. Children from a lower socioeconomic background
  0   B. Children whose burn injury matches the history given
  0   C. Children who have received all their immunizations
  0   D. Children who suffer a symmetrical burn injury

43. In infants, the head and neck represent what percent of the body surface area?
  0   A. 14%
  0   B. 36%
  0   C. 9%
  0   D. 18%

44. What type of ultraviolet radiation causes a sunburn?
  0   A. Ultraviolet C radiation
  0   B. Ultraviolet B radiation
  0   C. Ultraviolet A radiation
  0   D. Ultraviolet D radiation

45. Which of the following burns should be treated at a burn center?
  0   A. Inhalation injury with a burn injury
  0   B. Second- and third-degree burns less than 10%

    0   C.  Third-degree burns less than 3%

    0   D.  Noncircumferential burns of the chest

46. An 18-month-old girl is brought to the emergency department by her parents after having bitten into an electrical cord. The child has a large blister and a charred wound on the right side of her lip. A delayed consequence of this type of burn would be:

    0   A.  Cardiac dysrhythmia

    0   B.  Hypovolemic shock

    0   C.  Bleeding

    0   D.  Cataracts

## Electrical Injuries

*A 30-year-old construction worker is brought to the emergency department by the rescue squad after having sustained an electrical shock of 10,000 volts. On arrival, he is alert and oriented, complaining of tingling in his left foot. His vital signs are B/P 120/70, P 100, R 18.*

47. All of the following factors determine the nature and severity of electrical injuries except the:

    0   A.  Age of the patient

    0   B.  Amperage of the current

    0   C.  Type of current

    0   D.  Duration of contact with the current

48. During the initial evaluation of this patient, the emergency nurse should assess for:

    0   A.  Fractures of his lower extremities

    0   B.  Entrance and exit wounds

    0   C.  Injuries to his eyes

    0   D.  Amnesia and psychosis

49. The tissue in the body with the least resistance to current flow is:

    0   A.  Bone tissue

    0   B.  Muscle tissue

    0   C.  Nerve tissue

    0   D.  Cardiac tissue

50. Because of the effects of electricity on the cardiovascular system, the most appropriate nursing diagnosis that the emergency nurse could use in planning the care of this patient is:

    0   A.  Injury, high risk for

    0   B.  Infection, high risk for

    0   C.  Fear

    0   D.  Cardiac output, decreased

## Lightning Injuries

*Every day there are approximately 8,000,000 lightning flashes throughout the world. Between 200 and 300 people are killed each year by lightning strikes. However, 70% to 80% of people struck by lightning survive.*[3,15]

*Even though this is not a common environmental emergency seen by the emergency nurse, it is important to be aware of the possibility of a lightning strike occurring no matter where one works. People at risk include campers, golfers, farmers, forest rangers, and construction workers.*[3,15]

51. All of the following are early indications that a person may have been struck by lightning except:

    0   A.  Vaporized rainwater

    0   B.  Feathery skin burns

    0   C.  A ruptured tympanic membrane

    0   D.  Bilateral cataracts

52. The initial management of the patient who is suspected of having been struck by lightning includes:

    0   A.  Treating the burns with antibiotic ointment and loose dressings

    0   B.  Airway management with cervical spine immobilization

    0   C.  Inserting two large-bore IV needles for aggressive fluid resuscitation

    0   D.  Placing the patient on a cardiac monitor and treating any life-threatening dysrhythmia

## Bites and Stings

53. The majority of bites treated in the emergency department result from:

    0   A.  Human bites to the metacarpophalangeal joint

    0   B.  Cat bites to the fingers and hands

    0   C.  Snake bites to the feet and ankles

    0   D.  Dog bites to the face, hands, and legs

54. Complications from bites and stings include all of the following *except:*

    0   A.  Hepatitis virus

    0   B.  Tuberculosis

    0   C.  Lyme's disease

    0   D.  Rabies

55. For the patient who has suffered a dog bite wound to the hand, the most appropriate nursing diagnosis would be:

    0   A.  Ineffective airway clearance

    0   B.  Fluid volume deficit

    0   C.  Risk for infection

    0   D.  Ineffective thermal regulation

56. Injury prevention strategies that the emergency nurse may use to avert a dog bite would include:
   - O  A. Always run from a dog and scream when it chases you
   - O  B. If knocked over by a dog, roll into a ball and lie still
   - O  C. Always approach an unfamiliar dog to ascertain their intentions
   - O  D. Always look an unfamiliar dog directly in the eyes

57. The most common source of exposure of rabies virus in humans in the United States is from:
   - O  A. Dogs
   - O  B. Skunks
   - O  C. Raccoons
   - O  D. Bats

58. The HDCV (human diploid cell vaccine) should always be administered in adults and older children in:
   - O  A. Deltoid area
   - O  B. Outer aspect of the thigh
   - O  C. Directly into the wound
   - O  D. Gluteal area

59. A simple method that may be used to remove the stinger from an insect bite is:
   - O  A. Anesthetizing the affected area and using a scalpel
   - O  B. Scraping off with a hard surface like a credit card
   - O  C. Applying an over-the-counter salve to loosen the stinger
   - O  D. Pulling it with a set of eyebrow tweezers

60. A 15-year-old boy who was stacking wood 2 days ago presents to the emergency department complaining of painful ulceration on the dorsal surface of the second digit of his right hand. He has no other complaints. Based on this history the most likely thing that may have bitten him is:
   - O  A. A black widow spider
   - O  B. A blue scorpion
   - O  C. A brown recluse spider
   - O  D. A wolf spider

61. A 30-year-old female presents to the emergency department with complaints of fatigue, headache and fever and chills. She also states that she has a "ring-like" reddened area on her right arm. A tick bite is suspected. Important pieces of history related to tick bite that should be obtained from this patient would include all of the following except:
   - O  A. Season of onset of her symptoms
   - O  B. A description of her outdoor activities
   - O  C. Travel in known tick area
   - O  D. Type of stinger removed from any wounds

62. A simple method to remove a tick in the emergency department is:
   - O  A. Coat the tick with lidocaine jelly
   - O  B. Pull the tick out with a pair of tweezers
   - O  C. Suffocate the tick with gasoline or kerosene
   - O  D. Apply heat to the tick with a match to remove it

63. The primary treatment of Lyme disease is:
   - O  A. Methylprednisone IV for 3 days
   - O  B. Amoxicillin PO for 3 weeks
   - O  C. Tetracycline PO for the patient who is pregnant
   - O  D. Topical antibiotics to the lesions for 2 weeks

64. A 5-year-old child is brought to the emergency department by his parents. They state that he has been unable to walk for the last few days and has had a low-grade fever and lack of appetite. They state that they had been camping recently and noticed the symptoms after they returned. Tick paralysis is suspected. The primary treatment of tick paralysis is:
   - O  A. Admission to the ICU and methylprednisone IV for 1 month
   - O  B. Admission to the ICU and IV antibiotics for 3 weeks
   - O  C. Removal of the tick and supportive care
   - O  D. Removal of the tick and oral antibiotics for 2 months

65. A 16-year-old male was snorkeling in the ocean and was stung by a jellyfish. Wound care of this patient would include:
   - O  A. Immediately rinsing the wound with fresh water and administering epinephrine SQ
   - O  B. Rubbing the affected area to remove all the remaining nematocysts
   - O  C. Removing all the remaining nematocysts with ungloved hands to decrease the risk of skin irritation
   - O  D. Applying acetic acid 5% (vinegar) to deactivate the toxin from the nematocysts

## ANSWERS

1. **C. Assessment.** The patient with heat exhaustion and heat stroke may have similar symptoms. Symptoms of these heat-related illnesses include changes in mental status, hypotension, and tachycardia. The patient suffering from heat exhaustion, however, sweats freely and may even complain of chilling.[1,2]

2. **A. Intervention.** In addition to the initial management of the ABCs, the primary care of the patient with heat stroke includes rapid cooling. There are several methods available for cooling the patient, including using ice packs, wetting the patient down, and using large fans, cold-water immersion, and rectal and gastric lavage.[2]

3. **C. Analysis.** Because of the large volume of fluid that has been lost through sweating, the patient with heat stroke will develop hypotension. Defining characteristics of fluid volume deficit include hypotension, tachycardia, dry skin, dry mucous membranes, and decreased skin turgor.[4]

4. **B. Evaluation.** Even though all the patient's systems are affected during the cooling process, the pulmonary system displays the most frequent source of complications. These complications include the potential for aspiration and pulmonary edema.[2]

5. **C. Assessment.** There are several types of drugs that can contribute to a patient being at greater risk for developing heat stroke, including antipsychotic, anticholinergics, tricyclics, and major tranquilizers.[1,2]

6. **B. Evaluation.** Monitoring the patient for the development of rhabdomyolysis would include monitoring the patient's urinary output, color changes in their urine (dark or blood), complaints of muscle cramps, and hyperkalemia.[1]

7. **B. Assessment.** Heat cramps are related to the loss of salt in thermal sweat from working in a hot environment. Heat cramps differ from exercise cramps in that they tend to occur while the person is resting and do not resolve spontaneously.[1]

8. **C. Intervention.** Heat cramps are usually treated with oral ingestion of a salt solution. The emergency nurse must also keep in mind that the patient with heat cramps may be hypochloremic. Careful evaluation of all the patient's electrolytes is important.[1,2,3]

9. **B. Analysis.** The most appropriate nursing diagnosis on which to base this patient's discharge planning is knowledge deficit related to the causes of heat cramps.[5]

10. **A. Evaluation.** The best criterion to use in evaluating discharge instructions is to have the patient explain the instructions to the emergency nurse.

11. **C. Assessment.** The pediatric patient is at risk for developing heat-related emergencies because they have decreased subcutaneous fat, a higher metabolic rate, a decreased ability to protect themselves from environmental changes, the presence of a larger body surface area to volume, and the potential to be suffering from a predisposing chronic illness such as cystic fibrosis.[6]

12. **A. Intervention.** The affected part should be rewarmed in water with a temperature of 105° to 115° F. In addition, the patient's core temperature needs to be monitored for hypothermia.[2]

13. **D. Assessment.** Signs and symptoms of frostbite include firm to hard tissue, pale to erythemic tissue, and blistering and blackening of the injured tissues.[3]

14. **C. Assessment.** The mechanism of injury in frostbite involves three processes. These include:
    - Disruption of the cellular and tissue structure from the formation of ice crystals
    - Direct injury to tissue protoplasm from the cold, probably from dehydration
    - Injury from impaired circulation [7]

15. **A. Assessment.** When the patient's core body temperature is below 86° F, he or she is at greater risk of developing ventricular fibrillation. This dysrhythmia can be easily stimulated by such procedures as the insertion of monitoring lines. At temperatures between 82.4° and 86° F, ventricular fibrillation may not respond to drugs or countershock.[1,2]

16. **C. Intervention.** The patient who is intoxicated is at greater risk of developing hypothermia. Alcohol will dull the patient's response to the cold, as well as cause vasodilatation and increase the rapidity of heat loss.[1,2,3,5]

17. **C. Analysis.** During the rewarming process the patient is at great risk of being injured. Sources of injury include the rewarming process, the risk of developing seizures during rewarming interventions, and the risk of aspiration.[5]

18. **D. Evaluation.** Fluid resuscitation is best monitored by changes in the patient's CVP and urinary output. These parameters help prevent the possibility of fluid overload.

19. **A. Assessment.** Afterdrop may occur during the rewarming of a patient with moderate to severe hypothermia. It occurs when the periphery is rewarmed and acidotic blood is dumped into the central circulation. Signs and symptoms of after-

drop include hypotension and cardiac dysrhythmia.[5,8]

20. **B. Intervention.** Active external rewarming includes "buddy-warming," removing wet clothes, putting on dry clothes, using heated blankets, and heating pads.[1,3]

21. **D. Intervention.** Active internal rewarming includes airway rewarming with warm humidified oxygen by mask or to the endotracheal tube, peritoneal lavage with warm fluids, and cardiopulmonary bypass.[3,6]

22. **C. Intervention.** Because of the peripheral vasoconstriction that occurs with hypothermia, heating devices may cause burns.[1]

23. **D. Assessment.** Factors that affect the outcome of a near-drowning victim include the age of the victim, the amount of time spent immersed in the liquid, the development of hypothermia, and the immediacy of resuscitative efforts.[1,2,9-11]

24. **B. Intervention.** The cervical spine should be immobilized in the unconscious near-drowning victim until possible injury to the cervical spine can be evaluated. The child was initially found unconscious at the bottom of the pool. He could have fallen into the pool or struck his head on the bottom of the pool.[1]

25. **A. Analysis.** The defining characteristics of impaired gas exchange include hypercapnia and hypoxia. Because of the aspiration of water, the child's lungs have sustained an alteration in alveolar capillary membrane function.[5]

26. **C. Evaluation.** The Glasgow Coma Scale can be a useful tool for ongoing evaluation of cerebral function of the near-drowning victim. The coma scale includes verbal response, eye opening, and motor response.[10]

27. **A. Assessment.** Risk factors related to near-drowning incidents include inability to swim, use of alcohol, seizure history, hyperventilation, hypothermia, and child neglect or maltreatment.[1,10]

28. **C. Intervention.** The most appropriate intervention is to develop and implement community programs to teach prevention. Many pediatric drownings occur because of lack of adult supervision, lack of fences around swimming pools, and lack of swimming instructions for young children.[1,9-11]

29. **A. Analysis.** Favorable prognostic factors include:
- Age < 3 years
- Submersion (warm water) < 3 minutes
- Ice in water
- Conscious on arrival in the ED
- Presence of pulse in the ED[10]

30. **C. Assessment.** Even though many articles still point out that hypertonic or hypotonic solutions in and of themselves cause additional injury in drowning, research in animals has found that it would take a large amount of aspirated fluids to add any additional injury. Most near-drowning victims only aspirate a small amount of fluid. However, water containing chemicals such as caustic cleaning fluids or soapsuds may cause chemical pneumonitis and surfactant destruction.[10]

31. **D. Assessment.** Signs and symptoms of an injury to the respiratory tract from a thermal exposure include facial burns, singed nasal hairs, hypoxemia, intercostal retractions, rales, rhonchi, and a hoarse voice.[12,13,14]

32. **B. Intervention.** Because the patient was potentially involved in an enclosed space and because he is unconscious, a carboxyhemoglobin level should be obtained so that the patient can be evaluated for carbon monoxide poisoning. Carbon monoxide will bind with hemoglobin 240 times faster than will oxygen, causing the patient to become hypoxic.[12,13,14]

33. **D. Assessment.** Burn injury below the glottis is distinguished by symptoms of bronchial and bronchiolar injury, including bronchorrhea and expiratory wheezes.[12,13,14]

34. **D. Assessment.** Partial-thickness, or second-degree, burns cause injury to the upper portion of the dermis. First-degree burns cause injury to the epidermal layer of the skin. Full-thickness, or third-degree, burns cause injury through the epidermis, dermis, subcutaneous tissues, and muscles. These burns will damage the regenerative epithelial cells, destroy nerve endings, and cause vessel thrombosis.[8,9]

35. **A. Analysis.** Circumferential burns of the body—particularly the chest and neck—can impair respiratory function. A defining characteristic of this nursing diagnosis is altered chest excursion. Because of the constriction caused by the burn injury, the patient cannot ventilate properly.[12,13,14]

36. **B. Intervention.** This calculation would be:

$$4 \text{ ml} \times 75 \text{ kg} \times 35$$
$$\text{(percent total body surface area burned)}$$

One-half of this should be given in the first 8 hours. That would be 5250 ml.[12]

37. **C. Evaluation.** The most useful evaluative criterion for this patient would be his ventilatory patterns. Since this patient is at risk for ventilation problems from circumferential burns and for hypoxia from inhalation injury and carbon dioxide

poisoning, the pattern of his ventilatory efforts will need to be closely monitored.

38. **C. Evaluation.** Urinary output is one of the best methods available to monitor fluid resuscitation. Adult urinary output should be 30 to 50 ml per hour.[12]

39. **C. Intervention.** Ice or povidone-iodine (Betadine) directly on the wound would only cause additional damage to the skin. The skin is the largest organ system, and when it is intact, it prevents toxins from entering the body, in addition to regulating body temperature. When it has been damaged, as in a burn injury, these functions are compromised. Washing with mild soap will help remove any debris from the burn and help prevent infection.[12]

40. **C. Assessment.** Petroleum burns can lead to systemic toxicity because of absorption of hydrocarbons and, if the gasoline contains lead, lead toxicity. In addition, prolonged contact with gasoline can lead to full-thickness burns.[12]

41. **A. Assessment.** The most common type of thermal injury seen in children under age 3 are scald injuries. Children over age 3 are more commonly injured by a flame.[6,12]

42. **D. Assessment.** A symmetrical burn injury should alert the emergency nurse to the possibility that the burn injury was intentional. For example, symmetrical burns to the lower extremities are generally an indication that the child may have been held in hot water. Splash or scald burns that are unintentional are rarely symmetrical.[6,12]

43. **D. Assessment.** In infants, the head and neck represent 18% of the body surface area. In the adult, this is only 9% of the body surface area.[6,12]

44. **B. Assessment.** Ultraviolet B waves are the main cause of sunburn and skin cancer.[13]

45. **A. Assessment.** According to the American Burn Association the following burns should be treated at a burn center:
    - Second- and third-degree burns greater than 20%
    - Third degree burns greater than 5%
    - Electric burns, including lightning injuries
    - Inhalation burns with burn injury
    - Circumferential burns of the extremities and chest[12]

46. **C. Assessment.** A delayed complication of this type of burn would be bleeding. The labial arteries can begin bleeding 3 to 5 days after the injury. The emergency nurse will need to teach the parents to use direct pressure to control the bleeding and re-

turn the child for further evaluation if the bleeding does not stop.[12]

47. **A. Assessment.** There are six major factors that determine the nature and severity of an electrical injury: voltage, amperage, type of current, duration of contact, current path through the victim, and skin resistance.[12]

48. **B. Assessment.** Locating the entrance and exit wounds through which the electricity passed will help the emergency nurse determine on which path the current traveled. Effects from electrical current passage may interfere with the cardiac, respiratory, and neurological systems.[12,13]

49. **C. Assessment.** Bone is the tissue with the greatest resistance to current flow. Nerve tissue has the least resistance to current flow.[12]

50. **D. Analysis.** Because of the effects of electricity on the cardiovascular system, close monitoring of the cardiovascular system is important. Defining characteristics of this nursing diagnosis include dysrhythmia, ECG changes, hypotension, cold, clammy skin, and variations in hemodynamic readings.[5,15]

51. **D. Assessment.** Cataracts are a late sign of injury from a lightning strike. Four types of injuries initially occur after a lightning strike: cardiac injuries, neurological injuries, burns, and blunt trauma.[1,15]

52. **B. Intervention.** Many times when patients are struck by lightning, they are found to be apneic. Because of the possibility of cervical spine trauma, the patient's airway needs to be approached with cervical spine immobilization.[12,15]

53. **D. Assessment.** The majority of animal bites treated in the emergency department are from dogs. In 1994, approximately 4.7 million people were bitten by dogs.[16]

54. **B. Assessment.** Bites and stings can cause multiple complications, including anaphylaxis, envenomation, local tissue damage, and transmission of disease. Some of the diseases transmitted include hepatitis virus, rabies, Lyme's disease, and numerous bacteria such as *Staphylococcus aureus*.[1]

55. **C. Analysis.** Because of the location of the wound, the risk of infection increases.[1]

56. **B. Intervention.** The Centers for Disease Control and Prevention has issued guidelines for safety around dogs. These include:
    - Never approach an unfamiliar dog
    - Never run from a dog and scream
    - Stay still when an unfamiliar dog comes up to you

- If knocked over by a dog, roll into a ball and lie still
- Do not look a dog in the eye [17]

57. **D. Assessment.** Since 1980 there have been 36 cases of rabies diagnosed in the United States, and over 50% of them have come from bat variants. In most other countries, dogs remain the most common source of rabies exposures in humans. [18]

58. **A. Intervention.** HDCV (human diploid cell vaccine) and RVA (rabies vaccine absorbed) must be given in the deltoid area in adults and older children. For younger children, it may be given in the outer aspect of the thigh. [18]

59. **B. Intervention.** Many stingers will continue to secrete venom until removed. It is important to remove it without causing it to break apart. Using a hard surface such as a credit card and scraping it is one of the simplest methods to remove a stinger. [1]

60. **C. Assessment.** Black widow spiders live in secluded, dark areas such as garages, barns, and outhouses. The brown recluse spider resides in wood piles and storage areas. The bite of a black widow spider generally produces systemic symptoms such as abdominal pain, hypertension, nausea, vomiting and tachycardia. A brown recluse bite will produce a distinct type of wound that begins with a painful purpura and develops into a necrotic ulcerating wound. [1,19]

61. **D. Assessment.** History that should be obtained from a patient when a tick bite or tick-related disease is suspected should include:
- Season of onset, usually between May through September
- Outdoor activities—hiking in woods or fields
- Geography of outside activities—known tick areas
- Symptoms related to the tick bite
  - Fatigue
  - Weakness
  - Headache
  - Photophobia
  - Fever/chills
  - Muscle/joint pain
  - Rashes [20,21]

62. **A. Intervention.** Over the years, patients have used a variety of methods to remove ticks, including gasoline, kerosene, and matches (hopefully without the gasoline and kerosene). Pulling a tick out increases the risk of it coming apart and pieces remaining in the patient. Suffocating it with lidocaine jelly or Vaseline has been found to be safe and effective. [20]

63. **B. Intervention.** Lyme disease is treated with amoxicillin PO for 3 weeks. Tetracycline is not recommended for the patient who is pregnant. [20]

64. **C. Intervention.** The treatment for tick paralysis is immediate removal of the tick. As long as the tick is on the patient, it is secreting toxin, which blocks the release of acetylcholine. Symptoms of tick paralysis include symmetric weakness of the lower extremities that ascends and ataxia. Death can occur from respiratory arrest. Once the tick is removed, treatment is supportive. [21]

65. **D. Intervention.** Stings from jellyfish should be managed by:
- Immediately washing the wound with seawater because rubbing and freshwater will activate the remaining nematocysts
- Cleansing with vinegar 5% to inactivate the toxin
- Applying shaving cream or a paste of baking soda, flour, or talc and shaving off the remaining nematocysts
- Recuers and health care providers should always wear gloves to protect themselves [22]

## REFERENCES

1. Semonin-Holleran R: Environmental emergencies. In Jordan KS, editor: *Emergency nursing core curriculum,* ed 5, Philadelphia, 2000, WB Saunders.
2. Proehl JA: Environmental emergencies. In Kitt S et al, editors: *Emergency nursing: a physiologic and clinical perspective,* Philadelphia, 1995, WB Saunders.
3. Stewart C: *Environmental emergencies,* Baltimore, 1990, Williams & Wilkins.
4. Auerbach PS, Geehr EC: *Management of wilderness and environmental emergencies,* ed 3, St Louis, 1995, Mosby.
5. Kim MJ, McFarland GK, McLane AM: *Pocket guide to nursing diagnoses,* St Louis, 1993, Mosby.
6. Haley K, Eckles N, Baker P: *Emergency nursing pediatric course,* Park Ridge, IL, 1998, Emergency Nurses Association.
7. Mills W, Whaley R: Frostbite with rapid rewarming and ultrasonic therapy, *Wilderness Environ Med* 9(4):226-247, 1998.
8. Weissenberger EV: A 17-year-old with severe hypothermia and cardiac arrest from exposure, *J Emerg Nurs* 18:380-382, 1992.
9. Young L: A 22-month-old victim of near-drowning, *J Emerg Nurs* 18:197-198, 1992.
10. Dickison AE: Near-drowning, predictors of survival, *Wilderness Med Let* 16(2):1, 6-9, Spring, 1999.
11. Beyda DH: Childhood submersion injuries, *J Emerg Nurs* 24(2):140-144, 1998.
12. American Burn Association: *Prehospital burn life support,* Lincoln, NE, 1996, America Burn Association.
13. Bryant KK: Burn injuries. In Kitt S et al, editors: *Emergency nursing: a physiologic and clinical perspective,* Philadelphia, 1995, WB Saunders.

14. Dries DJ, Holleran R: Burn care pearls, *Air Med J* 16(3):68, 1997.

15. Lewis AM: Understanding the principles of lightening injuries, *J Emerg Nurs* 23 (6):535-541, 1997.

16. Dog-bite related fatalities in the United States, 1995-1996, *MMWR* 46:463-467, 1997.

17. Unintentional injury prevention fact sheet on dogs, National Center for Injury Prevention and Control, www.cdc.gov/ncipc/diup/dogbite2.htm, 1999.

18. Talan DA, Moran GJ, Pinner RW, editors: Update on emerging infections from the Centers for Disease Control and Prevention: updated postexposure prophylaxis guidelines, *Ann Emerg Med* 33(5):590-597, 1999.

19. Clowes TD: Wound assessment of the *loxoscles reclusa* spider bite, *J Emerg Nurs* 22(4):283-287, 1996.

20. Edlow JA: Lyme disease and related tick-borne illnesses, *Ann Emerg Med* 33(6):680-693, 1999.

21. Bruno R, Seannell D: Tick paralysis in a 2-year-old girl, *J Emerg Med* 24(1):13-15, 1998.

22. Auerbach P: Envenomations from jellyfish and related species, *J Emerg Nurs* 23:555-568, 1997.

# Chapter 7 _____

# Facial Emergencies

**REVIEW OUTLINE**

I. Anatomy and physiology
  A. Anatomical structures
    1. Mandible
    2. Maxilla
    3. Zygoma
    4. Zygomatic arch
    5. Nasal bones/structures
    6. Orbit
    7. Orbit rim
    8. Sinuses
      a. Frontal
      b. Maxillary
      c. Ethmoid
      d. Sphenoid
    9. Ethmoid
    10. Cranial nerves
    11. Cranial bones
    12. Oral cavity/contents
    13. Auditory bones/structures
    14. Major blood vessels
  B. Physiology
    1. Central nervous system
      a. Cranial nerves
      b. Functions of brain stem, cerebrum, and cerebellum
    2. Process of sight
    3. Process of speech
II. Assessment
  A. Primary survey
    1. A, B, C, D, E (airway, breathing, circulation, deficit [neurological], exposure)
    2. Stabilization
  B. Secondary survey
    1. History of illness or injury
      a. Mechanism and time
      b. AMPLE history
        (1) Allergies
        (2) Medications
        (3) Past medical history
        (4) Last meal

        (5) Events or treatment prior to arrival
    2. Chief complaint
      a. Pain: PQRST
        (1) Provocation
        (2) Quality
        (3) Radiation
        (4) Severity
        (5) Timing
      b. Bleeding
      c. Edema/ecchymosis
      d. Asymmetry
      e. Fever/chills
      f. Paresthesia
      g. Diplopia
      h. Malocclusion
      i. Trismus
      j. Deformity
    3. Physical examination
      a. General appearance
      b. Mental status/level of consciousness
      c. Glasgow Coma Scale score
      d. Vital signs
      e. Inspection
        (1) Symmetry of facial features
        (2) Ecchymosis
        (3) Edema
        (4) Eyes: subconjuctival hemorrhage, pupillary height, pupillary reaction, extraocular eye movements (EOMs)
        (5) Nose
        (6) Mouth malocclusion
        (7) Ears
        (8) Cranial nerves
        (9) Neck
        (10) Head
      f. Palpation
        (1) Symmetry
        (2) Localized point tenderness
        (3) Abnormal mobility

(4) Crepitus

(5) Temporomandibular joint (TMJ)

(6) Foreign bodies

(7) Lacerations/hematomas

III. Diagnostic methods for facial emergencies

    A. Radiology

        1. CT

        2. MRI

    B. Laboratory

IV. Related nursing diagnoses

    A. Airway clearance, ineffective

    B. Alteration in comfort, pain

    C. Anxiety

    D. Fluid volume deficit, high risk for

    E. Infection, high risk for

    F. Knowledge deficit

    G. Sensory-perceptual alteration

    H. Skin integrity, impairment of

V. Age-related changes

    A. Pediatric patient

        1. Facial bones in children are softer and more pliable than adults; therefore, facial fractures tend to be less severe[1]

    B. Geriatric patient

        1. Elderly have a decrease in pain perception

        2. Elderly tend to dismiss complaints as normal aging. All complaints should be investigated.

VI. Selected facial emergencies

    A. Sinusitis

    B. Trigeminal neuralgia

    C. Facial lacerations and soft tissue injuries

    D. Mandibular factures

    E. Maxillary fracture

    F. Zygomatic fractures

**M**axillofacial emergencies are common in any emergency department. Most injuries are not life-threatening, but the potential for disfigurement and emotional despair is great. The most common injury resulting in facial injuries is blunt trauma secondary to motor vehicle accidents. Other mechanisms of injury include those that produce both blunt and penetrating trauma such as altercations, domestic violence, falls, and sports-related accidents.

Maxillofacial emergencies produce life-threatening situations when they obstruct the airway and cause hemorrhagic shock. Mechanical obstruction of the airway occurs due to anatomical displacement of normal structures secondary to trauma or disease. Broken teeth or a swollen epiglottis are examples. Because the head is rich in vasculature, profuse bleeding is a natural occurrence with any injury. Maxillofacial trauma can cause severe hemorrhage, which may be occult because patients have a tendency to swallow blood rather than expectorate it.

Assessment and stabilization of clients with maxillofacial emergencies follow the same sequence, the ABCs, as for any trauma patient.

## REVIEW QUESTIONS
### Facial Trauma

**1.** The number one sign of the presence of facial fracture is:

  0  A. Edema

  0  B. Laceration

  0  C. Asymmetry

  0  D. Ecchymosis

*A 26-year-old woman is brought to your emergency department via life squad. She was the unrestrained driver of an automobile that ran into a bridge abutment. The car's windshield was reportedly cracked. The victim, Ms. Green, is awake and oriented. A large scalp laceration and facial trauma are obvious. Ms. Green's vital signs are B/P 90/60, P 100, and RR 28. Ms. Green has been appropriately immobilized on a backboard, with a cervical collar in place.*

**2.** Your first priority in the assessment of this patient is:

  0  A. Airway

  0  B. Breathing

  0  C. Circulation

  0  D. Deficit, neurologic

**3.** The most appropriate method for assessment of Ms. Green's airway would be:

  0  A. Ask the patient if she is getting enough air

  0  B. Auscultate the chest for normal breath sounds

  0  C. Draw arterial blood gases to evaluate oxygen saturation

  0  D. Have Ms. Green open her mouth and observe for foreign bodies

**4.** When assessing Ms. Green's airway, you discover that she has a large amount of bleeding into the oropharynx, which she is swallowing. Your immediate intervention would be:

  0  A. Prepare for intubation to protect the airway

  0  B. Insert a nasogastric tube to empty the stomach

0   C. Frequent suctioning and teaching the patient to expectorate the blood

0   D. Wait until the cervical spine is cleared and then place Ms. Green in a semi-Fowler's position

5. Based on the mechanism of injury and Ms. Green's vital signs, the most appropriate nursing diagnosis is:

0   A. Anticipatory grieving

0   B. Hyperthermia

0   C. Fluid volume deficit, high risk for

0   D. Impaired thought processes

*Ms. Green is diagnosed as having a bilateral LeForte III fracture, also known as "craniofacial dysjunction." As its name implies, the facial and cranial skulls become disjoined. A LeForte I fracture produces a horizontal detachment of the maxilla at the level of the nasal floor, leaving the maxillary alveolar ridge and hard palate mobile. A LeForte II, or "pyramid fracture," involves fractures of the maxilla, nasal bones, the medial half of the interior orbital rim, the orbital floor, and lacrimal bones.*

6. A common emergency nursing intervention is to monitor airway patency. What criterion is the first indicator of airway compromise?

0   A. Change in color

0   B. Change in mental status

0   C. Change in respiratory rate

0   D. Change in blood pressure and pulse

## Blowout Fractures

*The police bring Mr. Plant, a 32-year-old man, to your emergency department after his involvement in an altercation. He has sustained facial trauma and is diagnosed with a blowout orbital fracture on the right. He is awake and alert, with no obvious injuries. Mr. Plant's vital signs are B/P 120/80, P 84, R 18.*

7. Common signs and symptoms of a blowout orbital fracture include:

0   A. Blindness on the affected side

0   B. Flattened cheek on the affected side

0   C. Lowered pupil position on the affected side

0   D. Extraocular eye movements limited bilaterally

8. The most appropriate nursing diagnosis for Mr. Plant would be:

0   A. Hopelessness

0   B. Fluid volume deficit

0   C. Alteration in comfort, pain

0   D. Impaired thought processes

9. The patient who has sustained a blowout orbital fracture and has periorbital emphysema should have visual acuity monitored to evaluate for involvement of the:

0   A. Optic nerve

0   B. Intraorbital nerves

0   C. Central retinal artery

0   D. Extraocular eye muscles

10. If the patient with periorbital emphysema complains of a sudden decrease in visual acuity, the nurse should:

0   A. Prepare for immediate surgery

0   B. Reassess the patient's visual acuity

0   C. Have the patient lie flat and turn on the unaffected side

0   D. Prepare for a lateral canthotomy or intraorbital needle aspiration

## Bell's Palsy

*Mrs. Jones, a 45-year-old woman, presents with peripheral facial paralysis, fever, chills, and flulike symptoms. She is diagnosed as having Bell's palsy. This is Mrs. Jones' first episode of any type of disorder and she is very anxious.*

11. Bell's palsy affects which cranial nerve?

0   A. Seventh—facial

0   B. Fourth—trochlear

0   C. Fifth—trigeminal

0   D. Ninth—glossopharyngeal

12. Common signs and symptoms associated with Bell's palsy include:

0   A. Unilateral, flaccid facial paralysis

0   B. Onset of symptoms occurs gradually

0   C. Increased lacrimation on the affected side

0   D. Lid lag on the opposite side, especially noted when closing the eyes

13. The most appropriate nursing diagnosis for Mrs. Jones is:

0   A. Hopelessness

0   B. Infection, high risk for

0   C. Airway clearance, ineffective

0   D. Anxiety, related to knowledge deficit

14. The most appropriate nursing intervention related to the above nursing diagnosis involves education. Mrs. Jones should be taught that:

0   A. She must be admitted to the hospital to rule out a cerebrovascular accident (CVA)

O   B. Recovery is usually spontaneous and occurs within 3 weeks

O   C. To facilitate recovery, she must enter a rehabilitation program immediately

O   D. She will never recover and must learn to live with permanent Bell's phenomenon

## Facial Laceration

*A 10-year-old child, Tommy, is brought to the emergency department by his mother after a bicycle accident. Tommy fell headfirst on a gravel road. He was not unconscious and is awake and oriented. He has sustained a deep facial laceration extending from the forehead through the left eyebrow. He also has multiple facial abrasions. His vital signs are stable, and Tommy has no other obvious injuries.*

15. Assessment of all the wounds for the presence of foreign bodies is imperative to prevent:
    O   A. Potential infection
    O   B. Potential "tattooing" effect
    O   C. Improper wound closure (malalignment)
    O   D. All of the above

16. The primary nursing diagnosis related to Tommy's mechanism of injury is:
    O   A. Infection, high risk for
    O   B. Impaired gas exchange
    O   C. Fluid volume deficit, high risk for
    O   D. Potential alteration in body temperature

17. Preparation of Tommy's large laceration for suturing includes all of the following except:
    O   A. Anesthetize the wound prior to cleaning
    O   B. Shave the eyebrow to remove all surrounding debris
    O   C. Cleanse with the appropriate solution and rinse thoroughly
    O   D. Search thoroughly for foreign bodies with a magnification instrument (glasses or lens)

18. Tommy's mother is taught to observe for signs of infection. To evaluate the effectiveness of education, the emergency nurse should:
    O   A. Have Tommy's mother repeat what she has been taught
    O   B. Make an appointment for Tommy to return to the emergency department for a wound check
    O   C. Call Tommy's pediatrician the next day to make sure Tommy's mother has made an appointment for a wound check and suture removal

O   D. Make a written referral to the local public health department requesting follow-up information on Tommy

## Sinusitis

19. A 46-year-old male presents to the emergency department with a 1-week history of fever, cough, and thick, green nasal drainage. He is now complaining of a severe headache and facial pain. Based on clinical findings the patient is diagnosed with sinusitis. In addition to antibiotics what other treatments should be prescribed for this patient?
    O   A. A hand-held inhaler to decrease the possibility of asthma
    O   B. Lying flat in bed at night to promote sinus drainage
    O   C. Nasal or systemic decongestants
    O   D. Limited fluids to decrease nasal drainage

20. If a nasal decongestant is prescribed, the emergency nurse should caution the patient to not use it longer than 5 days because:
    O   A. Extended use of topical decongestants decreases sinus congestion
    O   B. Topical decongestants generally lose their effectiveness after 1 week
    O   C. The patient will not become dependent on the use of nasal decongestants
    O   D. The patient may develop an allergic reaction to the nasal decongestant

## ANSWERS

1. **D. Assessment.**[1,2,3]
2. **A. Assessment.** Obviously, the patient cannot survive without a patent airway. All other assessment parameters are secondary to airway assessment.[3]
3. **D. Assessment.** This is the best method to assess Ms. Green's airway for foreign bodies. The most common are broken teeth, the tongue, and blood. The tongue may obstruct the airway in patients with a decreased level of consciousness. It is important to look for broken teeth and occult bleeding, since fearful patients can easily hide both.[3]
4. **C. Intervention.** Swallowing blood needs to be prevented to keep the patient from vomiting and potentially aspirating.[3]
5. **C. Analysis.** Ms. Green's B/P is low and pulse is above average for the normal adult. Both are signs of hypovolemia.
6. **B. Evaluation.** A change in vital signs is a very late indicator of respiratory compromise. Color is a

poor assessment parameter in the adult. Frequently, patients will exhibit very subtle changes in mental status such as sudden anger, complaints, or sleepiness that the alert emergency nurse must be aware of to provide rapid diagnosis and intervention.[3]

7. **C. Assessment.** A blowout orbital fracture is a depressed fracture of the orbital floor in which the contents of the orbit protrude into the maxillary sinus. Thus the affected eye sinks into the maxillary sinus, producing a lowered pupil position and asymmetry of the eyes. Other common symptoms include conjunctival hemorrhage and eyelid ecchymosis due to blunt trauma, infraorbital nerve paresthesia due to a pinched facial nerve at the fracture site, and diplopia.[1,3]

8. **C. Analysis.** Blowout orbital fractures alone do not produce impaired thought process, hopelessness, or fluid volume deficit. They do, however, produce severe pain.[1]

9. **C. Evaluation.** Air may build up under pressure in the orbit, producing cessation of blood flow in the central retinal artery.[3,5]

10. **D. Intervention.** This is a true emergent procedure that must be performed in order to save the patient's sight by removing the trapped air.[3,5]

11. **A. Assessment.**[3]

12. **A. Assessment.** Other symptoms of Bell's palsy include rapid onset of symptoms, viral prodrome, lid lag on the affected side when closing the eyes, decreased lacrimation on the affected side, and Bell's phenomenon, which is an upward movement of the eyeball on the affected side when attempting to close the eye.[1]

13. **D. Analysis.** Bell's palsy does not affect the airway or have the potential for the patient to develop an infectious process. Most patients are extremely anxious due to a lack of knowledge concerning their medical diagnosis.[1]

14. **B. Intervention.** During the recovery phase, Mrs. Jones should be educated to rest and treat her flu-like symptoms appropriately. She will also be given eye drops, because of the decreased lacrimation on the affected side, and may require analgesics.[1]

15. **D. Assessment.** Infection, tattooing, and malalignment may all result from a missed foreign body.[1,3]

16. **A. Analysis.** Because Tommy sustained his injury on a gravel road, his potential for infection is high.[3,6]

17. **B. Intervention.** Eyebrows should never be shaved. They provide anatomical landmarks to ensure proper alignment of the wound, and they may not grow back.[3,6]

18. **A. Evaluation.** A return demonstration or repeat of verbal and/or written instructions is the best way to evaluate patient teaching.

19. **C. Intervention.** Nasal and systemic decongestants should be prescribed for the treatment of sinusitis to keep the sinuses open and decrease media for bacterial growth.[7,8]

20. **B. Intervention.** Nasal decongestants generally lose their effectiveness after 1 week. Longer or habitual use of nasal sprays can actually cause nasal tissue irritation that will result in increased nasal congestion.[8]

## REFERENCES

1. Revere CJ: Facial emergencies. In Jordan KS, editor, *Emergency nursing core curriculum,* Philadelphia, 2000, WB Saunders.
2. Rahman WM, O'Connor TJ: Facial trauma. In Barkin R, editor, *Pediatric emergency medicine,* St Louis, 1997, Mosby.
3. Jacobs BB, Baker P: *Trauma nursing core course,* Park Ridge, IL, 1995, Emergency Nurses Association.
4. Gerlock AJ: Facial trauma, *Trauma Q* 2(4):20-34, 1986.
5. Goldman R: For your eyes only, *Emergency* 19(12):27-29, 1987.
6. Gussack GS, et al: Pediatric maxillofacial trauma: Unique features in diagnosis and treatment, *Laryngoscope* 97:925-930, 1987.
7. Edlow J, Macnow L: Headache. In Davis M, Votey SR, Greenough PG, editors: *Signs and symptoms in emergency medicine,* St Louis, 1999, Mosby.
8. Kupcz D: Managing allergic rhinitis, *Nurs Pract* 24(5):107-120, 1999.

## ADDITIONAL READINGS

Kalish MA: Airway management in maxillofacial trauma, *Emerg Med Sci* 18(6):42-44, 1989.

Keresh JW: Ocular and periocular trauma, *Emerg Med Serv* 18(6):46-55, 1989.

Kitt S et al: *Emergency nursing: a physiologic and clinical perspective,* Philadelphia, 1995, WB Saunders.

Lee MJ, Martinez AJ: Focusing on facial and ocular injuries, *J Emerg Med Serv* 17(2):28-42, 1992.

Lower J: Maxillofacial trauma, *Nurs Clin North Am* 21(4):611-628, 1986.

Manson PN, Kelly KJ: Evaluation and management of the patient with facial trauma, *Emerg Med Serv* 18(6):22-30, 1989.

Newberry L: *Sheehy's emergency nursing principles and practice,* St Louis, 1998, Mosby.

# Chapter 8

# Genitourinary Emergencies

## REVIEW OUTLINE

I. Anatomy of the genitourinary tract
   A. Kidneys
   B. Ureter
   C. Bladder
   D. Urethra
   E. Renal vessels
   F. Urinary meatus

II. Male anatomy
   A. Penis
   B. Glans
   C. Prepuce
   D. Foreskin
   E. Urethra
   F. Scrotum
   G. Testes
   H. Epididymis
   I. Vas deferens
   J. Sexual maturity rating

III. Female anatomy
   A. Mons pubis
   B. Labia majora
   C. Labia minora
   D. Clitoris
   E. Posterior fourchette
   F. Fossa navicularis
   G. Vestibule
   H. Hymen
   I. Puberty
   J. Perineum
   K. Urethral meatus
   L. Vagina
   M. Cervix

IV. Assessment and collaborative care of the patient with a genitourinary emergency
   A. History
      1. Onset of problem (sudden or gradual)
      2. Last menstrual period
      3. Previous genitourinary diseases or surgeries
      4. Urinary symptoms
         a. Dysuria
         b. Frequency
         c. Urgency
         d. Burning
         e. Nocturia
         f. Hematuria
         g. Dribbling
         h. Incontinence
         i. Difficulty initiating urinary stream
      5. Gynecological related symptoms
         a. Vaginal discharge (color, amount)
         b. Vaginal bleeding (color, amount, clots, or tissue)
         c. Vaginal itching
         d. Vaginal burning
         e. Presence of sores, lumps
         f. Dyspareunia
      6. Medications
         a. Drugs that may interfere with urination
            (1) Antihistamines
            (2) Anticholinergics
            (3) Tricyclics
         b. Contraception
         c. Hormone therapy
         d. Sildenafil citrate (Viagra)
      7. Medical problems
         a. Diabetes
         b. Renal disease
         c. Thyroid disorders
         d. Sexually transmitted diseases
         e. Erectile dysfunction
   B. Physical assessment
      1. Location of pain
      2. Associated signs and symptoms: nausea, vomiting, change in bowel functions
      3. Fever, chills
      4. Signs and symptoms of septic shock
      5. External genitalia
         a. Inflammation
         b. Ulceration
         c. Discharge
         d. Swelling, nodules, lesions
         e. Discharge
      6. Color of patient's urine

7. Amount of urine
8. Evaluation of hematuria
9. Auscultation of bowel sounds
10. Palpation and pelvic examination
11. Palpation and male genital examination
12. Prostate examination
13. Rectal examination, male and female
C. Age-related changes
  1. Pediatric patient
    a. Bowel and bladder continence
      (1) Age
      (2) Stage of bowel and bladder training
      (3) Type of diapers used
    b. Tanner's classification of sexual development of the female[1]
      (1) Stage 1—Preadolescent—no pubic hair, fine body hair similar to hair on the abdomen
      (2) Stage 2—Sparse growth of long, slightly pigmented downy hair mostly along the labia
      (3) Stage 3—Darker, coarser hair, beginning to spread
      (4) Stage 4—Coarse, curly hair that looks like adult pubic hair, but not as much as an adult
      (5) Stage 5—Coarse, curly dark hair in the same amount as an adult
    c. Tanner's classification of sexual development of the male[1]
      (1) Stage 1—No pubic hair, penis and testicles the same size as childhood
      (2) Stage 2—Some growth of pubic hair, penis has slight enlargement, testes and scrotum begin to enlarge
      (3) Stage 3—Pubic hair darkens, spreads, penis increases in length, testicles and scrotum continue to enlarge
      (4) Stage 4—Pubic hair as in the adult, but not as much, penis increases in length and size, glans develop, scrotal skin darkens
      (5) Stage 5—Pubic hair in adult quantity, penis, scrotum, and testicles in adult shape and size
  2. Geriatric patient
    a. Bowel and bladder continence
      (1) May experience increase in incontinence
      (2) May experience increase in urgency and frequency
    b. Changes seen once the woman has gone through menopause
      (1) Decrease in pubic hair
      (2) Labia and clitoris decrease in size
      (3) Vagina becomes shorter
      (4) Mucosa in the vagina becomes pale, thin, and dry
    c. Changes in the male
      (1) Pubic hair decreases and grays
      (2) Penis decreases in size
      (3) Testicles hang lower in the scrotum
D. Collaborative care
  1. Stabilization of ABCs (airway, breathing, circulation)
  2. Intravenous fluids
  3. Diagnostic studies or procedures
    a. Complete blood cell count (CBC) with differential
    b. Blood cultures when a fever is present
    c. Electrolytes, blood urea nitrogen (BUN), creatinine
    d. Beta human chorionic gonadotropin (BHCG; female patients of childbearing age)
    e. Type and crossmatch
    f. Urinalysis and urine culture
    g. Urine stone analysis
    h. Dipstick urine
    i. Gram stain
    j. Wet mounts
      (1) Saline
      (2) KOH
    k. Cultures and blood tests for sexually transmitted diseases
      (1) Gonococcus culture
      (2) Chlamydia culture
      (3) Rapid plasma reagin (RPR) for syphilis
    l. Ultrasound
    m. Intravenous pyelogram (IVP)
    n. Retrograde urethrogram
    o. Cystogram
    p. CT or MRI of abdomen and selected organs
V. Collaborative care problems
  A. Anxiety
  B. Body image disturbance
  C. Dysreflexia
  D. Fluid volume deficit, high risk for
  E. Hyperthermia (related to infection)
  F. Incontinence, urge

G. Infection, high risk for

H. Knowledge deficit

I. Pain (acute and chronic)

J. Rape-trauma syndrome

K. Self-esteem disturbance

L. Urinary elimination, altered

M. Urinary retention

VI. Genitourinary and gynecological emergencies

A. Renal trauma

B. Bladder trauma

C. Foreign bodies

D. Kidney stone(s) (urolithiasis)

E. Urinary tract infection

F. Urinary retention

G. Benign prostatic hyperplasia

H. Pyelonephritis

I. Hematuria

J. Renal failure

K. Torsion of the testicles

L. Epididymitis

M. Priapism

    1. Sexual assault

    2. Foreign bodies

N. Sexually transmitted diseases

    1. Syphilis

    2. Gonorrhea

    3. Chlamydia

    4. Herpes simplex

    5. Condyloma acuminatum (venereal warts)

    6. Chancroid

    7. Granuloma inguinale

    8. Lymphogranuloma venereum

    9. Hepatitis B

    10. HIV

VII. Selected genitourinary emergencies

A. Urinary tract infection

B. Pyelonephritis

C. Urinary calculi

D. Testicular torsion

E. Epididymitis

F. Genitourinary trauma

    1. Sexual assault

    2. Urethral injury

    3. Renal trauma

    4. Bladder injury

    5. Foreign bodies

G. Priapism

The assessment and care of the patient who is suffering from a genitourinary emergency begins with obtaining a history of the patient's chief complaint and then performing an evaluation of the patient's back, abdomen, urine, external genitalia, and pelvis. When obtaining information related to urinary tract symptoms, the emergency nurse should include questions about dysuria, frequency, urgency, and hematuria. In addition, the emergency nurse should obtain a history of any related symptoms such as fever, chills, nausea or vomiting, or discharge. The age and sexual activity of the patient are additional pieces of information that may shed light on the nature of the patient's problem.

Certain disease processes such as diabetes, hypertension, gout, and spinal cord injury leave the patient at risk for developing a genitourinary problem. Trauma to the abdomen, back, or genitals may be specific sources of injury to the urethra, bladder, or kidneys.

The care of the patient with a genitourinary emergency may include diagnostic studies: CBC, electrolytes, BUN, creatinine, BHCG for female patients of childbearing age, urinalysis, urinary culture, ultrasound, IVP, and CT or MRI.

Many genitourinary emergencies cause the patient a great deal of pain, and pain patterns may provide clues to the basis of the patient's problem. Pain management may include oral, intramuscular, or intravenous administration of medications, as well as providing the patient with comfort measures such as a warm blanket or a place to lie down. Assisting the patient with the mangement of their pain will help the emergency nurse determine the cause of the patient's discomfort.

The incidence of sexually transmitted diseases continues to rise despite public awareness and education.[2] A disease such as syphilis, which was not routinely seen in the emergency department, has become more frequent and is now seen in its secondary and sometimes in its neuroleptic stages. Both hepatitis B and HIV are considered sexually transmitted diseases and pose particularly challenging problems for the emergency department, including infection control issues.

The emergency nursing care of the patient with a genitourinary emergency will depend on the origin of the emergency and the patient's response to it.

## REVIEW QUESTIONS
### Urinary Calculi

*A 32-year-old man comes to the emergency department complaining of abdominal and back pain. He states that he has been urinating frequently, but only a small amount of urine comes out. He states that he has seen some blood in his urine.*

1. The initial assessment of this patient should include:

    **0**  A. Palpation of the patient's bilateral femoral pulses

0   B. Determining the pattern of the patient's
       pain

0   C. Discovering what type of diet the
       patient is currently on

0   D. Obtaining a blood urea nitrogen (BUN)
       level and creatinine to rule out renal
       failure

2. The most common cause of kidney stones is:
   0   A. Oxalate
   0   B. Magnesium ammonium
   0   C. Uric acid
   0   D. Calcium oxalate

3. All of the following could contribute to this
   patient's inability to void except:
   0   A. Ingestion of eight glasses of water
   0   B. Taking 50 mg of amitriptyline (Elavil)
   0   C. Blunt trauma to the bladder
   0   D. Presence of a foreign body in the
          urethra

4. The patient is unable to void, and the emergency
   nurse will need to obtain a specimen through
   catheterization. What can the nurse do to make
   the procedure more comfortable?
   0   A. Give the patient some ice water to drink
          to increase his output
   0   B. Tell the patient to take slow, deep breaths
          as the catheter is inserted
   0   C. Obtain an order to use lidocaine
          (Xylocaine) jelly to lubricate the catheter
   0   D. Use the largest size catheter in order to
          drain the largest amount of urine

5. The patient's IVP reveals a kidney stone. Because
   it is a small stone, the patient will be discharged
   home to attempt to pass it. The patient will be
   given oxycodone (Percodan) for pain and a
   strainer to use while voiding. An appropriate
   nursing diagnosis for the patient's going-home
   instructions would be:
   0   A. Fluid volume deficit related to renal
          calculi and potential obstruction
   0   B. Pain related to penile discharge from the
          catheterization
   0   C. Urinary elimination, altered patterns,
          related to obstruction from a kidney stone
   0   D. Incontinence, urge, related to renal
          calculi and the patient's age

6. A nonurgent side effect of oxycodone is:
   0   A. Constipation
   0   B. An anaphylactic reaction

0   C. Respiratory depression
0   D. Hypotension

7. When teaching the patient about diet related to
   the development of renal calculi, the emergency
   nurse should instruct the patient to avoid which
   of the following foods?
   0   A. Orange juice
   0   B. Red meat
   0   C. Spinach
   0   D. Walnuts

8. Audit criteria for the chart of this patient (or any
   patient who has been treated in the emergency
   department for renal calculi) should include
   documentation of:
   0   A. Hemoptysis
   0   B. Urinalysis
   0   C. Hematochezia
   0   D. A CBC with differential

9. Criteria for admission of the patient with renal
   calculi would be:
   0   A. Small-diameter stones that can be easily
          passed
   0   B. Multiple kidney stones visualized on the
          IVP
   0   C. Absence of stones in the patient's
          bladder
   0   D. Need for intravenous pain medication

## Testicular Torsion

*An 10-year-old boy is brought to the emergency department
by his parents. They state that he had been climbing a tree
and began suffering severe pain in his groin. The child is
alert, diaphoretic, and obviously very uncomfortable.*

10. A history that may indicate testicular torsion
    would include:
    0   A. Age of the patient
    0   B. Sexual activity
    0   C. Gradual onset of scrotal pain
    0   D. Presence of nausea

11. The diagnosis of testicular torsion has been made
    by the urologist. Manual manipulation of the
    testicle has failed to reduce the torsion. The
    emergency nurse will now prepare the patient
    and his family for:
    0   A. Care of the testicular torsion at home
    0   B. Admission to the hospital for
           observation
    0   C. A barium enema to reduce the torsion
    0   D. Surgery for reduction of the torsion

12. The child becomes very upset when he is told that he must go to surgery for repair of the problem with his testicle. He becomes combative and states he will not go. The emergency nurse will plan the care of the patient using the following nursing diagnosis:
    - O  A. Growth and development, altered, related to surgery
    - O  B. Fear related to a potentially threatening situation
    - O  C. Sexual dysfunction (high risk for) related to testicular torsion
    - O  D. Mobility, impaired physical, related to having a surgical procedure

13. The emergency nurse provides the patient and his family with a private place in which to prepare for the surgery and spends time explaining the activities related to the surgery. The emergency nurse might observe which of the following if this intervention is effective?
    - O  A. The patient's pulse rate increases to 150 when the nurse enters the room
    - O  B. The patient turns his back when the nurse enters the room
    - O  C. The patient verbalizes his fear of the surgery
    - O  D. The patient's family takes the child home against medical advice

## Hematuria

14. A 66-year-old man presents to the emergency department complaining of blood in his urine. He states that he has also noticed an increased need to go to the bathroom at night, but he is having no pain with urination. The most probable cause of his hematuria is:
    - O  A. A congenital abnormality of his urethra
    - O  B. An asymptomic urinary tract infection
    - O  C. Benign prostatic hyperplasia
    - O  D. A pelvic neoplasm

15. Which of the following may cause pseudohematuria?
    - O  A. Phenytoin
    - O  B. Metronidazole
    - O  C. Rhubarb
    - O  D. All of the above

## Urinary Tract Infections

*An 18-month-old female is brought to the emergency department by her mother. Her mother states that she feels warm, has been drinking only small amounts of fluid, and periodically cries.*

16. In children, what symptom may be the only sign of a urinary tract infection?
    - O  A. Refusal to drink liquids
    - O  B. Fever without other associated symptoms
    - O  C. Nausea and vomiting and refusal to eat
    - O  D. Complaint of pain with urination and bowel movements

17. Risk factors that contribute to the potential for urinary tract infections include:
    - O  A. Length of the male urethra
    - O  B. A nulliparous female
    - O  C. Lack of sexual activity
    - O  D. Diabetes mellitus

18. A female patient diagnosed with a urinary tract infection (UTI) is being discharged from the emergency department and will be treated with ampicillin and phenazopyridine. The emergency nurse should instruct the patient that phenazopyridine will:
    - O  A. Decrease her needs for drinking additional fluids
    - O  B. Turn her urine orange
    - O  C. Treat her fever and chills
    - O  D. Take several days to be effective

19. Effectiveness of treatment for a UTI can be evaluated by the patient by:
    - O  A. An increase in urinary frequency 48 hours after treatment
    - O  B. A fever of 103° F with chills after 24 hours of treatment
    - O  C. A decrease in pain with urination after 24 hours
    - O  D. The formation of bruises on the patient's upper extremities

*An 80-year-old man is brought to the emergency department by his daughter. She states that he has had a fever and has been incontinent. She also states that he has been more confused than normal. He only has a history of hypertension, which is being managed with atenolol.*

20. The initial management of this patient in the emergency department would include:
    - O  A. Sending the patient to radiography for an abdominal film
    - O  B. Obtaining an atenolol level
    - O  C. Obtaining a urine to rule out a urinary tract infection
    - O  D. Drawing a prostate-specific antigen (PSA) level to rule out benign prostatic hypertrophy (BPH)

## Sexually Transmitted Diseases

21. A 22-year-old man comes to the emergency department complaining of scrotal swelling and pain. Epididymitis is diagnosed by the emergency physician. The organism that frequently causes epididymitis in sexually active males is:
    0   A. *T. vaginalis*
    0   B. *Chlamydia trachomatis*
    0   C. *Treponema pallidum*
    0   D. *Escherichia coli*

22. An 18-year-old male comes to the emergency department complaining of a rash on the palms of his hands. He is a runaway and has been sexually active with both men and women to earn money. He has never been treated for any sexually transmitted disease, but offers a history of nonpainful sores on the glans of his penis that have disappeared. What is the most likely cause of his rash?
    0   A. Diabetes mellitus
    0   B. Syphilis
    0   C. Gonorrhea
    0   D. Herpes simplex II

23. The current recommendations for the treatment of uncomplicated gonococcal infection from the Centers for Disease Control and Prevention (CDC) include:
    0   A. Parenteral penicillin G plus azithromycin IM
    0   B. IV tetracycline plus IV azithromycin
    0   C. Ceftriaxone IM plus azithromycin PO
    0   D. Aqueous penicillin plus azithromycin PO

24. An appropriate nursing diagnosis for the patient who is being treated for a sexually transmitted disease in the emergency department would be:
    0   A. Infection related to *Chlamydia trachomatis*
    0   B. Knowledge deficit related to the etiology and treatment of epididymitis
    0   C. Sexual dysfunction (high risk for) related to the diagnosis of gonorrhea
    0   D. Violence, high risk for, related to the diagnosis of a sexually transmitted disease

25. A patient diagnosed as having a sexually transmitted disease is treated with an IM antibiotic. To evaluate the patient for the potential of an anaphylactic reaction to the medication, the emergency nurse should observe the patient for:
    0   A. 24 hours
    0   B. 30 minutes

    0   C. 5 minutes
    0   D. No observation is needed

26. A 15-year-old boy comes to the emergency department complaining of a yellow penile discharge and burning with urination. He tells the triage nurse he will not stay if she has to call his parents. This emergency nurse assures him that she will not have to notify his parents for treatment because:
    0   A. Adolescents in the United States can consent for examination and treatment of a sexually transmitted disease (STD) without parental notification
    0   B. A 15-year-old is old enough to give his consent because he came to the emergency department unaccompanied
    0   C. An older brother or sister is allowed to give consent for evaluation and treatment of a sibling if the teenager does not want to notify parents
    0   D. There is no available treatment for the types of signs and symptoms that he is having

27. When discharging a patient being treated with metronidazole for a trichomoniasis infection, the emergency nurse should emphasize that the patient:
    0   A. Does not need to have his partner evaluated and treated if he takes all his medication as prescribed
    0   B. May continue to drink alcohol with all his meals as he has previously been doing before being prescribed the medication
    0   C. Sexual partners should use barrier contraception until the person who is infected has been seen again and cleared of infection
    0   D. Take the medication before he eats any type of food or at any meal

## Renal Problems

28. A 78-year-old man was found at home. He had fallen 3 days earlier and has been laying on the floor. Upon arrival in the emergency department, he is covered with urine and feces. His right arm and chest are purple from where he has been laying, and compartment syndrome is suspected. The patient is cleaned up, and an urinary catheter is inserted. A small amount of dark yellow urine is obtained and tests positive for

blood. The most probable cause of the blood in his urine is:

  0   A. Benign prostatic hypertrophy

  0   B. Chronic urinary tract infection

  0   C. Hypokalemia from dehydration

  0   D. Rhabdomyolysis from tissue injury

**29.** Acute tubular necrosis is a cause of:

  0   A. Prerenal failure

  0   B. Postrenal failure

  0   C. Intrarenal failure

  0   D. Urethral stricture

**30.** A major complications of continuous ambulatory peritoneal dialysis (CAPD) is:

  0   A. Peritonitis

  0   B. Catheter occlusion

  0   C. Renal calculi

  0   D. Rhabdomyolysis

## Genitourinary Trauma

*An 18-year-old man is brought to the emergency department after having been struck by a car while riding his bicycle. The patient was wearing a helmet. He is alert and oriented, complaining of back and abdominal pain. His vital signs are B/P 80/40, P 140, RR 28.*

**31.** A sign of severe injury to the pelvis or bladder is:

  0   A. Coopernail's sign

  0   B. Kehr's sign

  0   C. Homan's sign

  0   D. Chadwick's sign

**32.** Which of the following would be a contraindication to insertion of a urinary catheter?

  0   A. The patient has a pelvic fracture

  0   B. The patient complains of lower abdominal pain

  0   C. The patient is unconscious

  0   D. There is blood around the urinary meatus

**33.** The initial care of this patient would be based on the following nursing diagnosis:

  0   A. Injury, high risk for, related to blunt force to the flank

  0   B. Infection, high risk for, related to insertion of the catheter

  0   C. Fluid volume deficit related to hemorrhage

  0   D. Anxiety related to potential sexual dysfunction

**34.** Audit criteria for the chart of this patient (or any patient who has suffered genitourinary trauma) should include documentation of:

  0   A. Presence or absence of hematuria

  0   B. Presence of family in the emergency department

  0   C. Neurological assessment, including GCS

  0   D. History of a sexually transmitted disease

**35.** Signs and symptoms of a ruptured bladder include:

  0   A. Normal urinary output post injury

  0   B. Clear urine that dipsticked negative for blood

  0   C. Abdominal distention and pain with palpation

  0   D. A normal distribution of contrast during a cystogram

**36.** The most serious complication of a human bite to the genitals is:

  0   A. Bleeding from the wound

  0   B. Disfigurement from the wound

  0   C. Inability to reimplant lost tissue

  0   D. Infection from bacterial contamination

**37.** An indication of renal injury is:

  0   A. Balance's sign

  0   B. Kehr's sign

  0   C. Grey Turner's sign

  0   D. Cullen's sign

## Priapism

**38.** A 39-year-old African-American man presents to the emergency department with the complaint of a sustained erection. The patient states that he has had this problem in the past. What medical problem may be the cause of this patient's priapism?

  0   A. Sickle cell disease

  0   B. Diabetes mellitus

  0   C. Acute renal failure

  0   D. Systemic lupus

**39.** A common complication of priapism is:

  0   A. Gangrene of the penis

  0   B. Hemorrhagic shock

  0   C. Urinary retention

  0   D. Sexual impotence

**40.** A 33-year-old mentally retarded male is brought to the emergency department by his caregivers. They state he has a fever of 102° F , a foul-smelling penile discharge, and he is afraid to urinate because of pain. The family states he has never had any sexual contacts. A potential source of his symptoms probably is:

0    A.  Nongonococcal urethritis
0    B.  Foreign body
0    C.  Urinary calculi
0    D.  Pyelonephritis

41.  Accidental straddle injuries in the female pediatric patient are usually located:

0    A.  Above the 9-3 o'clock area of the vagina
0    B.  At the 8-2 o'clock area of the vagina
0    C.  Inside of the vaginal wall
0    D.  Near the mons pubis

## Sexual Assault

*A 20 year-old-male comes to the emergency department stating that he has been "raped." He had been hitchhiking and had accepted a ride. The driver hit him in the face and forced him to have anal intercourse. The patient is alert and oriented complaining of pain in his face and rectum.*

42.  Male victims of sexual assault:

0    A.  Sustain more physical trauma than female sexual assault victims
0    B.  Do not require evidence collection because sexual assault is unlikely
0    C.  Cannot become infected with sexually transmitted diseases
0    D.  Have to be aroused to sustain an erection

43.  The most common form of sexual assault in the male patient is:

0    A.  Forced oral intercourse of the assailant
0    B.  Forced manual genital stimulation of the assailant
0    C.  Forced masturbation of the assailant
0    D.  Receptive anal intercourse

## Pyelonephritis

*A 23-year-old woman comes to the emergency department complaining of a fever, chills, dysuria, and pain all over. The patient states that she has never had a kidney or bladder infection.*

44.  Based on the patient's urinalysis and CBC, the emergency physician makes the diagnosis of acute pyelonephritis. A common physical finding in the patient with pyelonephritis is:

0    A.  Tenderness over the affected flank area
0    B.  Tenderness behind both calves
0    C.  Tenderness in the upper extremities
0    D.  Tenderness over the sinuses

45.  The patient is to be discharged from the emergency department. Discharge teaching for the patient diagnosed with acute pyelonephritis should include all of the following except:

0    A.  Rest in bed as much as possible
0    B.  Increase fluid intake to 3500 to 4000 ml per day
0    C.  Only take the antibiotics until feeling better
0    D.  Return if the pain increases

## ANSWERS

1.  **B. Assessment.** Determination of the location and pattern of the patient's pain will help the emergency nurse discover the origin of the patient's problem. The complaint of inability to void would have already alerted the emergency nurse to the possibility of a kidney stone. The location and pattern of pain contributes additional information. The pain may be in different places, depending on the location of the stone. Classic pain patterns for renal stones include pain in the flank area radiating to the groin, pain in the lower quadrant, and low back pain.[3]

2.  **D. Assessment.** Seventy-five percent of renal stones result from calcium oxalate.[3]

3.  **A. Assessment.** All of the answers except ingestion of fluids could contribute to the patient's inability to void. It is important for the emergency nurse to get a detailed history from the patient in relation to any potential problem that could cause the patient to be unable to void. Drugs such as antihistamines, anticholinergics, and antidepressants can cause urinary retention. Bladder trauma and the presence of a foreign body in the urethra could also interfere with the patient's ability to void.[3]

4.  **C. Intervention.** Using copious amounts of lubricant—lidocaine jelly—can be helpful in making the procedure more comfortable for the patient. If the catheter will not pass, the obstruction site should be noted and the physician or urologist notified to prevent trauma to the urethra.[3]

5.  **C. Analysis.** The patient will need to be taught about the use of the strainer while voiding and the use of pain medication and its effect on urinary elimination. The defining characteristics of this nursing diagnosis are dysuria, frequency, urinary retention, and change in amount, color, or odor of the urine.[4]

6.  **A. Assessment.** Oxycodone may cause multiple side effects. However, emergent side effects would include an anaphylactic reaction, respiratory depression, and hypotension. Nonurgent side effects

are constipation, nausea and vomiting, and drowsiness. The emergency nurse needs to instruct the patient when it is indicated for them to return to the emergency department when side effects occur and how to manage other potential side effects such as constipation and nausea and vomiting.[5]

7. **C. Intervention.** Renal stones may form from oxalates. Foods rich in oxalates include tea, cocoa, grapefruit juice, almonds, and greens.

8. **B. Evaluation.** A urinalysis should be obtained on all patients with complaints of urinary symptoms. The color, amount, odor, and presence or absence of blood should be documented on the chart.

9. **D. Evaluation.** The need for intravenous administration of pain medication is a need for admission to monitor the patient for potential complications related to medication administration.[6]

10. **A. Assessment.** History related to testicular torsion includes the age of the patient, which is generally from newborn to 20 years of age; sudden onset of pain, and nausea and vomiting. Sexual activity would be related to the risk of epididymitis.[7]

11. **D. Intervention.** To ensure testicular salvage, the torsion needs to be reduced within 6 hours. If manual manipulation is attempted and fails, the patient will need to have surgery performed for detorsion of the testes.[6]

12. **B. Analysis.** The emergency nursing care of this patient would be planned using the nursing diagnosis of fear related to a potentially life-threatening situation, which would be the surgery. The defining characteristics of this nursing diagnosis include terror; fight behavior, flight behavior, and panic.[4]

13. **C. Evaluation.** The patient's ability to verbalize his fears about the surgery would help the emergency nurse evaluate the effectiveness of the interventions.[4]

14. **C. Assessment.** The most likely cause of his hematuria is benign prostatic hypertrophy (BPH), which is the most common cause of gross hematuria in men over 60.[8]

15. **D. Assessment.** There are multiple factors that may cause pseudohematuria, including medications and foods. It is important for the emergency nurse to obtain a history of the patient's diet and medications in relation to the onset of the hematuria.[8]

16. **B. Assessment.** Many times fever may be the only symptom of a urinary tract infection in young children. Almost 40% of children with a UTI may be asymptomatic.[3]

17. **D. Assessment.** Risk factors for the development of a UTI include diabetes mellitus, pregnancy, the shorter length of the female urethra, people over 50 years of age, and urological abnormalities.[3]

18. **B. Intervention.** Phenazopyridine is a nonnarcotic analgesic that has an analgesic action specific to the urinary tract system. Side effects of the drug include turning the urine orange. The drug may also cause hepatotoxicity and hematologic problems such as thrombocytopenia.[5]

19. **C. Evaluation.** Effectiveness of treatment can be evaluated by the patient experiencing a decrease in symptoms 24 hours after therapy has begun.[3]

20. **C. Intervention.** Urinary tract infections in the elderly manifest themselves with the symptoms of fever, incontinence, decreased appetite, confusion, and lethargy.[9]

21. **B. Assessment.** The most common organism causing epididymitis in a sexually active male patient is *Chlamydia trachomatis*. It may account for over two thirds of the cases of epididymitis.[3]

22. **B. Assessment.** The clinical manifestations of secondary syphilis include mucocutaneous lesions that occur in 80% of patients with the disease. The mucotaneous lesions appear on the palate, pharynx, glans of the penis, and vulva. The rashes that occur in secondary syphilis do not itch and can be macular, papular, pustular, or squamous lesions. They frequently appear bilaterally on the palms of the hands or soles of the patient's feet.[2,3,6]

23. **C. Intervention.** Current CDC recommendations for the treatment of uncomplicated gonococcal infections include ceftriaxone 125 mg IM or cefixime 400 mg orally, along with azithromycin 1g PO or doxycycline 100 mg orally for 7 days.[2]

24. **B. Analysis.** The most important care that the emergency nurse can provide for the patient being treated for a sexually transmitted disease in the emergency department is to provide the patient with information about the disease process and the appropriate treatment regimen that the patient should follow to prevent the problems that could result.

25. **B. Evaluation.** After the patient has been given an IM antibiotic, the patient should be instructed to remain in the emergency department area for 30 minutes so that if any complications should occur, the patient can be quickly treated.[5]

26. **A. Intervention.** All adolescents in the United States may consent for a confidential evaluation and for medical treatment of a sexually transmitted disease.[2]

27. **C. Intervention.** When taking metronidazole for the treatment of a trichomoniasis infection, the patient should not drink any alcohol, should have the partner checked and treated for the disease, should use barrier contraception, and should eat before taking the medication to avoid stomach upset.[2,5]

28. **D. Assessment.** One of the complications of tissue injury, immobility, and dehydration is rhadomyolysis, which will lead to the development of acute renal failure.[10]

29. **C. Assessment.** Intrarenal (intrinsic) failure is caused by acute tubular necrosis (ATN), exposure to nephrotoxins, renal artery or vein stenosis, or thrombosis. A urethral stricture would cause postrenal failure.[11]

30. **A. Assessment.** A major complication of continuous ambulatory peritoneal lavage (CAPD) is peritonitis. The patient will come to the emergency department with the complaint of diffuse abdominal pain, tenderness, fever, and chills. Gram-positive cocci are the most common cause of infection.[12]

31. **A. Assessment.** The emergency nurse should suspect the possibility of genitourinary trauma with the presence of Coopernail's sign (ecchymosis of the labia or scrotum), Grey Turner's sign (ecchymosis of the flank area), and costovertebral tenderness (fractures of the lower ribs and the vertebrae).[3]

32. **D. Intervention.** Blood at the urinary meatus is an indication of an injury to the urethra. Before the catheter is passed, a urethrogram should be obtained.[3,6]

33. **C. Analysis.** Based on the patient's vital signs on arrival in the emergency department, the initial care of this patient would be directed at correcting hemorrhagic shock.

34. **A. Evaluation.** The presence or absence of hematuria should be documented for all patients who have suffered genitourinary trauma.[3]

35. **C. Assessment.** Signs and symptoms of a ruptured bladder include inability to void, hematuria, abdominal distention, nausea and vomiting, low or absent urinary output, and extravasation of dye in the pelvis during the cystogram.[3,6]

36. **D. Assessment.** Human bites to the genitals can result in serious wound infections because of bacterial contamination from the human mouth. In addition, syphilis, herpes simplex, HIV, and hepatitis may be transmitted through human bites.[3]

37. **C. Assessment.** A Grey Turner's sign is an indication of bleeding in the retroperitoneal space.

38. **A. Assessment.** Sickle cell disease, the use of psychotropic drugs, anticoagulants, and spinal cord injury are some of the causes of priapism.[3]

39. **C. Assessment.** In 50% of the patients with priapism, urinary retention can occur. Sexual impotence is a potential complication, but not a common one.[11]

40. **B. Assessment.** Foreign body placement may be accidental, such as by a patient who does not realize the potential consequences of such behaviors, for example, a patient with a learning disability or mental retardation. It is important to include this possibility as a differential diagnosis in the care of this patient.[11]

41. **A. Assessment.** Accidental straddle injuries typically involve soft tissue injury to the vagina above the 9-3 o'clock line.[13]

42. **A. Assessment.** Males who suffer a sexual assault are more likely to sustain more physical injuries than female victims. They are at risk of becoming infected with STDs, require evidence collection, and do not have to be sexually aroused to sustain an erection.[13]

43. **D. Assessment.** Receptive anal intercourse is the most common form of male sexual assault. However, there is a significant number of male victims who experience more than one type of nonconsensual sexual contact during an assault.[13]

44. **A. Assessment.** Signs and symptoms of pyelonephritis include chills, fever, urinary urgency and frequency, and tenderness over the affected flank area.[3]

45. **C. Intervention.** The patient should be instructed to take all of the antibiotics prescribed.

## REFERENCES

1. Bates B: *A guide to physical examination,* ed 6, Philadelphia, 1995, Lippincott.
2. Centers for Disease Control and Prevention. 1998 guidelines for the treatment of sexually transmitted diseases. *MMWR* 47(No. RR-1), 1998.
3. Kidd P: Genitourinary emergencies. In Kitt S et al, editors: *Emergency nursing: a physiological and clinical perspective,* Philadelphia, 1995, WB Saunders.
4. Kim M, McFarland G, McLane A: *Pocket guide to nursing diagnoses,* St Louis, 1993, Mosby.
5. McKenny L, Salerno E: *Pharmacology in nursing,* St Louis, 1998, Mosby.
6. Baxter C: Renal and genitourinary emergencies. In Newberry L, editor: *Sheehy's emergency nursing principles and practices,* St Louis, 1998, Mosby.
7. Miura B: Scrotal pain. In Davis M, Votey S, Greengough P, editors: *Signs and symptoms in emergency medicine,* St Louis, 1999, Mosby.
8. Fickenscher L: Evaluationg adult hematuria, *Nurs Pract* 24(9):58-65, 1999.
9. Marchiondo K: A new look at urinary tract infection, *Am J Nurs* 98(3):34-38, 1998.
10. Carriere SR, Elsworth T: Found down: Compartment syndrome, rhabdomyolsis and renal failure, *J Emerg Nurs* 24:214-217, 1998.
11. Baxter C: Genitourinary emergencies. In Jordan KS, editor: *Emergency nursing core curriculum,* ed 5, Philadelphia, 2000, WB Saunders.
12. Breitfeller J: Peritonitis. *Am J Nurs,* 33, 1999.
13. Girardin B, Faugno D, Seneski P, et al: *Color atlas of sexual assault,* St Louis, 1997, Mosby.

# Chapter 9

# Medical Emergencies

## REVIEW OUTLINE

I. Anatomy
   A. Immune response system
   B. Genitourinary system
   C. Gastrointestinal system
   D. Neurologic system
   E. Hematologic system

II. Physiology
   A. Fluid and electrolyte balance
   B. Renin-angiotensin-aldosterone system
   C. Acid-base balance
   D. Renal function
   E. Hepatic function
   F. Glucose metabolism
   G. Blood-clotting mechanisms
   H. Immunity
   I. Inflammatory response

III. Assessment of the patient with a medical emergency
   A. Airway
   B. Breathing/ventilatory patterns
      1. Apnea
      2. Hyperventilation
      3. Cheyne-Stokes respirations
      4. Hypoventilation
      5. Biot's (cluster) breathing
      6. Central neurogenic hyperventilation (CNH)
   C. Circulation
      1. Heart rate, cardiac rhythm
      2. Skin color, temperature, and turgor
      3. Capillary refill
      4. Blood pressure
   D. Neurological assessment
      1. Level of consciousness
      2. Sensory/motor response
      3. Pupil reactions
      4. Oculocephalic reflex
      5. Oculovestibular reflex
      6. Corneal reflex
      7. Decorticate posturing

8. Decerebrate posturing
9. Flaccidity
   E. History related to the current medical emergency
      1. Onset of symptoms
      2. Medical history
      3. Medications
      4. Allergies
   F. Risk factors
      a. Lifestyle
      b. Exposure to illness
      c. Splenectomy
      d. Contact with infected materials
      e. Blood transfusions
      f. Recent travel (national and international)
      g. Inadequate immunizations
      h. Immigration status

IV. Collaborative care of the patient with a medical emergency
   A. Maintenance of airway, breathing, circulation
   B. Diagnostic studies or procedures
      1. Laboratory tests
         a. Complete blood count (CBC)
         b. Electrolytes
         c. Ethanol level
         d. Glucose level
         e. Creatinine, blood urea nitrogen (BUN)
         f. Urinalysis
         g. Drug screen
         h. Liver function tests
         i. Coagulation studies
         j. Test specific to the suspected disease or problem, i.e., thyroid levels, TB screen, Monospot
         k. Type and crossmatch
         l. Serum uric acid level
         m. Serum ammonia level
         n. Reticulocyte count
         o. Sedimentation rate
         p. Cultures

2. ECG

3. Chest radiograph

4. Arteriogram

5. Doppler studies

6. Ultrasound

7. CT scan

8. Magnetic resonance imaging (MRI)

C. Pharmacological agents to treat specific medical emergencies

V. Related nursing diagnoses

  A. Airway clearance, ineffective

  B. Aspiration, potential for

  C. Body temperature, altered, potential for

  D. Breathing pattern, ineffective

  E. Cardiac output, decreased

  F. Diarrhea

  G. Fatigue

  H. Fluid volume deficit

  I. Fluid volume excess

  J. Gas exchange, impaired

  K. Infection, potential for

  L. Injury, potential for

  M. Knowledge deficit

  N. Pain

  O. Anxiety

  P. Fear

VI. Selected medical emergencies

  A. Communicable infectious disease emergencies

  B. Endocrine emergencies

  C. Fever

  D. Rashes

  E. Coma

  F. Hematological emergencies

  G. Fluid and electrolyte imbalances

  H. Reye's syndrome

  I. Gout

  J. Dehydration

M edical emergencies may not be as dramatic as a cardiac arrest or multiple trauma, but they certainly can be as life threatening. They may present as a cluster of symptoms involving virtually every body system. Many medical conditions overlap with, or result in, other clinical problems. For example, a patient with sickle cell crisis may also have dehydration, fever, and an electrolyte imbalance. Sorting the present problem from other related medical emergencies presents the emergency nurse with a unique patient care challenge.

People who have emergent medical problems make up a large percentage of the emergency department patient population. As with any other patient, medical emergency patients need immediate assessment and stabilization of their airway, breathing, and circulation. The emergency nurse needs to have a thorough understanding of the anatomy and physiology of the involved system or systems. A complete history needs to be obtained, along with a complete assessment of the patient's physical state.

The care of the patient with a medical emergency continuously changes as medications and therapies change. This means that the emergency nurse needs to continuously review current literature directed at the treatment of medical emergencies such as diabetes and complications related to HIV infection.[1,2]

The cause of the medical crisis may sometimes be as important as the treatment. The emergency nurse is responsible for coordinating the necessary diagnostic procedures and instituting the appropriate therapy.

## REVIEW QUESTIONS

*A 19-year-old male presents to the emergency department complaining of shortness of breath, low-grade fever, and a recent weight loss. He also complains of watery diarrhea. The patient states he has been living on the street for the last 6 months and has engaged in prostitution for food and shelter. He states that he has no other significant medical history and that he has never used "illegal" drugs. The patient is alert, pale, and thin.*

1. This patient has significant risk factors for:

  0  A. Disseminated gonococcal infection

  0  B. Active mycobacterium tuberculosis

  0  C. Infection with the HIV virus

  0  D. Acute *Giardia lamblia* infection

2. The specific test used to measure the effectiveness of HIV management is:

  0  A. ELISA test for HIV antibodies

  0  B. HIV RNA (viral load)

  0  C. CBC with differential

  0  D. $CD_4$ counts

3. Side effects of antiviral medications that may cause patients to present to the emergency department for treatment include:

  0  A. Acute pancreatitis

  0  B. Peripheral neuropathy

  0  C. Insomnia

  0  D. All of the above

4. An emergency nurse stuck herself in the finger with a syringe of blood obtained from a known HIV-positive patient. The needle penetrated her gloves. The current basic treatment regimen for occupational exposure to HIV is:

   0   A. Report it to the infectious disease clinical specialist within 24 hours of exposure to a known HIV-positive patient

   0   B. Call an attorney to file a complaint about the unsafe work environment and the use of needles without protective guards

   0   C. Begin treatment with zidovudine 600 mg per day in two to three divided doses for 4 weeks and lamivudine, 150 mg twice a week for 4 weeks

   0   D. There is no need for treatment because the risk of infection from this type of exposure is minimal

*Robert B., a 20-year-old foreign exchange student, is transferred to the emergency department from the college infirmary. He was admitted for a sore throat, fever, and malaise. He was transferred to the emergency department when he became short of breath and cyanotic despite high-flow oxygen. He had never received any immunizations until he came to study in this country about 3 months ago.*

5. Physical findings that indicate diphtheria include:

   0   A. Dirty gray-white, rubbery membrane covering structures of the pharynx

   0   B. White blisters on the patient's tongue, tonsils, and pharynx

   0   C. Red, blotchy rash on the patient's trunk and lower extremities

   0   D. Trismus with difficulty in pronunciation and chewing of food

6. The only effective control of diphtheria is:

   0   A. Wearing masks when treating infected patients

   0   B. Washing hands with betadine after caring for patients

   0   C. Avoiding crowds when an outbreak of the disease occurs

   0   D. Assuring that everyone has received appropriate immunization

7. Hepatitis A is transmitted by:

   0   A. Fecal-oral contact

   0   B. Blood transfusions only

   0   C. Eating contaminated shellfish

   0   D. Sexual intercourse

8. Persons at high risk for the development of hepatitis B include all of the following except:

   0   A. Health care workers frequently exposed to blood

   0   B. Hemodialysis patients

   0   C. Day-care workers

   0   D. Sexually active individuals

9. The most common infection caused by disseminated herpes is:

   0   A. Hepatitis

   0   B. Meningitis

   0   C. Encephalitis

   0   D. Mononucleosis

10. Which is not a characteristic symptom of the measles?

    0   A. Koplik's spots on the buccal mucosa

    0   B. Projectile vomiting and diarrhea

    0   C. Fever, photophobia, and conjunctivitis

    0   D. Red, blotchy rash over the abdomen

11. Bacterial meningitis is confirmed by a lumbar puncture that reveals:

    0   A. Red blood cells in the fluid too numerous to count

    0   B. WBC less than 500, normal glucose and protein levels

    0   C. WBC up to 20,000, decreased glucose level, increased protein level

    0   D. Presence of viral antibodies in the fluid, decreased protein level

12. Which of the following signs would be evidence of condition improvement in a 3-month-old infant with bacterial meningitis?

    0   A. Takes half of formula feeding

    0   B. Generalized hyperreflexia

    0   C. Subnormal body temperature

    0   D. Blood glucose level 50 mg/dl

13. Pertussis (whooping cough) primarily occurs in:

    0   A. Long-term smokers who received their childhood immunizations

    0   B. Patients with emphysema or other COPD-like diseases

    0   C. Children under 4 who have not been immunized

0   D. Young children with asthma who have been immunized

14. A 33-year-old female presents to the emergency department complaining of profuse watery diarrhea and low abdominal pain. The patient states that she just returned from a backpacking trip. She and her friends did drink water out of a "clear" stream. Indications of dehydration in this patient would include:
0   A. Orthostatic vital sign changes of an increase blood pressure ≥ 20mm Hg
0   B. No changes in resting respiratory rate and rhythm or skin color
0   C. Orthostatic vital sign changes of a decrease in pulse rate ≥ 20 bpm
0   D. Orthostatic vital sign changes of an increase in pulse rate ≥ 20 bpm

15. The patient is diagnosed with *Giardia lamblia*. Definitive treatment for this infection includes:
0   A. Metronidazole 250 mg tid for 7 days and good infection control practice
0   B. Drinking plenty of fluids to decrease the risk of dehydration and reinfection
0   C. Fluid resuscitation and morphine for the related abdominal pain
0   D. Prescribing a bland diet and loperamide (Imodium) until the diarrhea stops

16. Common electrolyte abnormalities associated with an adrenal crisis include all of the following *except*:
0   A. Hyponatremia
0   B. Hypernatremia
0   C. Hypokalemia
0   D. Hypercalcemia

17. An insulin drip has been initiated to treat a patient whose whole blood sugar is 700 mg/dl. The target glucose is:
0   A. 600 mg/dl
0   B. 250 mg/dl
0   C. 100 mg/dl
0   D. 350 mg/dl

18. Which statement, made by the parent of a diabetic child in ketoacidosis, would indicate that more health teaching is needed?
0   A. "When he gets the flu, I need to take him to the doctor right away."
0   B. "I can still give him Tylenol when he gets a fever at home."

0   C. "I can't let him eat anything he wants."
0   D. "Hopefully he will grow out of this when he gets a little older."

19. The drug of choice for managing hyperglycemia in diabetic ketoacidosis is:
0   A. Regular insulin
0   B. Lente insulin
0   C. Glyburide
0   D. 70/30 insulin

20. Hyperglycemic hyperosmolar nonketotic coma occurs primarily in:
0   A. Noninsulin-dependent diabetics
0   B. Elderly diabetics who do not eat
0   C. Patients without endogenous insulin
0   D. New–onset type I diabetes mellitus

*His friends brought Mr. Deaton, a 28-year-old diabetic, to the emergency department after fainting while waiting for a table at a local restaurant. He is diaphoretic and lethargic. His whole blood glucose on arrival to the emergency department is 34 mg/dl. Vital signs are B/P 106/70, P 64, R 16, Temp 99.0° F.*

21. The next appropriate step would be to:
0   A. Give orange juice by mouth and have suction available in case he vomits
0   B. Start a lactated Ringer's IV and give one-amp glucagon IV push
0   C. Start a normal saline IV and give one-amp dextrose 50% IV push
0   D. Observe the patient closely and check vital signs every 15 minutes

*Five minutes after carrying out the above action, Mr. Deaton is awake and talking.*

22. The next most appropriate step would be to:
0   A. Discharge the patient from the emergency department
0   B. Admit the patient to the critical care unit
0   C. Recheck the vital signs
0   D. Give the patient something to eat

*A 50-year-old woman presents to the emergency department with symptoms of fever, weakness, nausea with vomiting, and diarrhea. She is tachycardic, hypotensive, febrile, and anxious and has obvious tremors. Bilateral exophthalmos is present. Medical history is positive for hyperparathyroidism and a two-pack-a-day smoking habit for 20 years.*

23. The most probable cause for the above symptoms would be:
    - 0   A. Acute adrenal insufficiency
    - 0   B. Adult respiratory distress syndrome (ARDS)
    - 0   C. Acute alcohol withdrawal
    - 0   D. Thyroid storm (thyrotoxicosis)

24. The medication used to manage the tachycardia associated with a thyroid storm is:
    - 0   A. Lidocaine 1 mg/kg IV
    - 0   B. Verapamil 10 mg IV
    - 0   C. Propranolol 1 mg IV
    - 0   D. Adenosine 6 mg IV

25. The nursing diagnosis applicable for a patient who is dehydrated is?
    - 0   A. Gas exchange, impaired related to fluid loss
    - 0   B. Fluid volume deficit related to fluid loss
    - 0   C. Fluid volume excess related to fluid shifting
    - 0   D. Altered oral mucous membrane related to fluid volume loss

26. A sign or symptom of hyponatremia is:
    - 0   A. Hypertension
    - 0   B. Hyperactivity
    - 0   C. Seizure activity
    - 0   D. Neck vein distention

27. In caring for patients with abnormal sodium levels, it is important for the emergency nurse to remember that:
    - 0   A. The similar signs and symptoms of sodium disorders make them virtually impossible to diagnose without laboratory data
    - 0   B. Abnormal sodium levels are very common in young healthy people and may occur with no apparent cause
    - 0   C. Sodium is the chief intracellular electrolyte and subject to changes due to fluid shifts
    - 0   D. Normal sodium levels can range from 110 mEq/dl to 160 mEq/dl, depending on what type of diet the patient is on

28. A person with a calcium level of 6.0 mg/dl may be likely to exhibit all of the following signs except:
    - 0   A. Trousseau's sign
    - 0   B. Chvostek's sign
    - 0   C. Grey Turner's sign
    - 0   D. Laryngeal stridor

29. The treatment of hypercalcemia includes which of the following?
    - 0   A. Sodium polystyrene sulfonate (Kayexalate) enemas
    - 0   B. Intravenous isotonic saline infusion and loop diuretics
    - 0   C. Charcoal and magnesium citrate per gastric tube
    - 0   D. Calcium chloride or calcium gluconate IV

**Disseminated Intravascular Coagulation**

30. Clinical conditions that can often lead to the development of disseminated intravascular coagulation (DIC) include all of the following except:
    - 0   A. Congestive heart failure
    - 0   B. Abruptio placentae
    - 0   C. Venomous snakebites
    - 0   D. Multiple trauma

31. The treatment of a patient with DIC includes which of the following:
    - 0   A. Infusions of packed red blood cells, platelets, and heparin
    - 0   B. Treating the underlying cause
    - 0   C. Monitoring the patient in a critical care unit
    - 0   D. All of the above

*A 7-year-old boy with hemophilia is brought to the emergency department after falling off his bike and sustaining a 2 cm knee laceration. His bleeding is controlled, and the laceration is sutured. No other injuries are noted.*

32. The next appropriate step would be to do which of the following?
    - 0   A. Discharge the child home with his parents for observation
    - 0   B. Administer one prophylactic dose of cryoprecipitate
    - 0   C. Observe the child in the emergency department for 4 hours
    - 0   D. Admit to pediatric hematology unit for continuous observation

33. If this same boy were to sustain major trauma and be transported to a community hospital emergency department, they would be wise to do which of the following?
    - 0   A. Contact his hemophilia treatment hospital and ask them for guidelines for his care and/or possible transfer
    - 0   B. Treat him as any other pediatric trauma

patient without consideration of the effects of his hemophilia on his injuries

   0  C. Refuse to accept the patient when he arrives, due to the specific treatment needed to stabilize him

   0  D. Ask the parents if they have any factor VIII that the emergency department staff can administer

*Mr. Thompson, a 36-year-old African-American man, comes to the emergency department in sickle cell crisis.*

**34.** Which of these symptoms should the emergency nurse be most concerned about?

   0  A. Bilateral knee joint pain

   0  B. Temperature of 101.4° F

   0  C. Chest pain

   0  D. Anxiety

**35.** All of the following treatment measures would be utilized during this crisis except:

   0  A. Factor XIII infusions

   0  B. Intravenous fluids

   0  C. Supplemental oxygen

   0  D. Intravenous analgesics

*Mr. McClurg is brought into the emergency department one morning after his friends were unable to wake him after "a night of partying." He is unconscious and responds only to deep, painful stimuli. His vital signs are B/P 108/58, P 60, R 12, Temp 96.0° F (rectally), SaO₂ 92%.*

**36.** Priorities of care for Mr. McClurg include all of the following except:

   0  A. Maintenance of a patent airway

   0  B. Determination of any injuries

   0  C. Obtaining a whole blood glucose level

   0  D. Sending him for a routine CT scan

**37.** The physician orders naloxone (Narcan) 2 mg IV push to be given. What might the emergency department nurse consider before giving this medication?

   0  A. Diluting it with a dextrose solution

   0  B. Applying protective restraints

   0  C. Asking the patient if he has allergies

   0  D. Refusing to give the medication

**38.** Which of the following patients may be at risk for an allergic reaction to latex?

   0  A. A child with spina bifida or with a physician-diagnosed allergy

   0  B. A patient who has had frequent urinary catheterizations

   0  C. Persons who have frequent occupational exposure to latex products

   0  D. All of the above persons are at risk of an allergic reaction to latex

*Amanda, age 2, is brought to the emergency department for fever and vomiting of 24 hours' duration. Vital signs are B/P 98/50, P 110, R 28, Temp 102.2° F (rectally). Acetaminophen (Tylenol) suppository gr. 2 was given upon arrival. One hour after arrival she has been assessed, the physician has examined the child, laboratory work has been drawn, and a chest radiograph has been done. Suddenly her mother screams for help. As you and another nurse enter the room, you note that Amanda is having a generalized tonic-clonic grand mal seizure, which lasts 60 seconds.*

**39.** After assessing that her airway is patent and she has a pulse, the next step should be to:

   0  A. Recheck the child's temperature

   0  B. Call for additional help

   0  C. Pad the side rails for patient protection

   0  D. Tell the mother to leave the room

**40.** A subtle manifestation of seizure activity in a neonate is:

   0  A. Absence of movement or lapses in awareness

   0  B. Unilateral brief muscle contractions of lower extremities

   0  C. Abrupt loss of muscle tone

   0  D. Eye deviation and fluttering, lip smacking

**41.** In caring for Amanda, you remember that vomiting in children:

   0  A. Is a normal reaction for children in her age group

   0  B. Is an ominous sign of impending cardiopulmonary arrest

   0  C. Is frequently related to a respiratory problem

   0  D. Is commonly a sign of child maltreatment or neglect

**42.** Amanda's temperature returns to normal and her tests are complete. The diagnosis is a viral illness, and she may now be discharged. After giving her mother discharge instructions, which comment would tell you that more teaching is needed?

   0  A. "If she gets a fever again, I'll give her aspirin every 4 hours until it's back down."

0   B. "I can let her eat or drink a little at a time as long as she isn't vomiting."

0   C. "I need to call our doctor and see him tomorrow or the next day."

0   D. "If she gets worse or has another seizure, I can bring her back here."

43. Based on the above response, the nursing diagnosis applicable to Amanda's mother would be:
   0   A. Knowledge deficit, fever control
   0   B. Feeding self-care deficit
   0   C. Altered health maintenance
   0   D. Health-seeking behavior

44. Reye's syndrome primarily affects which two organs?
   0   A. Brain and spleen
   0   B. Brain and heart
   0   C. Heart and kidneys
   0   D. Brain and liver

45. The cardinal symptoms of Reye's syndrome (altered level of consciousness and recurrent vomiting) typically:
   0   A. Are fatal
   0   B. Are unreliable
   0   C. Follow a minor viral infection
   0   D. Follow a urinary tract infection

46. A crucial diagnostic test in a child with Reye's syndrome would be:
   0   A. Ammonia level
   0   B. ECG
   0   C. Uric acid level
   0   D. Urinalysis

47. A common life-threatening complication of uremia is:
   0   A. Pancreatitis
   0   B. Gastric ulcers
   0   C. Hyperkalemia
   0   D. Renal calculi

48. Prophylaxis for the management of hepatitis exposure is available for all of the following *except:*
   0   A. Hepatitis type A
   0   B. Hepatitis type C
   0   C. Hepatitis type B
   0   D. All hepatitis viruses

49. A 7-year-old male was brought to an outlying emergency department for "flulike" symptoms.

His mother states her pediatrician told her to bring him to the emergency department if he did not feel better. The child is lethargic and pale, with skin cool to the touch. Purpura is noted on both his lower extremities. His vital signs are BP 80/40; HR 136R; RR 38; rectal temperature 97° F. Which medications may be initiated to maintain the child's blood pressure?
   0   A. Rocephin 1 g intravenously
   0   B. Nipride 0.3-0.5 µg/kg/min
   0   C. Dobutamine 2.5 µg/kg/min
   0   D. Norepinephrine 2 µg/min

50. A condition caused by inadequate excretion of uric acid is:
   0   A. Arthritis
   0   B. Gout
   0   C. Lupus
   0   D. Dehydration

## ANSWERS

1. **C. Assessment.** Although it is not confirmed, based on the significant history, risk factors, and symptoms, the nurse should give definite consideration to an HIV infection as being the cause of his problems. Disseminated gonococcal infections can include septicemia, arthritis, dermatitis, meningitis, endocarditis, and perihepatitis. Traveler's diarrhea usually does not involve a cough and such a profound weight loss.[1,3]

2. **B. Intervention.** $CD_4$ counts were the standard that was used by practitioners to evaluate the effectiveness of HIV treatment until 1996 when the FDA approved the use of a test that measured viral loading (HIV RNA).[1]

3. **D. Assessment.** The antiviral medications that are used to manage HIV infection cause multiple side effects that may prompt patients to seek treatment in the emergency department. Some of these can cause serious complications such as pancreatitis.[4]

4. **C. Intervention.** The CDC has provided recommendations for the management of significant HIV exposure, including initiating drug prophylaxis as soon as possible.[5]

5. **A. Assessment.** There is a dirty gray-white rubbery membrane covering the pharynx and larynx. The patient may have cutaneous lesions.[3]

6. **D. Intervention.** Diphtheria is contracted by airborne respiratory droplets or direct contact with respiratory secretions. The disease spreads more easily in crowded living conditions. However, the most effective management is to assure that every-

one is appropriately immunized, including booster shots.[3]

7. **A. Assessment.** Hepatitis A is commonly spread via the fecal-oral route. It is found in serum and stool and is infectious 2 weeks before and 1 week after jaundice. Hepatitis B is transmitted most commonly by blood and sexual contact. Hepatitis E is an enterically transmitted infection from shellfish and contaminated water.[3,6]

8. **C. Assessment.** Day-care children and their caregivers are not at risk for the development of hepatitis B. Those at highest risk include health care and public safety workers who have exposure to blood in the workplace, clients and staff at institutions for the developmentally disabled, hemodialysis patients, recipients of clotting factor concentrates, household contacts and sexual partners of hepatitis B carriers, adoptees from countries where hepatitis B is endemic (Pacific Islands and Asia), IV drug abusers, sexually active homosexual and bisexual men, sexually active men and women with multiple partners, and inmates of long-term correctional facilities.[3,6]

9. **C. Assessment.** Encephalitis is the most common infection caused by disseminated herpes.[3]

10. **B. Assessment.** Symptoms of the measles do not usually involve vomiting and diarrhea unless a concurrent GI problem exists. Patients (especially children) who have measles typically exhibit the following symptoms: fever, Koplik's spots on buccal mucosa, conjunctivitis, photophobia, harsh cough, and a red, blotchy rash that lasts 1 week.[3]

11. **C. Intervention.** Bacterial meningitis is confirmed by a lumbar puncture result that shows WBCs up to 20,000, a decreased glucose level, and increased protein levels. The appearance will also be cloudy, and the Gram stain will show that bacteria are present. Viral meningitis will be evidenced by clear cerebrospinal fluid, a WBC count less than 500, normal glucose and protein levels, and no evidence of bacteria. Clinical symptoms are also correlated with diagnostic indicators in the diagnosis of any type of meningitis.[3,8]

12. **A. Evaluation.** It is usually considered a good sign any time a child begins to eat after a serious illness. A 3-month-old who takes half of his formula is probably improving. Generalized hyperreflexia, subnormal body temperature, and hypoglycemia are signs that the condition is potentially worsening and the child should be closely watched.[3,9]

13. **C. Assessment.** Pertussis, better known as whooping cough, primarily occurs in infants and children up to 4 years of age who have not been properly immunized, although it may occur at any age.[3]

14. **D. Assessment.** Orthostatic vital sign changes of an increase in pulse of greater than 20 beats per minute indicate fluid loss.

15. **A. Intervention.** Giardia occurs all over the world and has become one of the most common causes of diarrhea. Water is the most widespread source of giardia. Management includes management of the patient's dehydration, metronidazole PO, and instructions about good handwashing techniques and appropriate treatment of water, especially when camping.[10]

16. **B. Assessment.** The sodium and potassium levels remain low in a state of adrenal crisis, as do the blood glucose and plasma cortisol levels. The calcium level increases, as does the BUN, which occurs from azotemia secondary to dehydration.[3]

17. **B. Intervention.** For a patient in diabetic ketoacidosis, started on an insulin drip, a goal of a whole blood glucose of 250 mg/dl is desired. If an attempt is made to get the level at 150 or 100 mg/dl, rebound hypoglycemia may quickly occur, and treating the hypoglycemia may lead to wide fluctuations in the blood glucose level. In other words, conservative treatment of hyperglycemia is recommended to prevent the patient from "bottoming out" their blood glucose too quickly.[11]

18. **D. Evaluation.** Children do not outgrow their diabetes. Young adulthood may bring about a more controlled (less brittle) diabetic state, but outgrowing the disease is not seen. The other statements regarding taking the child to the doctor for the flu, still giving acetaminophen (Tylenol) for fever, and not letting him eat anything he wants are true.[12]

19. **A. Intervention.** The drug of choice for managing hyperglycemia in diabetic ketoacidosis is regular insulin because of its rapid but short-duration actions. Lente insulin is considered a longer-acting form of insulin than regular and should not be used. Oral hypoglycemic agents are never used for the initial management of diabetic ketoacidosis.[13]

20. **A. Assessment.** Hyperglycemic hyperosmolar nonketotic (HHNK) coma occurs primarily in noninsulin-dependent diabetics. It may also be the initial presentation of new-onset type II diabetes mellitus. It results in profound dehydration due to hyperglycemia and resultant osmotic diuresis. Usually the patient is unable to drink enough fluids to prevent the dehydration. Ketoacidosis does not develop, probably because there is enough endogenous insulin present to inhibit ketogenesis. Usually there is underlying infection, stroke, or sepsis.[3]

21. **C. Intervention.** The priority is to immediately increase the blood glucose level. That would be accomplished by starting a normal saline IV and giving dextrose 50% 1 amp IV push stat. During the initial phase, nothing should be given by mouth due to the patient's impaired level of consciousness. Lactated Ringer's is not the preferred IV solution, and glucagon would not be used, either. Simply observing the patient's vital signs is not enough.[3]

22. **D. Intervention.** After the dextrose 50% injection, the patient should start to respond within 1 to 2 minutes. This should be followed with an additional food source, especially protein (milk, sandwich, and so on), to prevent a rebound hypoglycemia from occurring. It would be inappropriate to admit or discharge the patient based only on simple hypoglycemia until other potential problems can be ruled out.[2]

23. **D. Assessment.** The symptoms of fever, weakness, nausea, vomiting, diarrhea, tachycardia, hypotension, anxiety, tremors, and exophthalmus all point to thyroid storm or thyrotoxicosis. Additional symptoms that may be seen include abdominal pain, possible coma, delirium or confusion, rales secondary to congestive heart failure, hepatic tenderness, and periorbital edema. Many of these symptoms do resemble acute alcohol withdrawal, but not adult respiratory distress syndrome.[3,4]

24. **C. Intervention.** Propranolol 1 mg IV slowly for the tachycardia associated with a thyroid storm.[14]

25. **B. Analysis.** The applicable nursing diagnosis for this patient would be fluid volume deficit. Fluid volume excess is the exact opposite. Impaired gas exchange and altered oral mucous membranes would not apply.

26. **C. Assessment.** Hyponatremia is a well-known cause of seizures. Other signs of hyponatremia include altered mental status, poor skin turgor, sunken fontanels and eyes, dry mucous membranes and skin, flat neck veins, orthostatic vital sign changes, and hypotension and tachycardia. The patient may complain of a recent acute illness, nausea, vomiting, and diarrhea, immobility or inability to drink fluids, trauma or burns, lethargy, thirst, confusion, weight changes, muscle cramps, dizziness, fatigue, and headache. Cardiorespiratory arrest and hyperactivity are not normally signs of hyponatremia. A salty taste to the skin may be identified in a patient with hypernatremia or cystic fibrosis.[15]

27. **A. Assessment.** Sodium disorders are difficult to diagnose without the assistance of laboratory testing to determine the sodium status. Similar symptoms are seen in both hyponatremia and hypernatremia.

Sodium, the chief extracellular electrolyte, is normally 135 to 145 mEq/dl of plasma. Abnormal sodium levels are common in older people.[15]

28. **C. Assessment.** The normal serum calcium level is 8.5 to 10.5 mg/dl, so this patient would be considered hypocalcemic. Grey Turner's sign is ecchymosis in the flank areas, commonly seen in abdominal trauma from retroperitoneal bleeding. A positive Chvostek's sign is seen when the facial nerve is tapped and twitching of the upper lip is noted on the same side of the stimulation. A positive Trousseau's sign occurs when carpophalangeal spasms are seen after moderate pressure (i.e., blood pressure cuff inflation) applied to the upper arm. Both of these signs are indicative of hypocalcemia. The ECG changes commonly seen in hypocalcemia are a prolonged (lengthening) QT interval and decreased left ventricular contractility.[15]

29. **B. Intervention.** Hypercalcemia should be treated with normal saline infusions and loop diuretics. Sodium polystyrene sulfonate (Kayexalate) enemas are used to treat hyperkalemia. Charcoal and magnesium citrate (a potent cathartic) are given to flush the bowel, especially after drug overdoses.[15]

30. **A. Assessment.** Congestive heart failure is not well-known to lead to the development of DIC. Common disorders that are known to cause DIC are many. They include sepsis (the most common cause), obstetrical emergencies (abruptio placentae, placenta previa), multiple trauma (especially crush-type injuries), burns, fatty emboli, multisystem organ failure, all types of shock, hyperthermia or hypothermia, malignancies and leukemia, snakebites, transfusion reactions, and postcardiac arrest.[15]

31. **D. Intervention.** Although somewhat controversial, the treatment of a patient in DIC includes infusions of packed red blood cells, platelets, and IV heparin infusions. Treating the underlying cause should also be a top priority. Monitoring in a critical care unit is required due to the high mortality rate of 50% to 70%.[15]

32. **C. Intervention.** After any type of injury or procedure on a hemophiliac—no matter how minor—the child should be observed for up to 4 hours following the procedure. Cryoprecipitate is usually not administered except in extreme emergencies. An immediate admission or discharge would be inappropriate for this patient at this time.[15]

33. **A. Intervention.** Contacting the hemophilia treatment hospital and asking for guidelines on the patient's care is by far the best course of action. Hemophiliacs need very specialized care and treat-

ment, and preparing for transfer to the referral hospital should definitely be considered. Refusing to accept the patient because of his hemophiliac status is totally inappropriate and could cost the patient his life.[9,15]

34. **C. Assessment.** Chest pain, rather than a fever, knee pain, or anxiety, would be of the utmost concern and should receive the highest priority. Patients who are in sickle cell crisis may develop angina, myocardial infarction, pulmonary embolus, high-output cardiac failure, and life-threatening dysrhythmia due to anemia and profound hypoxia. Other complications include hemolytic anemia, cholelithiasis, priapism, renal disease, and a high risk of developing infections.[15]

35. **A. Intervention.** Factor XIII infusions are given to hemophiliacs, not to sickle cell crisis patients. Intravenous fluids, supplemental oxygen, and parenteral analgesics are all appropriate treatment measures.[15]

36. **D. Intervention.** The patient is unconscious; questions about suicide are not appropriate at this time. Maintaining airway patency, searching for any injuries, and obtaining laboratory specimens should be done in that order.[3]

37. **B. Intervention.** Consideration should be given to applying protective restraints prior to giving naloxone (Narcan). This drug, a potent narcotic antagonist, acts very rapidly. If the patient were a narcotic overdose, he may awaken quickly and possibly injure himself or the nurse, along with removing any therapeutic treatment measures (e.g., IVs, tubes, and so on). An allergy to a narcotic would not prohibit the administration of this drug, nor is it necessary to dilute it with a dextrose solution.[3]

38. **D. Assessment.** All of these persons are at risk of developing an allergic reaction to latex.[16]

39. **A. Assessment.** The child's seizure is probably due to a dramatic rise in her core body temperature. Generally febrile seizures are due to how quickly the temperature rises rather than how high. Knowing that the airway is patent and a pulse is present, it would be safe to recheck her rectal temperature at this point and initiate further temperature control measures. Calling for help is not necessary (two nurses are in the room). Padding the side rails is not a priority and can be done later. As long as the mother is physically and emotionally able to stay in the room, she should be allowed to do so.[9,15]

40. **D. Assessment.** Newborns may exhibit subtle signs of seizure activity, including eye deviation and fluttering, lip smacking, and bicycling.[9]

41. **C. Assessment.** Because of diaphragmatic irritation and coughing that trigger the gag reflex, infants and children may have a respiratory problem that presents as what appears to be a gastrointestinal problem. Many clinicians are confused by these presenting symptoms. Vomiting is not normal for any age group; nor is it an ominous sign or a sign of child neglect.[9]

42. **A. Evaluation.** Aspirin is contraindicated in children because of the increased incidence in the development of Reye's syndrome. Acetaminophen should be used instead. Small sips of fluids and small bites of food in the absence of vomiting, calling the family physician, and returning to the emergency department for further seizures are all appropriate discharge instructions for the mother to remember.[9]

43. **A. Analysis.** If the mother incorrectly stated that aspirin should be given for a fever, then the applicable nursing diagnosis would be knowledge deficit for fever control. Feeding self-care deficit, altered health maintenance, and health-seeking behavior nursing diagnoses would not apply.

44. **D. Assessment.** Reye's syndrome primarily affects the brain and liver. The primary defect is mitochondrial injury, which is present in all tissues. Elevated ammonia levels, hypoglycemia, and acidosis contribute to neurologic dysfunction, cerebral edema, and coma.[15]

45. **C. Assessment.** The recurrent vomiting and altered mental status typically follow a minor viral infection such as chicken pox, upper respiratory infection, or influenza. Reye's syndrome has a 10% to 20% mortality rate, and it can be a devastating illness, but it is not always fatal.[15]

46. **A. Assessment.** An elevated serum ammonia level is diagnostic for Reye's syndrome. The ammonia level rises because of defects in the liver enzyme system that converts ammonia to urea. This high ammonia level results in an altered level of consciousness, most often coma.[15]

47. **C. Assessment.** A common, life-threatening complication of uremia is marked hyperkalemia. This results from the inability of the kidney to excrete potassium and sodium. Hyperkalemia can cause sudden death due to life-threatening cardiac dysrhythmias.[17]

48. **B. Intervention.** Prophylaxis is available for hepatitis types A and B, including serum globulin, immune globulin, and vaccination.[3,5]

49. **D. Intervention.** Vasoactive support of the child with suspected meningococcemia must be aggres-

sive and a vasopressor such as norepinephrine (Levophed) will help maintain the child's blood pressure.[4,9]

50. **B. Assessment.**[15]

## REFERENCES

1. Klaus B, Grodesky M: HIV in 2000: Historical perspective and an outlook for the future, *Nurs Pract* 25(1):103-110, 2000.

2. Miller J: Management of diabetic ketoacidosis, *J Emerg Nurs* 25(6):514-519, 1999.

3. Peabody SP: General medical emergencies. Part I. In Jordan K, editor: *Emergency nursing core curriculum,* ed 5, Philadelphia, 2000, WB Saunders.

4. McKenry L, Salerno E: *Pharmacology in nursing,* St Louis, 1998, Mosby.

5. Kallenborn JC, Coleman R, Carrico R, et al: Occupational exposure: organizing ED care to determine rapid postexposure prophylaxis within hours instead of days, *J Emerg Nurs* 25(6):505-508, 1999.

6. Almeida S: Infectious and communicable diseases. In Newberry L, editor: *Sheehy's emergency nursing principles and practice,* ed 4, St Louis, 1998, Mosby.

7. Molitor L: A 15-year-old boy with a rash and fever, *J Emerg Nurs* 24(5):467-468, 1998.

8. Swartz M: Bacterial meningitis. In Goldman L, Bennett J, editors, *Cecil textbook of medicine,* ed 21, Philadelphia, 2000, WB Saunders.

9. Haley K, Eckles N, Baker P: *Emergency nursing pediatric course,* Park Ridge, IL, 1999, Emergency Nurses Association.

10. Coughlan L: *Giardia lamblia* in adults: a case study, *J Am Acad Nurs Pract* 11(10):431-434, 1999.

11. Miller J: Management of diabetic ketoacidosis, *J Emerg Nurs* 25(6):514-519, 1999.

12. Wood T: Endocrine emergencies. In Newberry L, editor: *Sheehy's emergency nursing principles and practice,* ed 4, St Louis, 1998, Mosby.

13. Sengewald J: Update on diabetes medications, *J Emerg Nurs* 25(1):28-30, 1999.

14. Dillman W: Thyroid. In Goldman L, Bennett J, editors: *Cecil textbook of medicine,* ed 21, Philadelphia, 2000, WB Saunders.

15. Newberry L: General medical emergencies. Part II. In Jordan K, editor: *Emergency nursing core curriculum,* ed 4, Philadelphia, 2000, WB Saunders.

16. Miller K, Weed P: The latex allergy triage or admission tool: an algorithm to identify which patients could benefit from "latex safe" precautions, *J Emerg Nurs* 24(2):145-152, 1998.

17. Huey TR: Gastrointestinal emergencies. In Newberry L, editor: *Sheehy's emergency nursing principles and practice,* ed 4, St Louis, 1998, Mosby.

# Chapter 10

# Mental Health Emergencies

## REVIEW OUTLINE

I. General patient assessment
- A. History
  1. Chief complaint
  2. Events leading to the patient seeking emergency care
  3. Medical history
  4. Social history
  5. Psychological/psychiatric history
  6. Current medications
  7. Allergies
  8. Previous emergency department visits
  9. History of physical and/or psychological abuse
  10. History of suicide/suicidal behavior
- B. Physical examination
  1. Primary assessment and critical interventions
  2. Secondary assessment
  3. Signs and symptoms of abuse
- C. Mental status examination
  1. Behavior and general appearance
  2. Speech and speech patterns
  3. Mood and affect
  4. Thought processes or mental content
  5. Perception
  6. Judgment
  7. Cognitive ability
     a. Attention and concentration
     b. Basic knowledge
     c. Abstract reasoning
     d. Orientation
     e. Memory
- D. Diagnostic procedures
  1. Rule out organic causes of altered mental status
     a. Drug screen
     b. Whole blood glucose
     c. Electrolytes
  2. ECG
  3. Radiographic imaging
     a. CT of the head
     b. MRI of head

II. Management of mental health emergencies
- A. Collaborative problems
  1. Altered family processes
  2. Ineffective individual coping
  3. Ineffective family coping
  4. Anticipatory grieving
  5. Dysfunctional grieving
  6. Risk for violence: directed at others
  7. Risk for violence: directed at self
  8. Posttrauma syndrome
  9. Anxiety
  10. Fear
  11. Powerlessness
  12. Sleep pattern, disturbance of
  13. Thought processes, alteration in
- B. Collaborative care for mental health emergencies
  1. Management of critical interventions for life-threatening illness or injury
     a. Provision of physical safety for the patient and health care providers
     b. Physical and chemical restraint
        (1) Benzodiazepines
        (2) Haloperidol
        (3) Neuromuscular blocking agents
     c. Rule out physical causes of altered mental status and/or behavioral changes
     d. Emotional support
        (1) Assess patient's potential for violence
        (2) Allow patient to ventilate
        (3) Set limits
     e. Provide patient and family with follow-up care and options

III. Age-related considerations
- A. Pediatric Patient
  1. Appropriate behavior varies with age and psychosocial development of the child
  2. Many pediatric patients may rely on acting-out behavior to express their needs
  3. Must consider child's psychosocial development when observing reactions to

specific mental health emergencies, i.e., grief

B. Geriatric patient
1. Always rule out organic causes of altered mental status or behavioral changes
2. Consider drug interactions as potential source of mental and behavioral changes

IV. Selected mental health emergencies
A. Anxiety and panic reactions
B. Ineffective coping
C. Crisis
D. Sudden loss and death
1. The concept of loss
2. Anticipatory grieving
3. Loss of bodily functions
4. Loss of family member or loved one
5. Loss of belonging
6. Loss of self-esteem (i.e., abuse, domestic violence)
E. Grief
1. Informing the family or significant others
2. Reactions
3. Anger
4. Cultural beliefs
5. Religious beliefs
F. Violence
1. Homicide
2. Suicide
3. Threatening behaviors
G. Psychosis
H. Bipolar disorder
I. Human abuse
1. Child maltreatment
a. Identification of children at risk
b. Identification of patterns of injury and neglect
c. History related to the injury
d. Notification of appropriate authorities
2. Elderly abuse
a. Identification of people at risk
b. Identification of patterns of injury and neglect
c. History related to the injury
d. Notification of appropriate authorities
e. Referral for support systems
3. Domestic violence
a. Identification of people at risk
b. Identification of patterns of injury and threats
c. Notification of appropriate authorities
d. JCAHO guidelines for emergency departments

Mental health emergencies encompass a vast expanse of psychological and psychiatric problems and disorders. Sudden loss triggers a cascade of generally normal human responses that emergency nurses must be prepared to deal with in order to provide the care and support patients or their families will need. The effect of politics on the American health care delivery system is illustrated beautifully in Curry's article published in the October 1993 issue of the *Journal of Emergency Nursing.*[1] The Community Mental Health Centers Act of 1963 essentially shut down many of the psychiatric institutions that provided housing and care for mentally ill patients. Many of the patients who previously were hospitalized were now referred to outpatient settings for care. Over the past 30 years, many of the federal and state funds for outpatient programs have been markedly decreased. Inpatient beds have also been drastically decreased. The emergency department continues to be one of the main sources of care for patients with psychiatric disorders. The patient who is confused, unkempt, homeless, anxious, or violent continues to begin his or her health care journey through the doors of the emergency department.

Any complaint of a mental health emergency must be evaluated for a potential organic cause. Hypoxia, hypoglycemia, and chemical intoxication provide examples of physiological reasons for mental and or behavioral changes.[2] The management of mental health emergencies involves not just the emergency department but also the communities these departments serve. Finally, emergency nurses need to recognize the need to care for themselves and their co-workers as well. Stress, grief, depression, and ineffective coping are not just matters limited to the patients and families we care for. Care of ourselves provides the energy and dedication needed to continue to care for others.

## REVIEW QUESTIONS

1. Ms. Pepper presents to the triage desk stating that "I know that I am going to die!" She is alert but is visibly shaking. Her skin is cool and diaphoretic. She is complaining of a "choking" feeling in her throat, shortness of breath, and numbness and tingling in both hands. She states that she has been awakened with similar feelings lately. Her family doctor has been unable to find a physical cause to her findings, but she knows something is wrong. Her physical examination reveals no physical cause of her symptoms. You suspect:

   O   A. Bipolar disorder

   O   B. Panic attack

0    C. Depression
0    D. Agoraphobia

2. An appropriate nursing diagnosis on which to base Ms. Pepper's plan of care is:
0    A. Spiritual distress related to her fear of death or impending disaster
0    B. Knowledge deficit related to problem-solving or coping strategies
0    C. Self-esteem disturbance related to her concern about her stress
0    D. Potential for violence related to her inability to control her anxiety

3. An effective intervention to manage hyperventilation related to a panic attack includes:
0    A. Administration of sedation, neuromuscular blocking agents, and endotracheal intubation to mechanically control the patient's ventilations
0    B. Encouraging the patient to increase respirations until he or she becomes hypoxic and passes out, which will then slow their breathing
0    C. Applying 100% oxygen through a nonrebreather mask and administering a beta-blocker in a handheld nebulizer to chemically control the patient's ventilations
0    D. Encouraging the patient to take slow deep breaths or teach other types of relaxation exercises to decrease the onset of feelings that trigger a panic attack

4. A 15-year-old female presents to triage complaining of insomnia, difficulty concentrating, and "thinking" about ways to die so that her pain goes away. She states that she moved to this area 6 months previously and had to leave her boyfriend behind. The patient is alert, speaking slowly with a flat affect. She says she came here because her teacher felt she needed some help. You suspect:
0    A. The patient is experiencing normal feelings related to leaving her boyfriend
0    B. The patient may be experiencing symptoms of depression and may attempt to hurt herself
0    C. The patient talked to her teacher so that she could be excused from school
0    D. The patient is trying to make her parents feel guilty because she had to leave her boyfriend

5. Mr. Ivey presents to the emergency department with signs and symptoms of ketoacidosis. He states that 3 weeks ago a mass was found on his neck and he is sure it is cancerous. Since then Mr. Ivey has stopped taking all of his medications. He is very quiet and withdrawn and speaks very softly. He does not make eye contact and relates that he has lost 30 pounds over the last 3 weeks because he has stopped eating. Upon further questioning, Mr. Ivey admits that he stopped taking his medication because he wants to die. Mr. Ivey is displaying signs and symptoms of:
0    A. An anxiety disorder
0    B. Depression
0    C. Psychosis
0    D. Bipolar disorder

6. The priority nursing diagnosis on which to base a plan of care for Mr. Ivey is:
0    A. Knowledge deficit related to his diabetes
0    B. Anxiety related to his possible cancer diagnosis
0    C. High risk for injury related to his depression
0    D. Sleep disturbance related to his diabetes

7. Mr. Ivey is treated for his ketoacidosis in an area of the emergency department where he can be observed at all times. The nursing staff allows him to ventilate his fears related to cancer. All therapies are aimed at correcting his medical problems while addressing his depression. Evaluative criteria for his plan of care includes:
0    A. Mr. Ivey agrees to hospitalization for further medical and psychological care
0    B. Mr. Ivey states that he is going to leave the hospital as soon as his blood sugar is under control
0    C. Mr. Ivey states that he would never go to the local mental health center for help
0    D. Mr. Ivey states that he would never ask his family for help because they do not understand about his disease

8. Major risk factors for suicide include:
0    A. Good physical health
0    B. Married couples
0    C. Ethanol use
0    D. An unorganized suicide plan

9. Jane, a 16-year-old girl, is brought to the emergency department by the life squad for superficial lacerations to her wrists. She is crying and states that she hates her mother for making her come to the hospital. Jane states that she cut her wrists because her boyfriend broke up with her. She is alert and oriented and has no history of any medical or psychological problems. Your assessment of the lethality of Jane's suicide attempt is:

    0   A. Low risk

    0   B. High risk

    0   C. No risk

    0   D. Acting-out behavior

*A 20-year-old male was brought to the emergency department by helicopter after having been pulled out of a running car and suffering carbon monoxide poisoning. His mother states that he recently returned home from school and had a particularly difficult quarter. The patient is intubated, hypotensive, and has a GCS of 3. His initial CO is 15.*

10. In addition to the critical lab values that need to be obtained, what other tests should be performed in the emergency department?

    0   A. CT to rule out neurological injury from his CO exposure

    0   B. Drug screen to identify other the presence of other toxins

    0   C. Abdominal CT to identify the presence of an ileus

    0   D. Liver function tests for potential transplant due to injury from CO exposure

*A 16-year-old boy is brought to the emergency department by helicopter after having been shot in the neck by a friend. He arrives in the emergency department in full arrest. History of the event reveals that the patient had been shot in his basement, but was able to walk up the stairs and ask his sister for help and then collapsed. His sister, a critical care nurse, administered CPR until the rescue squad arrived and the flight team transported him to the hospital. After 20 minutes of additional resuscitation, the trauma team pronounces the patient dead.*

11. The emergency nursing assessment of this patient's sister should include:

    0   A. Whether she has a history of allergies so that a sedative can be ordered to ease her grieving

    0   B. Whether her brother had any health insurance coverage so she will not have

to worry about his emergency department bills

    0   C. Whether she and her brother had ever discussed a particular funeral home where his remains may be sent

    0   D. Whether she has any family or friends who can come and be with her in the emergency department

12. The most appropriate intervention for the survivors of sudden death in emergency department is:

    0   A. Providing the family with a sedative to decrease their reaction to their grief

    0   B. Providing the family with a room where they can be with other members and make calls as needed

    0   C. Providing the family with the names of local funeral homes so they can begin to make arrangements

    0   D. Explaining to the family that their grief will decrease over time and they will soon forget this experience

13. After being told that her brother is dead, his sister begins screaming and states that she should have done more. Which of the following nursing diagnoses would be most appropriate to provide care for this patient's sister?

    0   A. Powerlessness related to her inability to save her brother's life

    0   B. Fear related to her inability to save her brother's life

    0   C. Anxiety related to inability to save her brother's life

    0   D. Injury, high risk for related to her inability to save her brother's life

14. One method that the emergency nurse may use to evaluate the effectiveness of her interventions related to the family who has suffered a sudden loss:

    0   A. Contact the family's chaplain by phone to see how the family is doing since the death

    0   B. Contact the family by phone and ask them how they are doing and if they have any questions the nurse may answer

    0   C. Evaluate the charting that was completed during the resuscitation process

    0   D. Consult the hospital's social service department for ideas related to evaluation of sudden loss

15. A crisis is:
    O  A. The mind's response to a demand or perceived threat
    O  B. An alarm reaction to a demand or perceived threat
    O  C. A sudden unexpected threat or loss of basic resources
    O  D. A stage of exhaustion to a demand or perceived threat

16. Mr. Red arrives in the emergency department by life squad after having had a generalized seizure at home. Mrs. Red reports that her husband has a history of seizures that had been well controlled with medications. However, he recently was placed on an antipsychotic drug for depression. Mr. Red's seizure activity is the result of:
    O  A. Stress related to his diagnosis of depression
    O  B. Neuroleptic medications decrease the seizure threshold
    O  C. Neuroleptic medications decrease sodium levels
    O  D. Neuroleptic medications decrease glucose levels

17. Mrs. Gray, a 44-year-old woman, is transported to the emergency department from the local long-term psychiatric facility. The nurse caring for her states that she has had a sudden mental change and has bilateral upper extremity rigidity. Her vital signs are a BP 186/102; HR 132R; and RR 28. All her signs and symptoms developed within the last 4 hours. Her current medications are haloperidol and eye drops. Her symptoms are probably indicative of:
    O  A. A cerebral vascular accident (CVA)
    O  B. Dehydration from decreased oral intake
    O  C. Neuroleptic malignant syndrome
    O  D. An acute psychotic disorder

18. Mr. Black, a well-kept, articulate 35-year-old man, presents with a chief complaint of severe lower back pain for the past 2 months. Mr. Black denies trauma but states that his pain began when his new neighbors starting shooting radar beams into his new apartment. Mr. Black is exhibiting symptoms of :
    O  A. Bipolar disorder
    O  B. Acute psychosis
    O  C. Paranoid disorder
    O  D. Dissociative disorder

19. A 36-year-old male is brought to the emergency department by the police after they were called to a grocery store to subdue him. The man went out-of-control after he was inadvertently struck by a display of paper towels that fell on him. He began screaming at the top of his voice, "They're trying to kill me." The police have the patient physically restrained. The patient refuses to communicate with the emergency department staff. This patient is exhibiting symptoms of:
    O  A. Acute psychosis
    O  B. Acute social phobia
    O  C. Acute hysteria
    O  D. Acute dementia

20. The patient is taken to a quiet room and placed in restraints for safety. When a restraint situation arises, the most important information to document is:
    O  A. Why the patient needs to be placed in restraints
    O  B. How the patient is to be restrained
    O  C. When the patient was placed in the restraints
    O  D. Where the restraints have been applied

21. The leading cause of delirium in the elderly is:
    O  A. Falls that result in injury
    O  B. Cardiovascular disease
    O  C. Urinary tract infection
    O  D. Small bowel obstruction

22. Nursing interventions to decrease agitation include:
    O  A. Shouting at the patient to be sure that he hears you
    O  B. Allowing the patient time to express himself
    O  C. Restraining the patient when trying to talk with him
    O  D. Expecting the patient to answer all of your questions at once

*Mr. White, a 24-year-old man, presents to the triage desk, pounds his fist on the desk, and states, "I need to see a doctor now!" You note the odor of alcohol on his breath. He has several abrasions on his face, and his clothing is soiled and torn. You ask Mr. White what happened, and he tells you "It's none of your ★@?/business."*

23. You determine that Mr. White's potential for violence is:
    O  A. High risk for violent behavior
    O  B. Low risk for violent behavior

O   C. No risk for violent behavior

O   D. No relationship to this patient's behavior

24. The triage nurse should:
O   A. Tell Mr. White to shut up and sit down until she has time for him because the waiting room is full
O   B. Tell Mr. White to immediately leave the emergency department before you hit him
O   C. Ask Mr. White to please wait while you place yourself in a safe place
O   D. Take Mr. White's hand and ask him if he would like to talk about his anger

*Mr. Johnson is a 66-year-old man who is brought to the emergency department by the life squad for uncontrollable behavior. Mr. Johnson reportedly boarded a bus and began yelling at the other passengers. The police were called when Mr. Johnson refused to leave the bus. Mr. Johnson is in restraints and continues to yell, "Let go of me!"*

25. Initial emergency nursing interventions should include all of the following except:
O   A. Obtaining a whole blood glucose level
O   B. Placing the patient on a pulse oximeter
O   C. Obtaining a set of vital signs
O   D. Sedating the patient with morphine sulfate

26. Mr. Johnson's whole blood glucose is 40. An intravenous line is inserted and an ampule of $D_{50}$ is administered. Mr. Johnson is now alert and oriented and embarrassed about his behavior. He states he is a diabetic and took his insulin, but did not eat enough for breakfast. Mr. Johnson should remain under observation for:
O   A. Agitation related to being a patient in the emergency department
O   B. Hypoglycemia because he has not eaten properly today
O   C. Elevated intracranial pressure (ICP)
O   D. Self-destructive behavior

27. A 16-year-old male is brought to the emergency department with the complaint of a "possible seizure." His head and upper torso are twisted to the right. He is having muscle spasms of the face and hands. He reports that he and his friends had taken some "little white pills" they received from a "friend." The paramedics report that they had given him some diazepam with little effect. The patient has symptoms of:
O   A. Status epilepticus
O   B. Acute psychotic reaction

O   C. Acute dystonic reaction

O   D. Acute conversion hysteria

28. Reversal of the patient's symptoms will occur with administration of:
O   A. Diazepam
O   B. Naloxone
O   C. Diphenhydramine
O   D. Etomidate

29. An 8-week-old girl is brought to the emergency department by her mother. She states that the child has been having vomiting and diarrhea for the past 24 hours. The mother states that the child also fell down the basement stairs. The triage nurse notes that the child has only been staring and is not moving her left side. Her BP is 70/palpation; HR 180; RR 32. Discoloration is noted around her right eye. When evaluating the history of the child's injuries, the emergency nurse must consider:
O   A. The child's growth and development
O   B. The child's past medical history
O   C. The child's immunization history
O   D. The child's current medications

30. When child maltreatment is suspected, the emergency nurse must:
O   A. Notify the parents about the nurse's concerns
O   B. Report the maltreatment to the appropriate authorities
O   C. Obtain the appropriate consent for further treatment
O   D. Consult with an attorney to protect herself from a lawsuit

31. A 5-year-old boy, brought to the emergency department by his teacher, is complaining about his stomach hurting. Initial evaluation reveals a child who will not make eye contact with the emergency nurse, is wearing diapers, and is clinging to his teacher. Of the following, which nursing diagnosis is most appropriate?
O   A. Functional urinary incontinence
O   B. Risk for altered parenting
O   C. Dressing/grooming self-care deficit
O   D. Caregiver role strain

*The life squad brings an 85-year-old man to the emergency department from a nursing home for problems with his urinary catheter. The patient is unable to verbally communicate. The nursing home staff reports that he can become agitated and they keep soft restraints on his extremities to prevent any injury to the patient or themselves. When the emergency nurse examines the catheter, it is found that there is a large laceration under the surface of the patient's penis. It appears that the catheter has eroded through the urethra and the body of the penis. There is a large amount of bloody drainage coming from the wound.*

**32.** The patient's condition suggests neglect. The secondary survey of this patient must include:

- 0 A. Documentation of any belligerent behaviors
- 0 B. Patterns of additional injury such as bruising
- 0 C. Documentation of blood in the patient's stool
- 0 D. Documentation about the patient's level of activity

**33.** One of the vital emergency nursing interventions for the elderly patient who has suffered abuse or neglect is:

- 0 A. Acting as a patient advocate for the elderly
- 0 B. Listening to the patient's caregivers
- 0 C. Planning for the patient's discharge
- 0 D. Teaching others about elderly abuse

**34.** Because of the large wound caused by the urinary catheter, the most appropriate nursing diagnosis on which to base this patient's care is:

- 0 A. Incontinence, functional related to an ineffective urinary catheter
- 0 B. Infection, high risk for related to the injury caused by the catheter
- 0 C. Knowledge deficit related to the patient's ability to care for his catheter
- 0 D. Communication, impaired related to the patient's inability to express what he needs

**35.** When reviewing documentation related to suspected abuse, the emergency nursing charting should reflect:

- 0 A. The financial and insurance status of the patient
- 0 B. Where the patient receives his primary health care
- 0 C. Appropriate referrals related to the reported abuse
- 0 D. The language the patient uses for verbal communication

**36.** Women who are victims of abuse often present to the emergency department with other complaints that mask the real problem. All of the following are common chief complaints related to battering *except*:

- 0 A. Sexual assault
- 0 B. Suicide attempts
- 0 C. Alcoholism
- 0 D. Positive self-esteem

**37.** You are caring for a 28-year-old mother of three children who admits her injuries are the result of battering. She informs you that she will be returning home to her suspected abuser. An appropriate reply to her announcement should be:

- 0 A. "I have not heard of anything so stupid in my life! You have wasted our time!"
- 0 B. "Have you heard of Nicole Brown Simpson? Maybe you should think about it!"
- 0 C. "Well, I am going to call the police and report this for you anyhow even if you will not."
- 0 D. "Do you have a plan in mind as to how you will protect yourself and the children if anything should happen?"

## ANSWERS

1. **B. Assessment.** Patients who are experiencing a panic attack complain of a feeling of impending doom or death. They manifest physical symptoms of tachypnea, tachycardia, shortness of breath, and numbness and tingling in their extremities related to hyperventilation. These symptoms can lead to physical and psychological dysfunction if the source of the patient's anxiety is not identified and managed.[3]

2. **B. Analysis.** This care of this patient should be directed at identifying ways to assist her to cope with her anxieties.

3. **D. Intervention.** Teaching the patient how to relax so that a panic attack can be averted is most the effective management of hyperventilation.[3]

4. **B. Assessment.** The patient's history suggests that her symptoms have persisted for several months and she has been unable to find an effective way to cope with the changes in her life. The expression of suicidal thoughts indicates the potential for her to hurt herself.[3]

5. **B. Assessment.** Depression is characterized by alteration in mood, weight loss, insomnia, agitation,

and overall negative self-concept. Mr. Ivey is also at great risk of causing further injury to himself because he has stopped taking his medications.[4]

6. **C. Analysis.**

7. **A. Evaluation.** The patient's ability to recognize that he needs both medical and psychological care indicates that he has an understanding of his current situation.[5]

8. **C. Assessment.** Major factors for suicide include age (less than 19, older than 45); depression; previous attempts; ethanol abuse; loss of rational thinking; lack of social support; organized plan; chronic illness; and no spouse.[5]

9. **A. Assessment.** Jane's suicide attempt ranks low in lethality because of age, sex, and lack of an organized plan. However, she will need to be carefully watched and taught appropriate coping strategies.[5]

10. **B. Intervention.** Patients who attempt suicide often use more than one method. A drug screen should be performed very early in this patient's evaluation to rule out other causes of his altered mental status and hypotension because his CO level may not completely explain these.[6]

11. **D. Assessment.** An individual who is facing a sudden loss, such as death of a loved one, will need the support of family, friends, or professional personnel.[7]

12. **B. Intervention.** Providing the family with a private place to be with other family members and make calls or arrangements away from the general distractions of the emergency department is one of the most appropriate interventions for survivors of sudden loss.[7]

13. **A. Analysis.** The nursing diagnosis of powerlessness would be the most appropriate for the care of this patient's sister. Defining characteristics of this nursing diagnosis include verbalization of the feeling that one has no control over a particular situation or its outcome, expression of doubt about one's role performance (particularly in this case, since the sister is a critical care nurse), and expressions of dissatisfaction and frustration over the inability to perform previous tasks and/or activities.[8]

14. **B. Evaluation.** Families have reported that talking with those who have been a part of the resuscitation and allowing them to ask questions has been of help in assisting them to cope with sudden death.[9]

15. **C. Assessment.** A crisis is a sudden, unexpected threat or perceived threat to or a loss of basic resources or life's goals. Stress is the body's response to a demand, change, or perceived threat. The stress response is divided into three stages: alarm, resistance, and exhaustion.[7]

16. **B. Analysis.** Neuroleptic medications decrease the seizure threshold.[4]

17. **C. Assessment.** The patient whose psychosis is being treated with an antipsychotic medication must be monitored for signs and symptoms of neuroleptic malignant syndrome (NMS). NMS is characterized by a sudden change in mental status, fever and muscular rigidity, tachycardia, and a labile blood pressure. The risk of NMS is most common in patients receiving haloperidol and may even occur when the patient has been on it for a long time.[10]

18. **C. Assessment.** Paranoid disorders are characterized by a logical, yet bizarre explanation of medical problems.[4]

19. **A. Assessment.** Acute psychosis is characterized by the patient's inability to recognize reality or communicate. The patient is at great risk for injuring herself or others.[4]

20. **A. Intervention.** When placing a patient in restraints, the reason why the patient has to be restrained needs to be carefully documented. The patient's behavior must be carefully described. All patients who are restrained must be carefully monitored.[11]

21. **C. Assessment.** A urinary tract infection (UTI) is one of the most common causes of delirium in the elderly. Other causes include pneumonia, sepsis, hypothermia, dehydration, renal failure, diabetes, and hypoxia.[12]

22. **B. Intervention.** Interventions to decrease a patient's agitation may include: approaching the patient in a calm manner; speaking to the patient in a gentle audible voice; and allowing the patient enough time to express himself.[12]

23. **A. Assessment.** Mr. White is exhibiting several signs of potentially violent behavior. He is pounding his fist on the desk, speaking loudly, cursing, has alcohol intoxication, and appears to have already been in a fight.[3]

24. **C. Intervention.** Answer A would further irritate Mr. White. Answer B would jeopardize the safety of other staff and patients. Answer D would also irritate Mr. White. You should never touch an angry patient. Answer C is the most appropriate because your first priority is your own physical safety.[3]

25. **D. Intervention.** The patient's altered mental status and behavioral changes should be evaluated before the patient is given any sedation.[4]

26. **B. Assessment.** Mr. Johnson should be observed for a reccurrence of hypoglycemia.

27. **C. Assessment.** Dystonic reactions are characterized by prolonged involuntary muscle spasms, usually in the head, neck, and tongue.[13]

28. **C. Intervention.** Diphenhydramine is administered intravenously to reverse the effects of haloperidol.[10]

29. **A. Assessment.** Knowledge about growth and development can provide the emergency nurse with important information about whether this child may have been maltreated. In this case study, for example, the history of what supposedly happened to the child should alert the emergency nurse to the possibility of abuse: an 8-week-old who is not ambulatory could not have "fallen down stairs." Signs of abuse include wounds in various stages of healing, specific patterns of injury incompatible with the reported incident, and injuries incompatible with the developmental level of the child.[14]

30. **B. Intervention.** In all 50 states, health professionals are required to report suspected child maltreatment and neglect to the children's services boards, department of public welfare, or local authorities.[14]

31. **B. Analysis.** The information presented in this question describes a child who is not displaying appropriate growth and development skills. There appears to be the potential for problems with the child's caregivers.

32. **B. Assessment.** From the state of the patient's catheter, it appears that the patient has evidence of neglect. The emergency nurse should perform a secondary assessment focusing on the patient's state of hydration, nutrition, hygiene, mental status, and the presence of any old or new injuries.[3]

33. **A. Intervention.** The most significant emergency nursing intervention that can be provided for this patient is becoming the patient's advocate. The emergency nurse has the opportunity to identify patients who are at risk for abuse and neglect and initiate the appropriate patient referrals and ensure that the patient is safe.[3]

34. **B. Analysis.** The presence of the wound from the urinary catheter puts him at greatest risk for infection and sepsis.

35. **C. Evaluation.** When abuse or neglect is suspected, referral to appropriate authorities and patient care service agencies must be reflected in the nursing documentation.[3]

36. **D. Assessment.** Women who are battered generally suffer from low self-esteem. They may present to the emergency department complaining of sexual assault, attempted suicide, and substance abuse.[3,15]

37. **D. Intervention.** Answers A, B, and C are examples of attempts to manipulate the patient. The patient must be ready to make a change in her life. She also needs to know that there are options available.[15]

## REFERENCES

1. Curry JL: The care of psychiatric patients in the emergency department, *J Emerg Nurs* 19(5):396-407, 1993.
2. Williams D, Dwyer BJ, editors: Safe strategies for recognizing and managing violent patients, *Reports Emerg Nurs,* Preview Issue: 1-8, 1990.
3. Polli GE, Lazear SE: Mental health emergencies. In Jordan K, editor: *Emergency nursing core curriculum,* ed 5, Philadelphia, 2000, WB Saunders.
4. Newberry L: Mental health emergencies. In Newberry L, editor: *Sheehey's emergency nursing principles and practice,* ed 4, St Louis, 2000, Mosby.
5. Robie D, Edgemon-Hill E, Phelps B, et al: Suicide prevention protocol, *Am J Nurs* 99(12):53-57, 1999.
6. Weintraub B: A fatal case of acid ingestion, *J Emerg Nurs* 23(5):414-416, 1997.
7. Jacobs BB, Hoyt S, editors: *Trauma nursing core course,* Des Plaines, IL, 2000, Emergency Nurses Association.
8. McFarland GK, McFarland EA: *Nursing diagnosis and intervention: planning for patient care,* St Louis, 1989, Mosby.
9. Fraser S, Atkins J: Survivors' recollections of helpful and unhelpful emergency nurse activities surrounding sudden death of a loved one, *J Emerg Nurs* 16:13-16, 1990.
10. McKenry LM, Salerno E: *Pharmacology in nursing,* St Louis, 1998, Mosby.
11. George JE, Quattrone MS: Restraining patients: Can you be sued? Part II, *J Emerg Nurse* 19(1):408-411, 1993.
12. Allen LA: Treating agitation without drugs, *AJN* 99(4):36-41, 1999.
13. Cahill JJ: A twist of face. Acute dystonic reactions, *J Emerg Med Serv* 18(7):46-54, 1993.
14. Haley K, Eckles N, Baker P: *Emergency nursing core course,* Park Ridge, IL, 1999, Emergency Nurses Association.
15. Muelleman RL, Feighny KM: Effects of an emergency department-based advocacy program for battered women on community resource utilization, *Ann Emerg Med* 33(1):62-66, 1999.

# Chapter 11

# Neurological Emergencies

## REVIEW OUTLINE

I. Anatomy and physiology[1-3]
  A. Anatomy
    1. Scalp
    2. Skull
    3. Meninges
      a. Dura mater
      b. Arachnoid
      c. Pia mater
    4. Brain
      a. Cerebrum
      b. Diencephalon
      c. Cerebellum
      d. Brain stem
      e. Spinal cord
        (1) Vertebrae
        (2) Ligaments
        (3) Fibrocartilaginous
      f. Gray matter
      g. White matter
  B. Physiology
    1. Neurons
    2. Neurotransmitters
      a. Epinephrine
      b. Serotonin
      c. Prostaglandins
      d. Acetylcholine
    3. Central nervous system
      a. Frontal lobe
      b. Parietal lobe
      c. Occipital lobe
      d. Temporal lobe
    4. Limbic lobe
    5. Basal ganglia
    6. Pons
    7. Medulla oblongata
    8. Reticular activating system
    9. Consciousness
    10. Spinal cord
      a. Ascending pathways
      b. Descending pathways
    11. Peripheral nervous system
      a. Cranial nerves
      b. Spinal nerves
    12. Autonomic nervous system
      a. Sympathetic
      b. Parasympathetic
    13. Circle of Willis
    14. Cerebrospinal fluid
  C. Intracranial pressure (ICP)
    1. ICP = volume of brain tissue + volume of blood + volume of cerebrospinal fluid
    2. Cerebral perfusion pressure = mean arterial blood pressure − mean intracranial pressure
  D. Nutrients of the brain and spinal cord
    1. Glucose
    2. Oxygen
  E. Age-related changes
    1. Pediatric patient
      a. Assessment based on the age of the child and what is age appropriate
      b. Denver Developmental Screening Test
      c. Include parental evaluation of child's behavior
      d. Motor assessment of newborn
        (1) Normal newborns lie with their limbs semiflexed, legs abducted at the hip, symmetrical posture
        (2) Infant reflexes
    2. Geriatric patient
      a. Changes in hearing, vision, and motor and sensory function will alter neurological examination in the older adult patient
      b. Hearing
      c. Vision
        (1) Loss of accommodative power
        (2) Corneal arcus or arcus senilis common
        (3) Pupils decrease in size
        (4) Cataract formation

      d. Motor function

        (1) Muscular atrophy

        (2) Speed of movement decreased

        (3) Decrease in muscle strength

        (4) Development of a benign essential tremor

        (5) Reflexes may be diminished

      e. Sensory

        (1) Vibratory sensation decreases

        (2) Position sense may decrease

        (3) May be altered by chronic diseases such as diabetes

        (4) Sensory perception of the extremities

II. Neurological assessment

  A. Level of consciousness

    1. Glasgow Coma Scale

      a. Eye opening

      b. Verbal response

      c. Motor response

    2. AVPU: alert, responds to verbal stimuli, responds to painful stimuli, unresponsive

  B. Pupillary response

  C. Motor response

  D. Sensory response

  E. Cranial nerves

    1. Eye movements (II, III, IV, VI)

    2. Speech musculature (VII, IX, X, XII)

    3. Protective reflexes

      a. Gag reflex (IX and X)

      b. Corneal (V and VII)

    4. Senses

      a. Smell (I)

      b. Hearing (VIII)

      c. Touch (V)

    5. Facial movements (VII)

  F. Vital signs, including a temperature

  G. History

    1. Mechanism of injury

    2. Medical history

    3. Medications

  H. Neurological function tests

    1. Doll's eyes

    2. Caloric testing

    3. Apnea test

III. Collaborative care of the patient with a neurological emergency

  A. Airway: neurogenic influences, seizure activity, oxygen

  B. Breathing: hypoventilation, hyperventilation, cervical spine injury

  C. Circulation: normotension, hypotension, hypertension

  D. Neurological deficit: baseline neurological assessment

  E. Immobilization of the cervical spine

  F. History of illness or injury, medical history, current medications

  G. Indications of injury and/or illness

    1. Periorbital ecchymosis (raccoon's eyes)

    2. Battle's sign

    3. Leakage of CSF

    4. Palpable depressions

    5. Hyperthermia

    6. Petechia

    7. Purpura

    8. Rashes

  H. Control of ICP

    1. Recognition of the signs and symptoms of increasing ICP

      a. Altered level of consciousness

      b. Pupillary changes

      c. Motor function changes

      d. Sensory function changes

      e. Cushing's response

        (1) Widening pulse pressure

        (2) Bradycardia

        (3) Ataxic respiration

    2. Elevation of the bed, decreased stimulation

    3. Airway management for oxygenation

    4. Medications

      a. Mannitol

      b. Furosemide (Lasix)

      c. Phenobarbital

      d. Phenytoin (Dilantin)

      e. Sedation

      f. Neuromuscular blocking agents

      g. Experimental agents

  I. Laboratory tests

    1. Drug screen

    2. ETOH (blood alcohol level)

    3. Glucose

    4. Hemoglobin and hematocrit

      a. Electrolytes

      b. Complete blood count

      c. HIV status

    5. Lumbar puncture

  J. Radiography

    1. Cervical spine evaluation

    2. CT scan

    3. MRI

    4. Carotid doppler studies

  K. Cervical traction

  L. ICP monitoring

IV. Related nursing diagnoses[4]

  A. Airway clearance, ineffective

  B. Anxiety

  C. Breathing pattern, ineffective

  D. Fear

E. Gas exchange, impaired

F. Grieving, anticipatory

G. Home maintenance management, impaired

H. Hopelessness

I. Hyperthermia

J. Hypothermia

K. Infection, high risk for

L. Injury, high risk for

M. Knowledge deficit

N. Pain

O. Powerlessness

P. Spiritual distress (distress of the human spirit)

Q. Swallowing, impaired

R. Tissue perfusion, altered (cerebral or spinal cord)

V. Specific neurological emergencies

A. Headache

B. CVA

C. Seizures

D. Coma

E. Infections

F. Aneurysms

G. Bell's palsy

H. Skull fractures

1. Basilar

2. Linear

3. Open skull fracture

I. Concussion

J. Mild head injuries

1. Coma scale: 13 to 15

2. No focal neurological signs or symptoms

3. Negative findings on the CT scan

K. Moderate head injury

1. Coma scale: 9 to 12

2. Focal neurological findings

3. Positive findings on the CT/MRI scan

L. Severe head injuries

1. Coma scale: 8 or less

2. Neurological findings

3. Injury noted on the CT/MRI scan

M. Contusion

N. Bleeds

1. Subdural hematoma

2. Epidural hematoma

3. Intracerebral hematoma

4. Subarachnoid hemorrhage

O. Surface trauma

1. Scalp lacerations

2. Facial abrasions

P. Low back pain

Q. Spinal cord injuries

1. Anterior cord syndrome

2. Posterior cord syndrome

3. Central cord syndrome

4. Brown-Sequard syndrome

5. Complete transection of the cord

6. Spinal shock

The care of the patient who is suffering from a neurological emergency can be very challenging to the emergency nurse. There are multiple sources of neurological emergencies that may present to the emergency department, including head and spinal cord injuries, headaches, cerebral vascular accidents, infections, and seizures.

One of the most frequent neurological emergencies encountered by the emergency nurse is head trauma. Head injuries account for approximately 600,000 emergency department visits each year.[5] Head injuries are the most common type of neurological injury seen in both the pediatric and adult emergency patients. Sources of injuries include motor vehicle crashes, falls, assaults, sports injuries, and recreational activities.

A common patient complaint that presents to the emergency department is headache. Headaches may result from extracranial causes such as dehydration, hypoglycemia, glaucoma, allergic reactions, ear infections, and poisonings. Intracranial causes of headache include migraine, tension, trauma, and stroke. The evaluation of headache pain may be one of the most challenging assessments performed in the emergency department.[6]

The initial stabilization and management of the patient who has suffered a neurological emergency is based on several factors, including airway and ventilation management to ensure adequate oxygenation, continuous neurological assessment, immobilization of the cervical spine (when trauma is suspected), and management of increased intracranial pressure (ICP). It is important to review both the physiology and pathophysiology of ICP, as well as its management. There are several references listed at the end of this chapter that would be useful to use as review sources.

A baseline neurological assessment consists of five components: level of consciousness (Glasgow Coma Scale, Modified Glasgow Coma Scale, AVPU method [alert, response to verbal and painful stimuli, unresponsiveness]), pupillary response, motor response, sensory response, and vital signs. Other information that can provide additional clues to the patient's neurological status include the patient's medical history, history related to the present illness or injury, and current medications. Collaborative interventions that are employed to manage the patient who has a neurological emergency include management of the ABCs (all patients with suspected spinal cord injuries should be immobilized), laboratory and radiographic evaluations, medication administration, specific interventions such as burr hole trephination or cervical traction application, and a continuous neurological assessment.

## REVIEW QUESTIONS

*A 50-year-old man is brought to the emergency department by ground ambulance. He has multiple abrasions on his face. On arrival in the emergency department, the patient is having a generalized seizure and is cyanotic. An IV line has been established.*

1. What drug should be administered first to control this patient's seizures?
   - O  A.  Phenytoin sodium
   - O  B.  Lorazepam
   - O  C.  Phenobarbital sodium
   - O  D.  Lidocaine

2. This patient has a documented history of seizures and alcohol abuse. What other pieces of history should be obtained about this patient during the initial assessment?
   - O  A.  Any recent falls or blows to the head
   - O  B.  Compliance related to his seizure medications
   - O  C.  The amount of alcohol he has ingested
   - O  D.  The last time he was seen by a physician

3. The patient begins having another seizure. What is the primary nursing diagnosis on which the emergency nurse should base care?
   - O  A.  Swallowing, impaired related to his seizure activity
   - O  B.  Thought processes, altered related to his seizure activity
   - O  C.  Airway clearance, ineffective related to his seizure activity
   - O  D.  Injury, high risk for related to his seizure activity

4. The emergency physician has ordered that the patient be given 500 mg of phenytoin intravenously. The patient is placed on a cardiac monitor, and the infusion is started. What criterion should the emergency nurse use to evaluate the toxic effects of this drug?
   - O  A.  No noted seizure activity once the drug begins
   - O  B.  Bradycardic dysrhythmia on the cardiac monitor
   - O  C.  Nausea and vomiting after initiation of the infusion
   - O  D.  Sinus rhythm on the cardiac monitor

*An 18-month-old boy is brought to the emergency department by his parents, who say that the child has been "shaking" and clenching his teeth for about 15 minutes. They also state that he has not been feeling well for the past 2 days. He has had a fever they have been treating with acetaminophen (Children's Tylenol) and fluids.*

5. All of the following would suggest that the child is suffering from a febrile seizure except a:
   - O  A.  Family history of seizures
   - O  B.  Recent upper respiratory tract infection
   - O  C.  Fall from his crib striking his head
   - O  D.  Recent vaccination injection

6. Because of his generalized tonic/clonic seizure activity, an IV line cannot be established. What other route would ensure a rapid response to the anticonvulsant?
   - O  A.  Oral absorption
   - O  B.  Intramuscular
   - O  C.  Subcutaneous
   - O  D.  Intraosseous

7. During the child's seizure activity, the emergency nurse observes that the child's lips are cyanotic. What is the most appropriate nursing diagnosis on which the emergency nurse could base care?
   - O  A.  Injury, high risk for related to his seizure activity
   - O  B.  Thought processes, altered related to his seizure activity
   - O  C.  Gas exchange, impaired related to his seizure activity
   - O  D.  Growth and development, altered related to his seizure activity

8. Phenobarbital elixir has been prescribed for the child by the emergency physician. What should the parents be taught about the side effects of this drug?
   - O  A.  The drug will initially cause drowsiness
   - O  B.  The drug may cause mental retardation
   - O  C.  The drug may cause overgrowth of the child's gums
   - O  D.  The drug may discolor the child's teeth

9. After 23 hours of observation, the child is discharged from the emergency department. Which of the following should the emergency nurse instruct the mother to do if the child's fever returns?
   - O  A.  Dress and wrap the child in wool fabrics to keep him warm

0   B. Administer aspirin 15 mg/kg for an increase in temperature

0   C. Sponge the child with tepid water to decrease the child's temperature

0   D. Sponge the child with alcohol to decrease the child's temperature

*A 24-year-old woman comes to the emergency department complaining of severe pain in her head. She states no history of any medical problems.*

10. Common signs and symptoms associated with migraine headaches include:

0   A. Unilateral pupillary changes

0   B. Generalized tonic/clonic seizures

0   C. Photophobia, nausea, and vomiting

0   D. Ventricular fibrillation

11. For any patient with the complaint of headache, in addition to an evaluation of the ABCs (airway, breathing, circulation), the following assessment should be performed:

0   A. Level of consciousness

0   B. Palpation of peripheral pulses

0   C. Deep tendon reflexes

0   D. Abdominal assessment

12. A drug that has been found to be effective in the acute management of migraine headaches is:

0   A. Meperidine (Demerol) intravenously

0   B. Acetaminophen (Tylenol) rectally

0   C. Naproxen (Anaprox) orally

0   D. Dihydroergotamine (DHE) intravenously

13. Other emergency nursing interventions that will help relieve the pain of a headache include:

0   A. Application of a hot pack to the patient's forehead

0   B. Application of a cold cloth to the patient's forehead

0   C. Having the patient sit in the waiting room after medication administration

0   D. Leaving the lights on in the examining room

14. DHE is effective in aborting a migraine headache because:

0   A. It activates neurotransmitters that respond to norepinephrine

0   B. It activates serotonin receptors that abort headaches

0   C. It activates the beta endorphins that control pain

0   D. It activates corticosteroids that decrease inflammation in the brain

15. A potential side effect common to both DHE and sumatriptan is:

0   A. Hypertension

0   B. Feeling of warmth

0   C. Nausea and vomiting

0   D. Chest tightness

16. A relevant nursing diagnosis for the emergency nursing care of the patient with a headache would be:

0   A. Social isolation

0   B. Tissue integrity, impaired

0   C. Pain (acute)

0   D. Knowledge deficit

17. The emergency physician has ordered that the patient be given IV prochlorperazine for her nausea. Before discharge, the patient should be evaluated for:

0   A. Changes in pupillary function

0   B. Orthostatic hypotension

0   C. Presence of a rash

0   D. Diaphoresis

18. A food trigger of migraine headaches is:

0   A. Oranges

0   B. Chocolate

0   C. Tuna fish

0   D. Lettuce

19. Which of the following headaches would be classified as emergent?

0   A. Headache with a sudden onset

0   B. Headache that occurred after taking nitroglycerin

0   C. Headache associated with a chronic subdural hematoma

0   D. Tension headache related to work and stress

20. Cluster headaches are usually treated with:

0   A. Morphine sulfate 4 mg intravenously

0   B. Sumatriptan by subcutaneous injection

0   C. Breathing 100% oxygen by mask

0   D. Placing an ice pack on the patient's forehead

*A 74-year-old man has been brought to the emergency department by his family. They state that he has been walking "funny," they cannot understand what he says, the left side of his face is drooping, and he is not using his left arm. The onset of his symptoms were within the last 2 hours.*

21. The emergency nurse performs a cranial nerve assessment on the patient during the initial neurological evaluation. Which cranial nerves control the motor and sensory function of the patient's facial movement?
    - O  A. I and II (olfactory and optic)
    - O  B. IV and V (trochlear and trigeminal)
    - O  C. X and XI (vagus and spinal accessory)
    - O  D. V and VII (trigeminal and facial)

22. The NIH Stroke Scale is utilized to establish a baseline neurological assessment. When scoring the patient using this scale, the emergency nurse:
    - O  A. Should coach the patient to answer questions and perform the tasks correctly
    - O  B. Score the patient based on what he actually does, not what she thinks he can do
    - O  C. Perform the assessment in whatever order is convenient for her and the patient
    - O  D. Allow the patient's family to answer questions when the patient cannot

23. The patient's CT reveals an acute ischemic stroke. The patient is eligible for treatment with tissue plasminogen activator (t-PA). He weighs 75 kg. The initial bolus of t-PA for this patient would be:
    - O  A. 67.5 mg of t-PA intravenously
    - O  B. 12 mg of t-PA intravenously
    - O  C. 6 mg of t-PA intravenously
    - O  D. 6 mg of t-PA intramuscularly

24. The most serious complication of t-PA administration to treat an ischemic stroke is:
    - O  A. Hemoptysis
    - O  B. Intracranial hemorrhage
    - O  C. Hematuria
    - O  D. Coagulopathy

25. Bell's palsy can be differentiated from a stroke by the motor involvement of which cranial nerve?
    - O  A. V (trigeminal)
    - O  B. VII (facial)
    - O  C. III (oculomotor)
    - O  D. XI (spinal accessory)

26. A nursing diagnosis that the emergency nurse may use to plan patient care for the patient with Bell's palsy is:
    - O  A. Fear related to the patient believing he/she is having a stroke
    - O  B. Injury, high risk for related to the patient's inability to swallow
    - O  C. Tissue perfusion, altered, cerebral related to the Bell's palsy
    - O  D. Thought processes altered, related to the medications with which the patient will be treated

27. When discharging the patient who is being treated for Bell's palsy, the emergency nurse should instruct the patient to:
    - O  A. Keep returning to the emergency department until symptoms subside
    - O  B. Remember that symptoms will subside in 2 or 3 days with treatment
    - O  C. Use an artificial tear solution to prevent eye dryness and injury
    - O  D. Wear a patch over the affected eye to hide its appearance from the public

*A 3-year-old boy is brought to the emergency department by his parents. They state that he has been lethargic, febrile, and vomiting. He was recently treated for an inner ear infection. The patient's vital signs are B/P 70/40, HR 160, RR 40, and Temp (rectal), 103° F.*

28. During the initial evaluation of the child, the emergency nurse should also assess for:
    - O  A. Positive Kernig's or Brudzinski's signs
    - O  B. Occulocephalic reflex (Doll's eyes)
    - O  C. Presence of deep tendon reflexes
    - O  D. Positive Romberg test

29. Based on the patient's history and physical examination, the initial care of this patient should be:
    - O  A. Preparation for a lumbar puncture
    - O  B. Administration of antibiotics
    - O  C. Management of his hypotension
    - O  D. Obtaining a CT scan of the head

30. A set of arterial blood gas is obtained. The results are H, 7.15; $PO_2$, 60; $PCO_2$, 20; and $HCO_3$, 18. These blood gases indicate:
    - O  A. Respiratory alkalosis
    - O  B. Metabolic acidosis

0   C. Respiratory acidosis

0   D. Metabolic alkalosis

31. The child's presenting blood pressure and pulse indicate that the emergency nurse should base the initial care on which of the following nursing diagnosis?

0   A. Thermoregulation, ineffective related to his rectal temperature of 103° F and failure of acetaminophen to decrease his temperature

0   B. Fluid volume, deficit related to vasodilation and blood pooling caused by endotoxins

0   C. Fluid volume, excess related to reflex hypertension in response to the vasodilation and blood pooling

0   D. Tissue integrity, impaired related to systemic hypotension and the response of the body to the shock state

32. A urinary catheter is inserted. What criteria should the emergency nurse use to evaluate adequate urinary output during the fluid resuscitation?

0   A. Urine output >1 ml/kg/hr

0   B. Urine output <1 ml/kg/hr

0   C. Urine output <0.5 ml/kg/hr

0   D. Urine output >0.5 ml/kg/hr

33. For children younger than 5 years of age, what prevention intervention could the emergency department use to decrease the risk of meningitis?

0   A. Participate in a community immunization program to decrease the risk of *H. influenzae* type B infection

0   B. Instruct pregnant women to have a chlamydia culture performed before delivery to prevent contamination during delivery

0   C. Discuss with parents the need for Heptovax to be given to young children to prevent hepatitis B

0   D. Teach parents to wear a mask around their infant children if the parents have a "cold"

34. A clinical indication of meningitis that may be seen in infants, but not older children, is:

0   A. Headache and altered mental status

0   B. Vomiting and poor feeding

0   C. Hyperthermia and hypothermia

0   D. Bulging anterior fontanelle

35. Who should receive chemoprophylaxis for an exposure to *H. influenzae?*

0   A. Hospital personnel taking care of an infected child without significant exposure

0   B. An 18-year-old pregnant woman exposed to the infected child

0   C. A sibling of the infected child younger than 6 years of age

0   D. An adult taking care of the infected child who has not had a significant exposure

*An 18-year-old man is brought by helicopter to the emergency department after a motorcycle accident. At the scene of the accident, the patient was awake but combative. His initial Glasgow Coma Scale rating was 12. On his arrival in the emergency department, the patient's Glasgow Coma Scale rating is 7. He has abrasions on his face, and both eyes are ecchymotic and swollen shut.*

36. The presence of periorbital ecchymosis in a patient with an altered mental status may indicate:

0   A. Maxillary fracture

0   B. Basilar skull fracture

0   C. Mandible fracture

0   D. Nasal fracture

37. An additional indication of a skull fracture would be:

0   A. A hemotympanic membrane

0   B. A fracture of the first rib

0   C. An eyebrow laceration

0   D. Hyperhidrosis

38. Because of the possibility of a skull fracture, the emergency nurse should avoid:

0   A. Placing a cervical collar on the patient

0   B. Placing an oral airway in the patient

0   C. Inserting a nasogastric tube

0   D. Placing the patient on a cardiac monitor

39. The patient is orally intubated by the emergency physician. He is being oxygenated, but his neurological condition does not improve. His pupils are now 6 mm bilaterally and slow to react. His Glasgow Coma Scale rating has decreased to 5. The emergency physician orders

mannitol to be infused. The patient weighs 100 kg. How much mannitol will be initially infused?

0   A. 100 g

0   B. 50 g

0   C. 500 g

0   D. 25 g

40. Intracranial pressure is the result of:

0   A. The volume of brain tissue, plus the volume of blood, plus the volume of cerebrospinal fluid

0   B. The mean arterial blood pressure minus the mean intracranial pressure

0   C. $O_2$ plus a glucose level above 100

0   D. An increase in the mean arterial pressure

41. The patient begins having copious amounts of pink, frothy sputum coming from his endotracheal tube. The emergency nurse should base the care for this complication on which of the following nursing diagnoses?

0   A. Cardiac output, decreased

0   B. Gas exchange, impaired

0   C. Hypothermia

0   D. Fluid volume deficit

42. An 18-year-old man who fell from his bicycle is brought to the emergency department by the rescue squad. The squad reports that he lost consciousness after his fall, but was awake, alert, and oriented during transport. Upon arrival in the emergency department, the patient is unresponsive to verbal stimuli. His right pupil is 6 mm and unreactive and his left pupil is 2 mm and unreactive. With painful stimuli, the patient flexes his arms, and rigidity extends to his lower extremities. What type of posturing is he exhibiting?

0   A. Flaccid response to painful stimuli

0   B. Extension (decerebrate) response to painful stimuli

0   C. Flexion (decorticate) response to painful stimuli

0   D. Normal motor response to painful stimuli

43. The history of this patient's injury suggests what type of intracranial bleeding?

0   A. Subdural hematoma

0   B. Intracerebral hemorrhage

0   C. Subarachnoid hemorrhage

0   D. Epidural hematoma

*A 2-year-old boy has been brought to the emergency department by EMTs. He was involved in a motor vehicle crash with his parents, and at the time was restrained on his mother's lap by a shoulder harness. On arrival of EMTs, the child was in full cardiac arrest. CPR was initiated and a pulse obtained. His vital signs now include BP 70 by palpation and HR 60. He is being ventilated with a bag-valve mask.*

44. What size endotracheal tube will be needed to intubate this child?

0   A. 6.0 cuffed tube

0   B. 2.5 uncuffed tube

0   C. 7.0 uncuffed tube

0   D. 4.5 uncuffed tube

45. The child's vital signs suggest that the child may be suffering from:

0   A. Anaphylactic shock

0   B. Cardiogenic shock

0   C. Spinal shock

0   D. Septic shock

46. The collaborative emergency management of the patient in spinal shock would include:

0   A. Administration of Ringer's lactate solution until the child's blood pressure is 80/40

0   B. Administration of packed red blood cells until the child's blood pressure is 80/40

0   C. Administration of ceftriaxone intravenously to prevent meningitis

0   D. Administration of a vasopressor intravenously until vasomotor control is restored

47. The initial emergency nursing care of this patient should be based on which of the following nursing diagnoses?

0   A. Injury, high risk for

0   B. Tissue perfusion, altered (spinal cord)

0   C. Growth and development, altered

0   D. Unilateral neglect

48. Young children are at risk of sustaining a cervical spine injury because:

0   A. Their heads are smaller in proportion to the rest of their body surface area

0   B. Their neck muscles are still undeveloped and initially are stiff

0   C. Their injuries do not show up on regular x-ray films

0 D. Their heads are the largest part of their bodies

49. An 8-year-old girl who has been diagnosed as having a concussion is going to be discharged from the emergency department. After having been given discharge instructions, her parents should be able to evaluate their daughter for what changes?
0 A. Changes in blood pressure
0 B. Changes in level of consciousness
0 C. Changes in hemoglobin and hematocrit
0 D. Changes in urinary output

*A 27-year-old construction worker fell 3 feet from a ladder, landing on his buttocks, prior to his arrival in the emergency department. He walks into the emergency department, but complains of pain in his lower back that is radiating down his legs. The only obvious signs of trauma are abrasions and bruising on his buttocks.*

50. The initial assessment of this patient should include a history of:
0 A. Loss of consciousness
0 B. Tetanus immunization
0 C. Pulmonary disease
0 D. Diabetes

51. An important intervention for the patient who has fallen and sustained a back injury is:
0 A. Obtaining a blood alcohol level
0 B. Obtaining an urinalysis
0 C. Obtaining a hepatic profile
0 D. Obtaining a drug screen

52. No acute injury was found in this patient. Based on his initial complaint, which of the following nursing diagnoses should the emergency nurse use for basing care?
0 A. Fluid volume deficit
0 B. Pain (acute)
0 C. Cardiac output, decreased
0 D. Infection, potential for

53. The patient is given discharge instructions for a low back injury. It is important that the emergency nurse question the patient about his understanding concerning which of the following possible signs of serious complications related to low back injury?
0 A. Presence of some pain for 7 to 10 days
0 B. Presence of soreness and stiffness in the lower back

0 C. Presence of progressive weakness and bladder dysfunction
0 D. Decrease in pain and stiffness

*A 62-year-old man is brought to the emergency department by his caretaker from the state mental facility. His caretakers noted that he suddenly became febrile. Despite treatment with acetaminophen, his fever has remained at 103° F. His only medication is haloperidol. He is diagnosed with neuroleptic malignant syndrome.*

54. Other signs and symptoms of neuroleptic malignant syndrome include all of the following except:
0 A. Tachycardia
0 B. Gradual change in mental status
0 C. Muscular rigidity
0 D. Hypertension

55. Which of the following medications is used to treat the symptoms of neuroleptic malignant syndrome?
0 A. Potassium chloride
0 B. Streptokinase
0 C. Neuromuscular blocking agents
0 D. Tricyclics

*A 16-year-old, unrestrained female driver is brought to the emergency department after having been involved in a high-speed crash. Her initial GCS at the scene of the crash was 12. She is now only responding to deep pain (GCS of 7). The emergency physician decides to intubate her to protect her airway and manage her intracranial pressure using rapid sequence intubation (RSI).*

56. Indications for the use of neuromuscular blocking agents include:
0 A. To decrease the success rate of intubation
0 B. To increase the patient's intracranial pressure
0 C. To control an alert and cooperative patient
0 D. To manage the hypoxia associated with severe head injury

57. Preparation for administration of RSI for this patient would include:
0 A. Lidocaine 100 mg and etomidate 20 mg
0 B. Atropine .02 mg/kg and etomidate 20 mg
0 C. Midazolam 10 mg and lidocaine 100 mg

**0** D. Atropine .02 mg/kg and lidocaine 100 mg

58. A 44-year-old female presents to the emergency department with the "worst headache of her life." A CT reveals a subarachnoid hemorrhage. The treatment of choice in the emergency management of this patient is:

**0** A. Initiation of a heparin drip at 1000 units per hour

**0** B. Administration of t-PA based on a weight-calculated dose

**0** C. Preparation for insertion of a ventricular catheter for ICP monitoring

**0** D. Administration of nimodipine 60 mg orally every 4 hours

59. A method that may be used to manage a patient's intracranial pressure in the emergency department after intubation is:

**0** A. Hyperventilation to maintain the patient's $PaCO_2 < 30$ mm Hg

**0** B. Administration of neuromuscular blocking agents and sedation

**0** C. Administration of high-dose steroids intravenously

**0** D. Administration of prophylactic anticonvulsant therapy

60. The advantage of administering fosphenytoin over phenytoin is:

**0** A. Phenytoin may be administered more rapidly than fosphenytoin

**0** B. Phenytoin is more costly than fosphenytoin to administer

**0** C. Fosphenytoin is less irritating to veins during administration

**0** D. Phenytoin achieves a peak level more quickly than fosphenytoin

## ANSWERS

1. **B. Intervention.** Lorazepam (a benzodiazepine) crosses the blood-brain barrier more quickly than phenytoin or phenobarbital sodium. The appropriate dose of lorazepam (Ativan) for anticonvulsant therapy is 1 to 2 mg IV, which may be repeated at 10- to 15-minute intervals as needed for a total of not more than 4 mg. Signs and symptoms of respiratory depression must be carefully assessed.[7]

2. **A. Assessment.** It is easy to assume that this patient's seizures are being caused by alcohol intoxication, alcohol withdrawal, or not taking his medi-

cation properly. However, it is important to rule out a history of recent trauma, because the alcoholic patient is prone to the development of intracerebral bleeding more frequently following an injury.[8,9]

3. **C. Analysis.** Because the patient is having a seizure, he is unable to maintain his airway. Even though the patient is at risk for injury, the emergency nurse's initial care should be directed at stabilizing the patient's airway. Related factors contributing to this nursing diagnosis include an increase in secretions and cognitive impairment.[4]

4. **B. Evaluation.** The toxic side effects of phenytoin are cardiac dysrhythmia, including bradycardia and heart block.[6,7]

5. **C. Assessment.** A fall indicates that the seizure could be from trauma and not a medical cause.[9]

6. **D. Intervention.** Studies have demonstrated that the intraosseous route is comparable to giving the drug through an IV line. The other routes could be used, but the patient's response would be much slower.[10,11] An additional route (rectal) for diazepam has been evaluated in Europe and Canada, but rectal diazepam has not yet been approved by the Food and Drug Administration in the United States.[12]

7. **C. Analysis.** One of the related factors contributing to this nursing diagnosis is an altered oxygen supply. During the seizure activity, gas exchange may be impaired by airway obstruction and central nervous system depression.[4]

8. **A. Evaluation.** The most common side effects of this drug are drowsiness, lethargy, and depression. It is important to point this out to the child's parents. These effects will generally decrease after continued therapy.[6,7]

9. **C. Intervention.** Tepid water should be used to decrease the child's fever. Aspirin is not recommended to manage fevers in young children because of the risk of Reye's syndrome. Using alcohol to sponge the child may cause toxicity from the alcohol being absorbed into the child's skin, as well as shivering, which will only increase the child's temperature.[13,14]

10. **C. Assessment.** Signs and symptoms associated with migraine headaches are many and varied. Visual disturbances, including homonymous hemianopsia, transient blindness, and photophobia are seen. Other signs and symptoms include nausea and vomiting, vertigo, chills, cold hands and feet, abdominal distention, and cardiac dysrhythmia. However, unilateral pupillary changes and seizures would more likely suggest an expanding lesion.[15]

11. **A. Assessment.** Performing a baseline neurological assessment is imperative in the initial evaluation of a patient who is complaining of a severe headache. It is important to evaluate the patient for focal neurological symptoms that could indicate an expanding lesion requiring immediate neurosurgical evaluation and intervention.[15]

12. **D. Intervention.** Dihydroergotamine, which is a semisynthetic derivative of ergot alkaloid, has been found to be effective in the acute management of migraine headaches. Because it is more rapid acting than ergotamine, it can offer the patient quicker pain relief. Meperidine and other opiates are not as effective as dihydroergotamine in treating patients suffering pain from severe migraine headaches, because these patients generally have a depletion of serotonin, which is required for opiates to be effective.[7]

13. **B. Intervention.** Application of a cold cloth, along with the prescribed medical regimen, has been found to be helpful in the care of the patient with a headache. In addition, placing the patient in a quiet, dimly lit environment can also help decrease headache pain.[15]

14. **B. Intervention.** DHE (dihydroergotamine) works by activating serotonin-1 receptors. The result of this is the abortion of the migraine.[15]

15. **D. Assessment.** A potential side effect common to both DHE and sumatriptan is chest tightness. Hypertension, nausea, and vomiting are more common to the use of DHE. Sumatriptan may cause tingling and feelings of warmth. Both may cause chest tightness.[15]

16. **C. Analysis.** The emergency nursing care for the patient with a headache would include helping the patient with the management of his or her acute pain. Defining characteristics of pain include a verbal report of intense pain experience, narrowed focus, restlessness, unusual posture, diaphoresis, and increased muscle tension.[4]

17. **B. Evaluation.** IV prochlorperazine can cause postural hypotension because of its adrenergic blocking activity. The patient should be kept supine while in the emergency department and evaluated for postural hypotension before leaving.[6,7]

18. **B. Assessment.** Food triggers of migraine headaches include chocolate, bananas, avocados, nuts, onions, and caffeine.[16]

19. **A. Assessment.** A headache that has a sudden onset should be considered an emergent problem. Other emergent headaches include headache with an elevated temperature and a headache associated with hypoxia, hypercapnia, carbon monoxide poisoning, and trauma.[17]

20. **C. Intervention.** Cluster headaches are usually treated with administration of 100% oxygen by mask.[15]

21. **D. Assessment.** The motor function of the fifth cranial nerve (trigeminal) allows the patient to open and close his jaw. The sensory function of the fifth cranial nerve allows the patient to identify sharp and dull sensations on the forehead and cheek. The motor function of the seventh cranial nerve (facial) allows movement of the face, scalp, and eyelids. The sensory function of the seventh cranial nerve allows the patient taste for the anterior two thirds of the tongue.[18]

22. **B. Intervention.** The NIH Stroke Scale was developed to provide an organized and fairly comprehensive assessment tool for the patient who has suffered a stroke. It also helps to trend changes or improvements when specific therapies are initiated to manage an acute stroke. The NIH Stroke Scale should be administered in the order listed, and the patient should not be coached. The emergency nurse needs to score the patient based on what the patient does, not what she believes he can do.

23. **C. Intervention.** The initial bolus of t-PA is based upon 0.9 mg/kg up to a maximum of 90 mg. The initial bolus of this is 10% of the maximum dose. In this case the total patient dose is 67.5 mg. The initial bolus is 6 mg intravenously. The remaining 61.5 mg should be infused over 60 minutes.[19,20]

24. **B. Evaluation.** The most serious complication of t-PA administration to treat acute ischemic stroke is intracranial hemorrhage. The patient must be carefully evaluated for risks of bleeding before the drug is administered and then carefully monitored during and after its administration.[19,20]

25. **B. Assessment.** Bell's palsy affects the motor function of the seventh cranial nerve. This results in the patient's inability to wrinkle his or her forehead. Because of crossover of motor innervation of the seventh cranial nerve, the patient who has had a stroke with facial symptoms will still be able to wrinkle the forehead.[6]

26. **A. Analysis.** Because the symptoms of Bell's palsy are similar to the facial symptoms of a stroke, patients fear that they may be having a stroke. In addition, it generally takes 3 months for the symptoms to disappear. Defining characteristics of fear include apprehension, decreased self-assurance, and sympathetic stimulation.[4]

27. **C. Intervention.** Because Bell's palsy affects the eyelid, it may not close, and blinking will be de-

creased. The emergency nurse needs to instruct the patient how to keep the eye from drying out. Symptoms related to Bell's palsy generally take 3 weeks to 3 months to resolve.[6]

28. **A. Assessment.** Because of the history given by the child's parents, and based on the initial vital signs of the child, the emergency nurse should highly suspect that the child may be suffering from meningitis. Kernig's and Brudzinski's signs indicate meningeal irritation. The test for Kernig's sign is performed while the patient is lying flat. The patient's leg is flexed and then extended. If pain is elicited by this maneuver, meningeal irritation is indicated. Brudzinski's sign is elicited by flexing the patient's neck forward. Again, pain with this movement indicates meningeal irritation.[21]

29. **C. Intervention.** From the initial vital signs obtained, it is obvious that the child is in shock. It is probable that it is septic shock. The initial care of the child should thus be directed at correcting his shock state. Administration of antibiotics and a lumbar puncture may be indicated later, but the initial emergency nursing interventions need to be based on stabilizing the patient's airway, breathing, and circulation.[21]

30. **B. Assessment.** The child's pH of 7.15 and $HCO_3$ of 18 indicate metabolic acidosis. In addition, the $PCO_2$ of 20 indicates that the child is hyperventilating in an attempt to compensate for this metabolic state.

31. **B. Analysis.** Defining characteristics of fluid volume deficit include hypotension, increased pulse rate, narrowed pulse pressure, and decreased urinary output.[4]

32. **A. Evaluation.** Adequate fluid resuscitation for a 3-year-old would be indicated with a urinary output of greater than 1 ml/kg.[21]

33. **A. Intervention.** Since the development and implementation of the Hib vaccine, the incidence of Hib disease has decreased. One of the most common causes of meningitis in children under 5 years of age is *H. influenzae* type B.[21]

34. **D. Assessment.** Because the infant's anterior fontanelle remains open until 9 to 18 months, when an infant has meningitis and an indication of an increase in ICP that may accompany the infection, the result is a bulging anterior fontanelle.[3,21]

35. **C. Intervention.** Children less than 6 years of age are the most susceptible to *H. influenzae* and should be treated. Rifampin is the drug that is given. Rifampin should never be given to a pregnant woman. Adults are generally not susceptible to *H. influenzae* unless they incur a significant exposure.[21]

36. **B. Assessment.** Basilar skull fractures occur at the base of the skull. They are not usually seen on x-ray examination but are diagnosed clinically. The signs of a basilar skull fracture are periorbital ecchymosis (raccoon's eyes), rhinorrhea, and otorrhea.[22]

37. **A. Assessment.** Additional indications of a skull fracture include a unilateral or bilateral hemotympanic membrane, mastoid ecchymosis (Battle's sign), and conjunctival hemorrhage without evidence of direct trauma to the eye(s).[22]

38. **C. Intervention.** When a basilar skull fracture occurs, the cribriform plate of the ethmoid bone may be fractured. This could potentially allow passage of such things as nasogastric tubes directly into the brain.[22]

39. **A. Intervention.** Mannitol is given to the adult patient in dosages of 1 to 2 g/kg body weight. Mannitol is generally infused over a period of 30 to 90 minutes.[7]

40. **A. Assessment.** Intracranial pressure is the result of the volume of brain tissue, plus the volume of blood, plus the volume of cerebrospinal fluid.[1,2]

41. **B. Analysis.** The appearance of pink, frothy sputum may indicate neurogenic pulmonary edema. These excessive secretions could potentially interfere with the patient's ability to be oxygenated. A related factor contributing to this nursing diagnosis is alveolar capillary membrane changes.[4]

42. **C. Assessment.** Flexion response or decorticate posturing in response to painful stimuli is exhibited by arm flexion and adduction. The patient's lower extremities are rigid and extended.[23,24]

43. **D. Analysis.** In 40% of the patients who develop epidural hematomas, a classic history may be collected. This includes a loss of consciousness, followed by a lucid period, and then further neurological changes including altered mental status, lethargy, and unresponsiveness.[20]

44. **D. Intervention.** The formula that can be used to determine the appropriate tube size needed is 16 plus the age in years divided by 4. This would give an approximate size of 4.5. Other measures that can be used to estimate tube size include looking at the size of the child's little finger or nasal opening. It is important to note that an uncuffed tube should be used for a 2-year-old child.[10,28]

45. **C. Assessment.** Hypotension and bradycardia in a patient after a traumatic injury indicate that the patient may be in spinal shock. In addition, a child will normally be tachycardic. In this case, the child's pulse is 60 instead of 100. Spinal shock results when there is an injury or edema that blocks the sympathetic outflow tract, causing disruption of

the vasomotor center, which causes loss of sympathetic tone.[22]

46. **D. Intervention.** Because the patient has suffered an injury that compromises his ability to control vasomotor tone, vasopressors are needed. Some of the drugs that are used include dopamine, norepinephrine, isoproterenol, and dobutamine.[22] Recent research has demonstrated that high-dose methylprednisone is an important adjunct in the treatment of spinal cord injury. This is used in both adult and pediatric patients. The initial dosage of the drug is 30 mg/kg body weight diluted in normal saline and infused over a period of 15 minutes.[26]

47. **B. Analysis.** The initial care of this child should be based on providing both nursing and medical interventions to treat the complications of spinal shock and to prevent further injury. Defining characteristics of this nursing diagnosis include hypotension, decreased capillary filling, and alteration in mental status.[4]

48. **D. Assessment.** The largest part of the young child's body is the head. Their neck muscles are weaker. Because of these anatomical changes, young children are more likely to suffer higher cervical spine injuries.[24]

49. **B. Evaluation.** Since the child has suffered a concussion, the child's parents need to know the signs and symptoms of possible neurological compromise following injury. The initial sign or symptom of neurological compromise is a change in mental status. It is important that the emergency nurse instruct the family on what to look for and to be sure that the family understands the importance of this assessment.[24]

50. **A. Assessment.** For any patient who has fallen and sustained possible neurological or spinal injury, a history of whether there was a loss of consciousness should be obtained. This would alert the emergency nurse to the possibility of any additional injury or injuries.[26]

51. **B. Intervention.** When a patient has sustained a fall resulting in back pain, the possibility of renal injury needs to be evaluated. This is done by obtaining a urine specimen and submitting it for urinalysis or using a dipstick to determine the presence of blood.[26]

52. **B. Analysis.** Because of the muscle spasms and tenderness that have resulted from the fall, the patient's care will need to be directed at relieving the acute pain he is suffering. Pain management may include prescribed medications, the use of hot or cold compresses, and bed rest.[26]

53. **C. Evaluation.** A serious complication of low back injury would be a disk herniation. Signs and symptoms of this complication include progressive weakness and bladder dysfunction.[26]

54. **B. Assessment.** Symptoms of neuroleptic malignant syndrome include a sudden change in mental status, fever, muscular rigidity, and autonomic dysfunction.[27]

55. **C. Intervention.** Neuromuscular blocking agents have been used to manage the muscular rigidity that can lead to rhabdomyolisis.[29]

56. **D. Assessment.** Indications for the use of neuromuscular blocking include:
   - Management of the hypoxia from head injury
   - Status epilepticus management
   - Drug overdose requiring gastric lavage for airway protection
   - Status asthmaticus
   - Enhance success rate of intubation
   - Decrease struggle against the ventilator
   - Manage a combative patient for safe transport
   - Facilitate diagnostic procedures [28-32]

57. **A. Intervention.** Premedication for the patient with a head injury includes lidocaine 1.0-1.5 mg/kg and a medication that produces sedation and amnesia, such as etomidate. Atropine is indicated for premedication for pediatric patients. [28-32]

58. **D. Intervention.** Fibrinolytic therapy is contraindicated in the management of hemorrhagic stroke. Nimodopine (a calcium channel blocker) 60 mg orally has been found to improve outcomes after a subarachnoid hemorrhage.[19]

59. **B. Intervention.** The management of intracranial pressure includes ensuring that the patient is oxygenated and not agitated. Guidelines that were published in 1995 entitled *Management of Severe Head Injury,* sponsored by the Brain Trauma Foundation and endorsed by the American Association of Neurologic Surgeons, recommend that hyperventilation, high-dose steroids, and anticonvulsant therapy not routinely be used to manage ICP.[32]

60. **C. Evaluation.** Fosphenytoin may be administered more quickly, achieves peak level sooner, and is less irritating to veins during administration.[7]

## REFERENCES

1. Bickley LS: *Bates' guide to physical examination and history taking,* Philadelphia, 1999, Lippincott.
2. Neff J, Kidd P: *Trauma nursing: The art and science,* St Louis, 1993, Mosby.
3. Engel J: *Pocket guide to pediatric assessment,* St Louis, 1993, Mosby.

4. Kim M, McFarland G, McLane A: *Pocket guide to nursing diagnoses,* St Louis, 1993, Mosby.

5. Dietrich A, et al: Pediatric head injuries: Can clinical factors predict an abnormality on computed tomography? *Ann Emerg Med* 22(10):1535-1540, 1993.

6. Begley D, Newberry L: Neurologic emergencies. In Newberry L, editor: *Sheehy's emergency nursing principles and practice,* ed 4, St Louis, 1998, Mosby.

7. McKenry L, Salerno E: *Pharmacology in nursing,* St Louis, 1998, Mosby.

8. Adams S, Camarista L, Chadwick L: Neurologic emergencies. In Kitt S et al, editors: *Emergency nursing: a physiologic and clinical perspective,* Philadelphia, 1995, WB Saunders.

9. Mitchell P: Central nervous system I: Closed head injuries. In Cardona V et al, editors: *Trauma nursing,* Philadelphia, 1994, WB Saunders.

10. Kelley J: Seizure emergencies and disorders. In Kelley S, editor: *Pediatric emergency nursing,* Norwalk, CT, 1994, Appleton & Lange.

11. Chameides L, Hazinski M: *Pediatric advanced life support,* Dallas, TX, 1997-1999, American Heart Association.

12. Manley L, Haley K, Dick M: Intraosseous infusion: Rapid vascular access for critically ill or injured infants and children, *J Emerg Nurs* 14:63-69, 1988.

13. Rectal diazepam for acute seizures, *Emerg Med,* 35-38, 1990.

14. Soud T: The febrile child in the emergency department, *J Emerg Nurs* 19:355-358, 1993.

15. Foley J: Pharmacologic treatment of acute migraine and related headaches in the emergency department, *J Emerg Nurs* 19:225-229, 1993.

16. Minirth F: *The headache book,* Nashville, TN, 1994, Thomas Nelson.

17. Glaxo: *Which headache? A guide to diagnosis and management of headache,* Liverpool, England, 1990, Professional Postgraduate Services.

18. Snyder J: Neurological emergencies. In Jordan K, editor: *Emergency nursing core curriculum,* ed 5, Philadelphia, 2000, WB Saunders.

19. Kothari R, editor: *Acute stroke.* Dallas, TX, 1998-2000, American Heart Association.

20. Blank SJ, Keyes M: Thrombolytic therapy for patients with acute stroke in the ED setting, *J Emerg Nurs* 26(1); 24-30, 2000.

21. Reynolds E, Kelley S: Infectious disease emergencies. In Kelley J, editor: *Pediatric emergencies,* Norwalk, CT, 1994, Appleton & Lange.

22. Oman K, Drury T: Head trauma. In Kitt S et al, editors: *Emergency nursing,* Philadelphia, 1995, WB Saunders.

23. Proehl J: The Glasgow Coma Scale: Do it and do it right, *J Emerg Nurs* 18:421-423, 1992.

24. Semonin Holleran R: Head, neck, and spinal cord trauma. In Kelley J, editor: *Pediatric emergencies,* Norwalk, CT, 1994, Appleton & Lange.

25. Nayduch D, Lee A, Butler D: High-dose methylprednisone after acute spinal cord injury, *Crit Care Nurs* 8:69-78, 1994.

26. Jaworski M, Wirtz K: Spinal trauma. In Kitt S et al, editors: *Emergency nursing: a physiologic and clinical perspective,* Philadelphia, 1995, WB Saunders.

27. Foley J: Recognition and treatment of neuroleptic malignant syndrome, *J Emerg Nurs* 19:139-141, 1993.

28. Walls R: *Course manual national emergency airway management course,* Wessley, MA, 1998, Airway Management Education Center.

29. Munford B: Practical pharmacology of neuromuscular blockade, *J Air Med Trans* 17(4):149-156, 1998.

30. Silverman DG: *Neuromuscular block in preoperative and intensive care,* Philadelphia, 1994, WB Saunders.

31. Vender JS: Sedation, analgesia, and neuromuscular blockade in critical care: an overview, *New Horizons:* 2-7, 1994.

32. Bullock R, Chestnut RM, Clifton G et al: Guidelines for the management of severe head injury, *J Neurotrauma* 13:639-734, 1996.

# Chapter 12

# Obstetrical and Gynecological Emergencies

**REVIEW OUTLINE**

I. Female anatomy
   A. External
      1. Mons pubis
      2. Labia majora
      3. Labia minora
      4. Clitoris
      5. Posterior fourchette
      6. Fossa navicularis
      7. Hymen
      8. Perineum
      9. Urethral meatus
   B. Vagina
      1. Cervix
      2. Uterus
      3. Ovaries
      4. Fallopian tubes
      5. Bladder
      6. Ovarian arteries

II. Physiology
   A. Menstrual cycle
   B. Sexual act
   C. Stages of labor

III. Collaborative care of the patient with an obstetrical emergency
   A. Assessment of the pregnant patient
      1. Physiological changes from pregnancy
      2. Cardiovascular
         a. Heart rate
         b. Cardiac output
         c. Blood pressure and pulse changes
         d. Maternal circulation
         e. ECG changes
         f. Anemia of pregnancy
      3. Pulmonary
         a. Diaphragm elevation
         b. Respiratory alkalosis
         c. Oxygen consumption
      4. Anatomical changes
         a. Pelvic changes
         b. Pressure on inferior vena cava from gravid uterus
      5. ABCs (airway, breathing, circulation)
      6. History related to chief complaint
      7. Last menstrual period
      8. Estimated date of confinement
      9. Vaginal discharge and/or bleeding
      10. Para, gravida, abortions
      11. Abdominal tenderness
      12. Height of the fundus
      13. Ultrasound
      14. Beta human chorionic gonadotropin (BHCG), complete blood cell count (CBC), type and screen or crossmatch
   B. Assessment of the nongravid female patient
      1. Last menstrual period
      2. Gynecological symptoms
         a. Vaginal discharge (color, amount)
         b. Vaginal bleeding (color, amount, clots or tissue)
         c. Vaginal itching
         d. Vaginal burning
         e. Presence of sores, lumps
         f. Dyspareunia
      3. Medications
         a. Oral contraceptives
         b. Intrauterine device
         c. Norplant
         d. Depoprovera
         e. Diaphragm
         f. Spermicides, condoms
         g. Hormones (estrogen use)
         h. Exposure to DES (diethylstilbestrol)
      4. Medical problems
         a. Diabetes
         b. Renal disease

c. Thyroid disorders

d. Sexually transmitted diseases

C. Associated signs and symptoms

1. Nausea and vomiting

2. Fever, chills

3. Signs and symptoms of sepsis

D. Assessment of external genitalia

1. Inflammation

2. Ulceration

3. Discharge

4. Swelling, nodules, lesions

5. Color of patient's urine

E. Diagnostic studies

1. Laboratory

a. BHCG

b. CBC with differential

c. Electrolytes

d. BUN and creatinine

e. Type and crossmatch

f. Rh factor

g. Rapid plasma reagin (RPR)

h. Sexually transmitted disease (STD) cultures as indicated by the patient's history and signs and symptoms

i. Urinalysis

j. Urine culture

k. Gram stain

l. Wet mounts

(i) Saline

(ii) KOH

2. Ultrasound

a. Abdominal

b. Transvaginal

F. Interventions

1. ABCs

2. Administration of blood and blood products

3. Medications as indicated by the patient's problem

4. Emergency delivery

5. Perimortem cesarean section

6. APGAR scoring

7. Neonatal resuscitation based on PALS (pediatric advanced life support)

8. Measurement of fetal heart tones

9. Dilation and curettage

10. Culdocentesis

11. Ultrasound (abdominal, transvaginal)

12. Emergent surgery

13. Grief counseling

IV. Related nursing diagnoses

A. Anxiety

B. Family processes, altered

C. Fluid volume deficit, high risk for

D. Grieving, anticipatory

E. Infection, high risk for

F. Injury, high risk for

G. Pain

H. Spiritual distress (distress of the human spirit)

I. Trauma, high risk for

V. Obstetrical emergencies

A. Ectopic pregnancy

B. Abortion

1. Threatened abortion

2. Incomplete abortion

C. Hydatidiform mole

D. Hyperemesis gravidarum

E. HIV in the pregnant patient

F. Preterm labor

G. Abruptio placentae

H. Placenta previa

I. Pregnancy-induced hypertension

1. Preeclampsia

2. Eclampsia

3. Chronic hypertension

J. Emergency delivery

K. Neonatal resuscitation

L. Maternal trauma

M. Perimortem delivery

VI. Gynecological emergencies

A. Vaginal bleeding

B. Dysfunctional uterine bleeding

C. Genital trauma

D. Pelvic pain

E. Pelvic inflammatory disease

F. Sexually transmitted diseases

G. Sexual assault

Many women seek care for obstetrical and gynecological problems in the emergency department. These emergencies range from treatment for sexually transmitted diseases to life-threatening difficulties such as a ruptured ectopic pregnancy or abruptio placentae.

As women continue to work and lead the same life before and after childbirth, the likelihood that they may become a patient in the emergency department increases. Trauma is the most common cause of death for women of childbearing age.[1] Pregnant women are at risk for both illness and injury that will affect not only the mother but also the infant.

When caring for the patient who has an obstetrical emergency, there are several important points that the emergency nurse needs to consider. Pregnancy has both a physiological and psychological impact on a woman that will influence her response to both trauma and other disease states. The pregnant patient will experience changes in her cardiovascular, pulmonary, and nervous systems. Pregnancy may alter the pattern or the severity of trauma or disease states; pregnancy may alter laboratory results; and pregnancy can have its own complications, such as abruptio placentae, amniotic fluid embolism, or eclampsia.[2,3]

An emergency delivery will tend to increase the level of excitement in the emergency department. The emergency nurse should be familiar with the care of the delivering mother, as well as with the initial resuscitation and stabilization of the infant. The Pediatric Advanced Life Support course available from the American Heart Association and the Emergency Nursing Pediatric Course developed by the Emergency Nurses Association provides in-depth information related to the resuscitation of the neonate.

Finally, the care of the patient who is suffering from an obstetrical emergency can be very stressful for the patient, her family, and the emergency department staff. Unfortunately, many women suffer a miscarriage while in the emergency department, or they may lose their child as a result of a traumatic injury. Helping the family to deal with the sudden loss of their child can be very difficult. The emergency nurse needs to be aware of support sources for patient, family, and staff.

When obtaining a history related to a gynecological emergency, specific information that should be asked includes the date of the patient's last menstrual period and if there were any abnormalities. Information to consider when evaluating a patient's menstrual period involves the age of the patient when her period began, the intervals between her periods, the duration of her period, and the intensity of her flow. The type of contraception the patient uses should also be examined.[3]

If the patient is experiencing vaginal discharge, the color and amount of the discharge should be described and examined. Related symptoms such as fever, chills, nausea, and vomiting may indicate pelvic inflammatory disease. Vaginal discharge may also be a sign of a systemic disease such as diabetes mellitus.

The incidence of sexually transmitted diseases has been on the rise over the past 10 years and the complications of these diseases are seen more frequently in women. A serious complication from sexually transmitted diseases is pelvic inflammatory disease, which can cause not only sepsis but also infertility.

The care of specific obstetrical or gynecological emergency is based on the particular emergency the patient is experiencing. For the patient with an obstetrical emergency, the care of these patients needs to be appropriate and organized so that both the mother and the child may benefit. Gynecological emergencies must be recognized early and treated, and appropriate follow-up offered.

## REVIEW QUESTIONS
### Vaginal Bleeding

*A 23-year-old woman who is 30 weeks pregnant comes to the emergency department complaining of vaginal bleeding that started 1 hour earlier. She is a gravida of 1 and para of 0. She states that she is not having any pain or contractions with this bleeding.*

1. In the third trimester of pregnancy, the most likely cause of this woman's vaginal bleeding is:
   - O  A. Abruptio placentae
   - O  B. Placenta previa
   - O  C. Ruptured uterus
   - O  D. Incompetent cervix

2. The initial management of this patient may include all of the following *except:*
   - O  A. Insertion of a large-bore IV needle for fluid resuscitation
   - O  B. An abdominal ultrasound to evaluate the fetus
   - O  C. Type and crossmatch for possible blood loss
   - O  D. Pelvic examination by the emergency physician to evaluate cervical dilation

3. The patient with severe vaginal bleeding related to either placenta previa or abruptio placentae is at risk for developing:
   - O  A. Disseminated intravascular coagulation (DIC)
   - O  B. Adult respiratory distress syndrome
   - O  C. Pregnancy-induced hypertension
   - O  D. Trauma from a vaginal delivery

4. An 8-week pregnant female comes to the emergency department complaining of "heavy" bleeding. The patient's initial vital signs are B/P 80/40, P 120, and R 23. The appropriate nursing diagnosis on which to plan this patient's care is:
   - O  A. Airway clearance, ineffective, related to the patient's respiratory rate
   - O  B. Fluid volume deficit related to vaginal bleeding
   - O  C. Grieving, anticipatory, related to potential loss of pregnancy
   - O  D. Infection, high risk for, related to retained products of conception

5. Which of the following lab values would indicate DIC?
   - O  A. A hemoglobin level of 14 m/dl
   - O  B. A hematocrit of 40
   - O  C. White blood cells in the urine
   - O  D. A platelet count of 50,000

6. A risk factor for spontaneous abortion is:
   0   A. Cigarette smoking
   0   B. Bicycle riding
   0   C. Vegetarian diet
   0   D. Practicing meditation

7. The greatest fear related to a spontaneous abortion experienced by many women and men is:
   0   A. The mother dying because of excessive vaginal blood loss
   0   B. The child will not go to heaven unless it is baptized
   0   C. Their families will think they did something to cause the miscarriage
   0   D. That they will never be able to carry a child to term

## Ectopic Pregnancy

*A 29-year-old female presents to triage complaining of moderate abdominal pain, dizziness, and sweating. She states that her symptoms have been progressively worse over the past few days. She has no significant medical history, and her last menstrual period was 8 weeks earlier. She and her husband have been trying to get pregnant.*

8. The triage nurse places the patient in a pelvic examination room. The primary nurse should perform which of the following interventions during the initial assessment of this patient?
   0   A. Obtain orthostatic vital signs
   0   B. Perform a five-part neurological assessment
   0   C. Measure the patient's peak expiratory flow
   0   D. Obtain a cath urine for culture and sensitivity

9. The patient is complaining of pain in her right shoulder. This sign, associated with intraperitoneal bleeding, is known as:
   0   A. Kernig's sign
   0   B. Kehr's sign
   0   C. Cullen's sign
   0   D. Brudzinski's sign

10. The emergency nurse should obtain which of the following laboratory studies when evaluating this patient?
   0   A. Renal profile
   0   B. Quantitative BHCG
   0   C. Hepatic profile
   0   D. Drug screen

11. A transvaginal ultrasound shows a ruptured ectopic pregnancy. While the nurse is preparing the patient for surgery, she begins to cry and states that she does not want to lose her baby. The emergency nurse should base the nursing care on which of the following nursing diagnoses?
   0   A. Spiritual distress (distress of the human spirit) related to a lifestyle change
   0   B. Grieving, anticipatory related to the loss of her baby
   0   C. Grieving, dysfunctional related to the loss of her baby
   0   D. Thought processes, altered related to her hypotension and tachycardia

12. The patient demonstrates acceptance of the need for her surgery, even though there will be a loss, by:
   0   A. Signing out against medical advice, stating that she will be all right once she gets home
   0   B. Refusing to talk to her family when they enter the room
   0   C. Stating that she knows that she may die if she does not have surgery
   0   D. Stating that she will never get pregnant again if she consents to this surgery

13. The most common cause of maternal death in the first trimester of pregnancy in the United States is:
   0   A. Trauma from domestic violence
   0   B. Ruptured ectopic pregnancy
   0   C. Bleeding from placenta previa
   0   D. Bleeding from abruptio placentae

*An 18-year-old female presents to the emergency department complaining of irregular vaginal bleeding and mild abdominal pain. She states her last menstrual period was 6 weeks ago. She is sexually active and has not been using any contraceptives. A transvaginal ultrasound shows an intact ectopic pregnancy.*

14. Indications for the medical management of an ectopic pregnancy includes:
   0   A. A ruptured fallopian tube
   0   B. Profuse vaginal bleeding
   0   C. Severe abdominal pain
   0   D. No fetal heart activity

15. The patient is given methotrexate 50 mg/m$^2$. Methotrexate enhances the expulsion of the ectopic pregnancy by:
   0   A. Blocking the ability of the fetal tissue to implant
   0   B. Blocking the effect of progesterone on the fetal tissue
   0   C. Blocking the ability of rapid growth cells to reproduce

0   D. Blocking the effect of estrogen on the fetal tissue

## Pregnancy-Induced Hypertension (PIH)

*The paramedics bring a 34-year-old woman who is a gravida of 4 and a para of 3 to the emergency department. She has been nauseated, vomiting, and complaining of a headache with blurred vision for 3 days. There have been no problems with her pregnancy until now. Her B/P is 160/120, P 110, and R 20.*

16. The diagnosis of preeclampsia has been made. The emergency nurse should continually assess this patient for signs and symptoms of:
    0   A. Seizure activity
    0   B. Pulmonary emboli
    0   C. Renal failure
    0   D. Congestive heart failure

17. The patient's blood pressure continues to go up. She is now irritable, complaining of severe pain in her head and in her upper right quadrant. The patient has bilateral clonus. Which of the following medications is used to manage this patient's symptoms?
    0   A. Phenytoin, 1 to 5 g in 250 ml of normal saline
    0   B. Lorazepam, 3 to 5 mg IV push
    0   C. Magnesium sulfate, 4 to 6 g in 250 ml of normal saline
    0   D. Fentanyl, 2 to 5 ml IV push

18. A magnesium sulfate infusion is begun. The emergency nurse should evaluate which of the following as a symptom of toxicity?
    0   A. Normal deep tendon reflexes
    0   B. Urinary output greater than 30 ml/hr
    0   C. Magnesium level of 4 to 7 mEq/L
    0   D. Respiratory rate of less than 10

19. The patient is placed in a quiet room with dimmed lights. The side rails are padded and up on all sides of the bed. The patient's room is within sight of the nurse's station. These interventions are derived from which of the following nursing diagnoses?
    0   A. Infection, high risk for related to a potential for ruptured membranes
    0   B. Thought processes, altered related to the use of magnesium sulfate
    0   C. Injury, high risk for related to the potential of seizure activity
    0   D. Knowledge deficit related to the development of eclampsia

20. Magnesium sulfate is used in the treatment of preeclampsia because:
    0   A. It exerts an antihypertensive action to decrease the patient's blood pressure
    0   B. It affects neurotransmission of acetylcholine to decrease seizure activity
    0   C. It exerts a sedative effect so that the patient's headache pain is decreased
    0   D. It affects neurotransmission to decrease the occurrence of diplopia

21. A hydatidiform mole may cause all of the following *except:*
    0   A. PIH
    0   B. Hyperthyroidism
    0   C. A full-term delivery
    0   D. Coagulapathies

## Preterm Labor

*A 29-year-old woman who is at 28 weeks gestation comes to the emergency department complaining of regular uterine contractions, back pain, and a bloody vaginal discharge. She has a history of delivering a baby at 26 weeks 2 years earlier who did not survive.*

22. Risk factors for preterm labor do not include:
    0   A. Mother's age greater than 15 years
    0   B. Use of alcohol and cigarettes while pregnant
    0   C. No or inadequate prenatal care
    0   D. History of uterine bleeding

23. The emergency nurse has the patient lay on a stretcher until the emergency physician can see her. What is the most beneficial position for both the mother and the child while supine?
    0   A. Lying flat on her back with a pillow under her lower back
    0   B. Lying on her abdomen with a pillow under her chest
    0   C. Lying in the left lateral recumbent position
    0   D. Placing the patient in the lithomy position

24. The patient's contractions continue after a fluid bolus is given and the emergency physician orders a dose of terbutaline 0.25 mg to be administered subcutaneously every hour until her contractions decrease. What common side effect may the patient experience while receiving this drug?
    0   A. Tremors and anxiety
    0   B. Palpitations and tachycardia
    0   C. Hypertension
    0   D. Headache and dizziness

## The Pregnant Trauma Patient

*A 22-year-old woman who is 8 months pregnant has been involved in a motor vehicle crash. She was an appropriately restrained passenger (shoulder and lap belt) whose side of the car was struck by another vehicle going approximately 50 miles per hour. The patient is brought to the emergency department by helicopter with full cervical spine immobilization. Her vital signs are B/P 70/40, P 160, and R 32.*

25. The most common type of fracture found in the pregnant trauma patient is:
    - O  A. Fractured pelvis
    - O  B. Femur fractures
    - O  C. Lower rib fractures
    - O  D. Cervical spine fractures

26. When the mother has suffered a ruptured uterus as a result of blunt abdominal trauma, the infant may die because of:
    - O  A. Abdominal trauma
    - O  B. Head trauma
    - O  C. Pelvic trauma
    - O  D. Chest trauma

27. The primary survey of the pregnant trauma patient includes all of the following except:
    - O  A. Airway assessment
    - O  B. Ventilatory assessment
    - O  C. Abdominal ultrasound
    - O  D. Circulatory assessment

28. In addition to fluid and blood resuscitation, what other intervention could the emergency nurse perform to help increase the patient's blood pressure?
    - O  A. Position the patient with her head elevated to 30 degrees
    - O  B. Position the patient on her right side with her hips flexed
    - O  C. Position the patient in a left lateral position
    - O  D. Place the patient in Trendelenburg position

29. Because the diaphragm is elevated by a gravid uterus and decreases the mother's oxygen reserve, the mother and fetus are at risk for hypoxia. The emergency nurse would base their nursing care on which of the following nursing diagnoses?
    - O  A. Airway clearance, ineffective related to a full stomach
    - O  B. Gas exchange, impaired related to ineffective inspiration

    - O  C. Fluid volume deficit, high risk for related to increased volume
    - O  D. Mobility, impaired physical related to the size of the fetus

30. The pregnant patient demonstrates knowledge about the prevention of blunt trauma during pregnancy by:
    - O  A. Proper use of her lap and shoulder harness throughout her pregnancy
    - O  B. Not wearing her seat belt when she is in her third trimester
    - O  C. Wearing only a lap belt when she is in her third trimester
    - O  D. Not driving at all until she delivers in her third trimester

31. A pregnant female is at greater risk for intentional injury from:
    - O  A. Motor vehicle crash
    - O  B. Falling
    - O  C. Drug ingestion
    - O  D. Human abuse

32. A 23-year-old pregnant female suffers a cardiac arrest after a head-on motor vehicle collision. The patient arrives at the hospital 10 minutes after cessation of vital signs. A perimortem cesarean section should only be considered if:
    - O  A. The fundal height is 24 cm
    - O  B. The fundal height is 22 cm
    - O  C. The fundal height is 20 cm
    - O  D. The fundus is above the symphysis pubis

33. When the pregnant woman is injured, factors that do not contribute to fetal death include:
    - O  A. Direct injury to the fetus from penetrating abdominal trauma
    - O  B. Maternal anoxia from traumatic arrest
    - O  C. Fetal head injury from blunt impact to the abdomen
    - O  D. An intact placenta after the injury

34. Indications for a perimortem caesarian section include:
    - O  A. Maternal arrest greater than 15 minutes
    - O  B. Fetal age less than 20 weeks
    - O  C. Unsuccessful closed cardiac massage
    - O  D. Presence of adequate maternal vital signs

## Emergency Delivery

35. A 17-year-old teenager called her mother home from work when she delivered a 30-week fetus at home alone. The teenager's mother called the

paramedics, who have brought the teenage mother and infant to the emergency department. The mother's vital signs are stable on arrival. The emergency nurse should next assess:

0   A.  The status of the placenta

0   B.  Whether the patient has any vaginal tears

0   C.  Whether the mother wants to breastfeed

0   D.  The height of the fundus

36. The infant is cyanotic and making little respiratory effort. The paramedics have suctioned the infant, applied oxygen by mask, dried the infant, and attempted tactile stimulation to improve the infant's respiratory function. The emergency nurse should:

0   A.  Prepare equipment for intubation

0   B.  Give epinephrine through an umbilical catheter

0   C.  Perform chest compressions

0   D.  Bag-mask ventilate the infant's lungs with high-flow oxygen

37. Chest compressions should be performed on the newborn:

0   A.  When the infant's pulse is less than 60 to 80 beats per minute

0   B.  When the infant's pulse is greater than 90 beats per minute

0   C.  When the infant's pulse is 160 beats per minute

0   D.  After the infant has been given atropine

38. A location for emergent vascular access in the newborn is:

0   A.  Sternal intraosseous

0   B.  Umbilical vein

0   C.  Scalp vein

0   D.  Femoral artery

## Missed Abortion

39. The most common complication of a missed abortion is:

0   A.  Sepsis

0   B.  Pulmonary emboli

0   C.  Clotting abnormalities

0   D.  Infertility

## Gynecological Emergencies

40. A 20-year-old presents to the emergency department complaining of a rash on the palms of her hands and the soles of her feet. She states it does not itch. She states she is sexually active and generally uses a diaphragm for contraception.

She reports having several sexual partners over the last few months, but has had no symptoms of sexually transmitted diseases in the past few months. What sexually transmitted disease may be causing this rash?

0   A.  Herpes simplex II

0   B.  Nongonococcal urethritis

0   C.  Gonorrhea

0   D.  Syphilis

41. A 40-year-old female comes to the emergency department complaining of an increase in vaginal discharge, itching, vaginal irritation, and dsypareunia. She states that she has been married for 15 years and has had no other sexual partners. She describes the discharge as white and thick. The most probable cause of her symptoms is:

0   A.  *Lactobacilli acidophilus*

0   B.  Vulvovaginal candidiasis

0   C.  *Trichomoniasis vaginalis*

0   D.  *Neisseria gonorrheae*

42. A predisposing factor of candidiasis that requires additional referral for follow-up from the emergency department is:

0   A.  Multiple sexual partners

0   B.  Douching with commercial products

0   C.  Diabetes mellitus

0   D.  Use of an IUD

43. A 22-year-old female presents to the emergency department complaining about a thin, frothy, malodorous discharge. She states that her last menstrual period was 2 weeks ago and she has just recently begun a new relationship. She does take oral contraceptives. The most probable cause of her discharge is:

0   A.  Bacterial vaginosis

0   B.  Vaginal trichomoniasis

0   C.  Urethral chlamydia

0   D.  Vulvovaginal candidiasis

44. When discharging a patient who has been given metronidazole for vaginal trichomoniasis, the emergency nurse should instruct the patient that:

0   A.  She does not need to have her sexual partners treated for this sexually transmitted disease

0   B.  She may continue to drink alcohol with all her meals while taking this medication

0   C.  Her sexual partners should use barrier contraception until she has been seen again and cleared of all infection

O  D. She should always take the medication on an empty stomach because it never causes nausea

45. A 16-year-old girl brings her 10-day-old infant to the emergency department for care. She states that her child has had an eye infection since birth. Both of the infant's eyes are red and there is white drainage noted along the outside edges of the baby's eyes. The mother states the baby was born at home and she did not receive any prenatal care. The most likely cause of this child's eye infection is:

O  A. Congenital syphilis
O  B. Trachomatis
O  C. Chlamydia
O  D. Candidiasis

46. The child's eye infection should be treated with:
O  A. Ceftriaxone 125 mg IM for 10 days
O  B. Ceftriaxone 1 g ophthalmic ointment for 5 days
O  C. Erythromycin 50 mg/kg/day qid for 10 days
O  D. Spectinomycin 2 g IM for 10 days

47. A 42-year-old woman has been prescribed clindamycin cream for the treatment of bacterial vaginosis. Her discharge instructions should include which of the following information?
O  A. Her partner will need to be treated for infection so that she does not become reinfected
O  B. Caution should be used when using a condom or diaphragm since clindamycin cream weakens latex
O  C. She should not drink any alcohol before or after meals when using clindamycin cream
O  D. Bacterial vaginosis is usually caused by a gonococcal infection so her partner should be treated with penicillin

48. A positive whiff test is indicative of which form of vaginitis?
O  A. Vulvovaginal candidiasis
O  B. Vaginal trichomoniasis
O  C. Vaginal chlamydia
O  D. Bacterial vaginosis

49. A 17-year-old girl presents to the emergency department complaining of severe diffuse lower abdominal pain. Her vital signs are: BP 92/50;

HR 130R; RR 28 and she has an oral temperature of 103.6° F. She is pale, ambulating slowly, and is more comfortable with her hips flexed when she lays down. Which of the following information would assist the emergency nurse to differentiate the cause of the patient's hypotension and tachycardia?
O  A. A history of previous abdominal surgery
O  B. Last menstrual period and sexual activity
O  C. A history of previous urinary tract symptoms
O  D. The current diet she is on

50. Risk factors for the development of PID include:
O  A. Females age 30 to 45 years of age
O  B. Monogamous sexual relationship
O  C. Use of an IUD for contraception
O  D. No history of previous pelvic surgery

51. In addition to providing care for the patient's infection and fluid volume deficit, which nursing diagnosis would be appropriate for the care of the patient with PID?
O  A. Pain, acute, related to her pelvic inflammatory disease
O  B. Sexual dysfunction related to her complaint of abdominal pain
O  C. Activity intolerance related to the pain she experiences with movement
O  D. Anxiety related to whether her pregnancy test may be positive

52. Which of the following antibiotics are used to treat the patient with acute PID who requires hospitalization?
O  A. Cefoxitin 2 g IM plus doxycycline 100 mg orally two times a day
O  B. Cefoxitin 2 g IV plus doxycycline 100 mg IV or orally q 12 hours
O  C. Ofloxacin 400 mg orally bid for 14 days after discharge from the hospital
O  D. 4.8 million units of aqueous PCN IM three times a day

53. When counseling the patient who has been treated for PID, the emergency nurse should emphasize which of the following?
O  A. The emergency department is not where you should be treated for severe abdominal pain
O  B. Becoming pregnant will decrease your risk of developing PID in the future

O  C. Follow-up care is not necessary because you were treated in the emergency department

O  D. Reinfection may recur if you do not have your sexual partner(s) evaluated and treated

*An 18-year-old girl is brought to the emergency department by the police. She states that she had been hitchhiking and was picked up by a man who gave her something to drink. She woke up with her underwear off and she thinks he had intercourse with her before he left her about 6 hours ago.*

54. The initial assessment of a survivor of sexual assault should include:

O  A. Identification and treatment of any physical injuries the patient may have suffered

O  B. The patient's emotional response to the sexual assault

O  C. How the people with the victim are responding to the sexual assault

O  D. The amount of time it took for the patient to report the sexual assault

55. Clothing collected as evidence from the survivor of sexual assault should be:

O  A. Labeled and left outside of the patient's room

O  B. Labeled and placed in a plastic bag

O  C. Examined and given back to the patient

O  D. Labeled and placed in a paper bag

56. The patient stated that she had been given something to drink and has no memory of what has happened to her. Indications that a drug may have been given to a survivor of sexual assault include all of the following *except:*

O  A. Appearance of intoxication with no evidence of alcohol ingestion

O  B. Explained memory loss related to the incident

O  C. Unexplained patient drowsiness

O  D. Complaints of dizziness and confusion

57. Which of the following nursing diagnoses is most appropriate for the management of the survivor of sexual assault?

O  A. Post trauma syndrome

O  B. Social isolation

O  C. Rape-trauma syndrome

O  D. Powerlessness

58. Before ethinyl-estradiol-norgestrel (Ovral) can be administered as postcoital contraception for the survivor of sexual assault, the emergency nurse must:

O  A. Obtain written consent from the patient and her spouse

O  B. Assure that the patient's pregnancy test is negative

O  C. Determine if the patient is allergic to oral hormones

O  D. Obtain written consent from the patient

59. The most common cause of gonococcal infection in the preadolescent child is:

O  A. Sexual experimentation with other children

O  B. Sexual abuse by a known caregiver

O  C. Exposure to another infected child

O  D. There is no known cause

60. A 5-year-old girl is being prepared in the emergency department for a sexual abuse evaluation. What interventions may the emergency nurse use to help decrease the child's anxiety?

O  A. Separate the child and her caregiver before the examination

O  B. Tell the child, she is a "big girl" if she does not cry

O  C. Allow the child to pick which arm the blood may be drawn from

O  D. Take away all the child's toys before the examination begins

## ANSWERS

1. **B. Assessment.** The most likely cause of painless vaginal bleeding in the third trimester of pregnancy is placenta previa. Vaginal bleeding during pregnancy can occur for multiple reasons, including placenta previa, abruptio placentae, and preterm labor. If the bleeding is associated with pain, a board-like rigidity of the abdomen, and signs and symptoms of hemorrhagic shock, the patient may have an abruptio placentae. Painless vaginal bleeding (usually after 28 weeks of gestation) and uterine contractions are symptomatic of placenta previa.[2,5]

2. **D. Intervention.** The patient who has a placenta previa or abruptio placentae should not have a vaginal examination unless the appropriate physicians and nursing teams are available to manage the potential delivery that could occur.[2,5]

3. **A. Assessment.** Because of the potential for the mother to lose a large amount of blood from both

of these conditions, the patient is at risk for developing DIC.[2,3]

4. **B. Analysis.** The patient's vital signs indicate that she is suffering from some type of shock. Her vaginal bleeding could be the source of her blood loss. The initial care of this patient needs to be directed at identifying and treating her shock.[7]

5. **D. Evaluation.** Excessive or sudden blood loss can leave the patient at risk for developing DIC. Laboratory values that indicate DIC include a decreased platelet count (normal 150,000 to 400,000); hemoglobin is decreased (normal 12 to 15 ml/dl) and hematocrit is decreased (normal 36 to 45 ml/dl).[2]

6. **A. Assessment.** Cigarette smoking, alcohol consumption, stressful life events, drug use, and infection are risk factors for spontaneous abortion.[5]

7. **D. Assessment.** The greatest fear experienced by both women and men experiencing a spontaneous abortion is that it may recur and they will never be able to carry a child to term. The emergency nurse needs to reassure them that even though this is a possibility, 10% to 20% of pregnancies end in spontaneous abortion, and people do go on to carry pregnancies to term.[5]

8. **A. Assessment.** Obtaining orthostatic vital signs will provide information about whether or not the patient is bleeding. Based on the patient's chief complaint, there is a possibility of a ruptured ectopic pregnancy. In any young woman with the complaint of abdominal pain and amenorrhea, the emergency nurse should suspect the possibility of an ectopic pregnancy and base the initial assessment of the patient on this suspicion.[2]

9. **B. Assessment.** When the patient has significant intraperitoneal bleeding, the pain in the patient's abdomen from this bleeding may radiate to either shoulder. This sign is known as Kehr's sign and has also been associated with splenic injury.[3]

10. **B. Intervention.** A quantitative BHCG is obtained, along with a CBC, because both contribute information about the patient's condition.[2] Several other disease states can "mimic" an ectopic pregnancy, including spontaneous abortion, ovarian cyst, PID, and appendicitis. Other tests used to differentiate the diagnosis of ectopic pregnancy include pelvic ultrasonography and the patient's history.[2]

11. **B. Analysis.** The defining characteristics of this nursing diagnosis include the expression of distress because of a potential loss, and the realization or resolution of an impending death or loss.[7]

12. **C. Evaluation.** By acknowledging that she may die if she did not have the surgery, the patient is in

the stage of developing awareness related to her loss. The emergency nurse should encourage the patient to continue to discuss her feelings.[4]

13. **B. Assessment.** A ruptured ectopic pregnancy is the most common cause of maternal death in the first trimester of pregnancy. Fifteen percent of in vitro fertilizations result in an ectopic pregnancy, which makes this an important piece of history to be obtained from any woman complaining of abdominal pain and vaginal bleeding.[5]

14. **D. Assessment.** Indications for medical management of an ectopic pregnancy include unruptured fallopian tube, no active bleeding, and no fetal heart activity.[5,9]

15. **C. Intervention.** Methotrexate is a folic acid antagonist and it blocks the ability of cells to reproduce. It particularly targets cells with a rapid growth rate.[9]

16. **A. Assessment.** Because seizures are a frequent complication of preeclampsia, the patient needs to be continually assessed while in the emergency department for signs and symptoms of seizures.[2,3,6]

17. **C. Intervention.** Magnesium sulfate is given in a loading dose of 4 to 6g as a 10% solution in 250 ml of IV fluid. It is infused rapidly over 15 minutes.[5]

18. **D. Evaluation.** Magnesium toxicity can cause respiratory depression. Respiratory failure can occur with magnesium sulfate levels of 12 to 15 mEq/L.[8]

19. **C. Analysis.** One of the goals of the emergency nursing care for this patient would be to prevent the potential injuries that could occur from seizures, a potential complication of preeclampsia.[2,7]

20. **B. Intervention.** Magnesium sulfate directly affects the neurotransmission of acetylcholine to decrease the incidence of seizures.[8]

21. **C. Assessment.** A hydatidiform mole will not yield a full-term delivery. It is tissue where the fetus is missing and all chromosomes are derived from the father. It can cause pregnancy-induced hypertension, hyperthyroidism, and coagulapathies.[5]

22. **A. Assessment.** Risk factors for preterm labor include a mother younger than 15 years of age, use of alcohol and cigarettes while pregnant, history of uterine bleeding, and inadequate prenatal care.[10]

23. **C. Intervention.** The lateral recumbent position allows the gravid uterus to be displaced from the inferior vena cava and increase cardiac output.[2,3,6]

24. **A. Intervention.** Tremors and anxiety are common side effects that patients may experience while being treated with terbutaline. Hypertension, persistent tachycardia, and palpitations are less frequent and the patient should be monitored closely.[8]

25. **A. Assessment.** The most common type of fracture found in the pregnant trauma patient is a pelvic fracture. The most frequent mechanism that causes injury in the pregnant patient is the motor vehicle, which generally results in the patient suffering some type of blunt trauma.[1,11]

26. **B. Assessment.** When the mother suffers enough impact from blunt trauma to rupture her uterus, fetal death is usually the result of a skull fracture with intracranial hemorrhage.[1,11,12]

27. **C. Assessment.** Saving the life of the mother is the primary objective during the initial management of the pregnant trauma patient. If the mother does not survive, the possibility that the fetus may survive—particularly depending on the fetus's gestational age—is limited. An abdominal ultrasound should be a part of the secondary assessment.[11,12]

28. **C. Intervention.** Because the gravid uterus compresses the vena cava when the patient is on her back, the patient will experience supine hypotension. Supine hypotension, or vena cava syndrome, is the result of the gravid uterus compressing the vena cava and aorta. The patient should be placed on the left lateral side as soon as the cervical spine has been cleared. If the cervical spine has not been cleared, a pillow can be placed under the right side of the backboard.[6,11,13]

29. **B. Analysis.** A defining characteristic of this nursing diagnosis is hypoxia. A related factor contributing to this nursing diagnosis is an altered oxygen supply.[7]

30. **A. Evaluation.** The most common cause of fetal death during pregnancy is death of the mother. Women need to be educated about the proper way to wear safety restraints while they travel. The proper way to wear a restraint while pregnant is as follows: the lap belt is worn across the pelvis, and the shoulder harness is worn between the breasts and off the shoulder.[6,11]

31. **D. Assessment.** The incidence of intentional injury from human abuse increases during pregnancy. Connolly found a 24% increase, particularly resulting in injury to the fetus.[1]

32. **A. Assessment.** After 20 weeks of gestation, the fundus can be measured in centimeters. The number of centimeters is roughly equal to the age in weeks. Perimortem cesarean section is not recommended for the fetus less than 24 to 26 weeks because of the decreased chances of survival.[3,6,14,15]

33. **D. Assessment.** Factors that contribute to fetal death include maternal death and anoxia, direct injury to the fetus, and fetal head injury.[6,14,15]

34. **C. Intervention.** Indications for a perimortem cesarean section include maternal arrest of 5 minutes or less, fetal age of greater than 20 weeks, and inadequate maternal vital signs.[14,15]

35. **A. Assessment.** The status of the placenta should be assessed once the mother's ABCs have been assessed. A lengthening of the cord and a gush of blood indicate the delivery of the placenta. Once the placenta has been delivered, the emergency nurse should place it in a basin or a plastic bag, label it with the patient's name, and send it with the mother to the obstetrical unit.[2,3]

36. **D. Intervention.** Using the inverted pyramid for neonatal resuscitation, the emergency nurse should try bag-mask ventilation with high-flow oxygen. If this should fail to improve the infant's status, chest compressions would be indicated, followed by intubation and the administration of medications.[16]

37. **A. Intervention.** Chest compressions are performed on a newborn when the pulse rate is less than 60 to 80 beats per minute and when, despite adequate ventilation with 100% oxygen after 30 seconds, the infant's condition does not improve.[16]

38. **B. Intervention.** Locations for emergent vascular access in the newborn include umbilical vein and intraosseous route such as the proximal tibia or distal femur.[6,16]

39. **C. Evaluation.** Because of the retained products of conception, the patient is at risk of developing hypofibrinogenemia.[2]

40. **D. Assessment.** The clinical manifestations of secondary syphilis include mucocutaneous lesions that occur in 80% of patients with this disease. The lesions appear on the palate, pharynx, glans of the penis, and vulva. Rashes that occur in secondary syphilis do not itch and can be macular, papular, pustular, or squamous lesions. They frequently appear on the palms of hands or the soles of the feet.[4]

41. **B. Assessment.** Based on the signs and symptoms described by this patient, the most probable cause of her discharge is candidiasis. About 25% of vaginal discharge is caused by candidiasis whose signs and symptoms include white cottage cheese discharge, vaginal irritation, and itching and painful sexual intercourse.[17]

42. **C. Assessment.** Predisposing factors related to the development of vulvovaginal candidiasis include: antibiotic use, HIV, oral contraceptive use, pregnancy, and diabetes. If a patient is suspected of having diabetes, they should be referred for follow-up.[17]

43. **B. Assessment.** The signs and symptoms of vaginal trichomoniasis include: thin, frothy, copious,

green-yellow or gray, malodorous discharge. The predisposing factor of this disease is sexual activity.[17]

44. **C. Intervention.** The patient who has been treated for trichomoniasis with metronidazole should not drink any alcohol with the medication, have their partner checked and treated; use barrier contraception until the disease is cleared; and take the medication with food.[4]

45. **C. Assessment.** Chlamydia is one of the most common causes of conjunctivitis in the newborn less than 30 days of age.[4]

46. **C. Intervention.** The child should be treated with an oral medication, not eye drops. Erythromycin 50 mg/kg per day divided into four doses.[4]

47. **B. Intervention.** Clindamycin cream is oil-based and has been found to weaken latex products. Women diagnosed with bacterial vaginosis are the only ones treated, because treatment of male partners has not been found to be of benefit.[4,17]

48. **D. Assessment.** The whiff test indicates the presence of amines in the vaginal discharge, which is characteristic of bacterial vaginosis. Vaginal discharge is mixed with one or two drops of KOH, and if a foul or fishy odor is noted, the test is positive.[4,17]

49. **B. Assessment.** Differential diagnosis for the origin of this patient's hypotension, tachycardia, and abdominal pain include a ruptured ectopic pregnancy or pelvic inflammatory disease (PID). Date and description of the patient's last menstrual period will assist the emergency nurse to identify the possible causes of her hypotension, tachycardia, and abdominal pain.[4,6]

50. **C. Assessment.** Risk factors for the development of PID include females between the ages of 14 and 24; women with a history of PID; previous pelvic surgery; multiple sexual partners; use of cigarettes, alcohol, illegal drugs; and a history of using an intrauterine device for contraception.[4,6]

51. **A. Analysis.** The patient is experiencing acute pain related to the inflammation from her pelvic infection. Defining characteristics of this nursing diagnosis include guarding and protective behaviors, which can make a physical evaluation difficult. The patient's tachycardia may not only be the consequence of infection, but pain as well.[7]

52. **B. Intervention.** The treatment for acute PID that requires hospital admission is initially IV antibiotics. If the patient can tolerate it, doxycycline should be administered orally because IV administration is painful.[4]

53. **D. Intervention.** When counseling patients with PID who have been treated in the emergency de-

partment, the emergency nurse should emphasize that if her partner(s) is not evaluated and treated, reinfection is likely to continue. In addition, the nurse should discuss the need to return if the patient experiences increasing abdominal pain. PID in pregnancy can leave both the mother and fetus at risk for serious complications. Finally, the patient needs to follow-up to see if her treatment has been effective.[4,6]

54. **A. Assessment.** The initial assessment of any survivor of a violent crime should be focused on the identification and treatment of any physical injuries that could be potentially life-threatening.[3,6,18,19,20]

55. **D. Intervention.** All evidence that is collected needs to be labeled with the patient's name, date, time of collection, and who collected the evidence. A description of the evidence submitted should also be documented. Evidence such as clothing should be placed in a clean paper bag. Plastic bags collect moisture and destroy evidence.[18,19]

56. **B. Assessment.** Indications of drug ingestion in a sexual assault include appearance of intoxication without evidence of alcohol or drugs; unexplained drowsiness; and dizziness and confusion.[20]

57. **C. Analysis.** Unfortunately, the occurrence of sexual assault remains one of our society's major social ills. Nurses interact with the survivors of sexual assault not only in the emergency department, but within the hospital and community as well. Because of the complex care required by these survivors (females, males, children, young and older adults), specific nursing diagnoses have been developed. These include Rape-Trauma Syndrome; Rape-Trauma Syndrome-Compound Reaction; and Rape-Trauma Syndrome: Silent Reaction.[6,7]

58. **B. Intervention.** Before any postcoital contraception can be administered, a negative pregnancy test must be documented. Informed consent is necessary before the drug is administered only after it is determined that the patient is not pregnant.[18,19]

59. **B. Assessment.** The most common cause of gonococcal infection in preadolescent children (except the neonate) is from sexual abuse by a known caregiver.[18,19]

60. **C. Intervention.** Allowing the child to have some control over her care in the emergency department will help decrease her anxiety. Keeping everything as simple as possible, inlcuding allowing a caregiver to remain as long as possible with the child (obviously not the one responsible for the abuse), holding on to a favorite toy, or in some cases using sedation, will contribute to a less stressful examina-

tion for both the child and the emergency department personnel.[18]

## REFERENCES

1. Connolly AM, Katz VL, Bash KL, et al: Trauma and pregnancy, *Am J Perinatol* 14(6):331-336, 1997.
2. Reedy N, Brucker M: Emergencies in gynecology and obstetrics. In Kitt S et al, editors: *Emergency nursing: a physiologic and clinical perspective,* Philadelphia, 1995, WB Saunders.
3. Rita S: Obstetric emergencies. In Newberry, L, editor: *Sheehy's emergency nursing principles and practice,* ed 4, St Louis, 1998, Mosby.
4. Centers for Disease Control and Prevention: 1998 guidelines for the treatment of sexually transmitted diseases, *MMWR* 47(No. RR-1), 1998.
5. Carter S: Overview of common obstetric bleeding disorders, *Nurs Pract* 24(3):50-73, 1999.
6. Jordan KS: Obstetrical and gynecological emergencies. In Jordan KS, editor: *Emergency nursing core curriculum,* ed 5, Philadelphia, 2000, WB Saunders.
7. Kim M, McFarland G, McLane A: *Pocket guide to nursing diagnoses,* St Louis, 1993, Mosby.
8. McKenry L, Salerno E: *Pharmacology in nursing,* St Louis, 1998, Mosby.
9. Weinman S: Nonsurgical treatment of an ectopic pregnancy with methotrexate, *J Emerg Nurs* 22(6):597-599, 1996.
10. Peterson D: Preterm labor: Update on assessment and management, *J Emerg Nurs* 20(5): 373-376, 1994.
11. Southard P: The pregnant trauma patient: Special considerations in emergency department care, *J Emerg Nurs* 18(3):283-285, 1992.
12. Gerber-Smith L: The pregnant trauma patient. In Cardona V et al, editors: *Trauma nursing: from resuscitation through rehabilitation,* Philadelphia, 1994, WB Saunders.
13. Kloeck W, editor: *ILCOR advisory statements: Special resuscitation situations,* Dallas, TX, 1999, American Heart Association.
14. Strong T, Lowe R: Perimortem cesarean section, *Am J Emerg Med* 5:489-494, 1989.
15. Henderson S, Mallon W: Trauma in pregnancy, *Emerg Med Clin North Am* 16(1):209-228, 1998.
16. Chameides L, Hazinski M: Textbook of pediatric advanced life support, Dallas, TX, 1997-99, American Heart Association.
17. Cullins V, Dominquez L, Guberski T: Treating vaginitis, *Nurs Pract* 24(10):46-60, 1999.
18. Girardin B, Faugno D, Senski P: *Color atlas of sexual assault,* St Louis, 1997, Mosby.
19. Sexual Assault Protocol. Cincinnati, OH, 1999, University Hospital.
20. Armstrong R: When drugs are used for rape, *J Emerg Nurs* 23(4):378-381, 1997.

# Chapter 13

# Ocular Emergencies

## REVIEW OUTLINE

I. Anatomy and physiology
   A. Anatomical structures
      1. Anterior chamber
      2. Aqueous humor
      3. Canthus
      4. Central retinal artery
      5. Choroid
      6. Ciliary body
      7. Cornea
      8. Conjunctiva
      9. Crystalline lens
      10. Frontal bone
      11. Iris
      12. Lacrimal duct and glands
      13. Limbus
      14. Macula
      15. Maxilla
      16. Nasal bone
      17. Optic nerve
      18. Orbits
      19. Posterior chambers
      20. Punctum
      21. Pupil
      22. Sclera
      23. Sinuses
      24. Retina
      25. Tarsal plate
      26. Vitreous body
      27. Zygomatic bone
   B. Physiology
      1. Vision
      2. Accommodation
      3. Extraocular eye movements (cranial nerves II, III, IV, VI)

II. Ocular assessment
   A. History of illness or injury
      1. Risk factors for illness and injury
         a. Age of the patient
         b. Environment where patient lives, works, plays
         c. Occupation and hobbies
      2. Mechanism and time
      3. AMPLE history
         a. Allergies
         b. Medications
         c. Past medical history
         d. Last meal
         e. Events or treatment prior to arrival
      4. Change in condition from onset of symptoms to arrival in emergency department
   B. Pain
      1. Provocation
      2. Quality
      3. Radiation
      4. Severity
      5. Time
   C. General appearance of eye
      1. Edema/erythema
      2. Bleeding/tearing/discharge
   D. Visual acuity
      1. Test with and without glasses or contact lenses
      2. Use a Snellen eye chart, if possible
      3. Determine if patient can see fingers if unable to see eye chart. Start at approximately 10 feet and see if patient can count the number of fingers you are holding up. Continue to move closer to patient until patient can see the fingers. This is recorded as "Count fingers at X feet." If within 2 to 3 feet and patient still cannot see fingers, determine if patient can see hand motion. Record as "Hand motion at X feet." If patient has only light perception, use a penlight to see if patient can determine which direction light is coming from.
      4. Visual changes include
         a. Blindness
         b. Blurring
         c. Diplopia
         d. Cloudy or smoky
         e. Photophobia

E. Visual fields

Face the patient. Patient and examiner occlude opposite eyes. Examiner moves to bring his/her hands into the visual field from the periphery. Assess all four quadrants. The absence of vision in any quadrant is recorded.

F. Extraocular eye motion (EOM)

Face the patient. Have patient focus on an object such as a pencil. Move pencil up, down, to the left, and to the right. Observe patient's ability to move the eyes equally in all directions.

G. Pupil reactivity

Test for direct and consensual pupillary response when light is shined in the eye.

H. Pupil accommodation

Have the patient focus on a near, and then distant, object. Accommodation causes convergence of the eyes and pupillary constriction.

I. Medical history
1. Glaucoma
2. Chronic eye disease/past eye trauma
3. Diabetes
4. Cardiovascular disease
5. Hypertension

III. Diagnostic methods used for ocular emergencies
A. Intraocular pressure measurement with a Schiotz tonometer
B. Fluorescein stain
C. Slit lamp exam
D. Laboratory
E. Radiology
F. Visual acuity charts
G. Eversion of the eyelid

IV. Related nursing diagnoses
A. Alteration in comfort, pain
B. Anxiety
C. Fear
D. Knowledge deficit
E. Tissue perfusion, alteration in: optic nerve
F. Uncompensated sensory deficit, vision

V. Age-related changes
A. Pediatric patient
1. Visual acuity
a. 200/400 for infants at 2 months, reaching 20/100 by 1 year, and 20/20 by 4 or 5 years of age
b. Infant vision can be tested by observing the reach for a familiar object and fixation on light sources and objects
c. Charts and cards for older children include the Allen card, kindergarten test card, and Child Recognition Test

d. Children at risk for contagious eye illness because of close contact with others at school, daycare
e. Children at risk for injury by running with objects, lack of safety concerns

B. Geriatric patient
1. Changes associated with aging, such as a decrease in visual acuity, should be taken into consideration with exam
2. Medical history and medication history are important when assessing the elderly with an alteration in vision

VI. Selected ocular emergencies
A. Conjunctivitis
B. Glaucoma
C. Central retinal artery occlusion
D. Corneal abrasions
E. Foreign bodies
F. Retinal detachment
G. Chemical burns
H. Hyphema
I. Eyelid laceration
J. Globe rupture

Eye injuries and eye illnesses are common emergencies evaluated and treated in the emergency department.[1] The eyes represent only 0.275 of the total body surface area, yet they account for approximately 10% of all bodily injuries.[2] Eye injuries can be a result of blunt or penetrating trauma. Blunt trauma is most frequently the result of physical violence secondary to altercations. Penetrating trauma is usually caused by industrial accidents but can also be the result of an assault. Both blunt and penetrating trauma can be caused by motor vehicle accidents, sports-related injuries, and falls.

Conjunctivitis, a common ocular emergency, is caused by multiple things including infection, irritants, and burns. It is also associated with systemic illnesses such as upper respiratory infections. Millions of Americans suffer from chronic eye disease such as glaucoma. They, too, can present to our emergency departments with an exacerbation of an existing illness. The symptom of blurred vision may be an indication of an ocular problem or a symptom of diseases processes such as TIA or CVA.[3]

Whether the patient presents with a traumatic or medical ocular emergency, the emergency nurse must rapidly assess and intervene to prevent permanent visual loss. Patients will present with anxiety due to fear of disfigurement and loss of vision. Therefore, the emergency nurse must also be skilled in providing emotional support as well as physical care.

## REVIEW QUESTIONS

Match the terms in column A to the definitions in column B.

| A | B |
|---|---|
| 1. Blepharitis | A. Inflammation of the cornea that is light-sensitive, red, and painful. |
| 2. Hordeolum | B. Also known as a sty, infection of the upper or lower eyelid at the accessory gland. |
| 3. Chalazion | C. Inflammation of the lid margin, usually caused by *Staphylococcus aureus.* |
| 4. Keratitis | D. A sebaceous cyst that forms on the inside surface of the eyelid. |

*Mr. Lord, a 22-year-old construction worker, presents to the emergency department with complaints of pain, redness, and drainage from the left eye, which has worsened over the past 2 days. His visual acuity is normal. He is diagnosed as having conjunctivitis.*

5. Upon assessment of Mr. Lord's visual acuity, you would expect to find:
   0   A. A decrease in visual acuity in the affected eye due to the conjunctivitis
   0   B. A decrease in visual acuity in both eyes due to the conjunctivitis
   0   C. No change in the patient's visual acuity due to the conjunctivitis
   0   D. An improvement in visual acuity in both eyes due to the conjunctivitis

6. An appropriate nursing diagnosis for the patient with conjunctivitis would be:
   0   A. Sensory-perceptual alteration, input deficit
   0   B. Infection, high risk for
   0   C. Alteration in comfort, pain
   0   D. Tissue perfusion, alteration in, optic nerve

7. Initial nursing interventions for Mr. Lord should be aimed at providing comfort. One method for this would include:
   0   A. Providing cold compresses to the affected eye
   0   B. Providing warm compresses to the affected eye
   0   C. Cleansing the eye the diluted antiseptic solution
   0   D. Irrigate the affected eye with warm saline until clear

8. Discharge instructions for Mr. Lord should include patient teaching about conjunctivitis being:
   0   A. Permanent
   0   B. Contagious
   0   C. Self-limiting
   0   D. Nontransmissible

9. The anterior chamber of the eye is that space between the pupil and cornea filled with:
   0   A. Natural tears
   0   B. Aqueous humor
   0   C. Vitreous humor
   0   D. Interstitial fluid

10. A hyphema is bleeding into the:
    0   A. Lens of one eye
    0   B. Posterior chamber
    0   C. Anterior chamber
    0   D. Canal of Schlemm

*Mr. Gordon, an 18-year-old, presents to the emergency department with a chief complaint of eye pain as the result of an altercation. Mr. Gordon states he was punched in the eye by his opponent. Upon medical evaluation, he is diagnosed as having a hyphema. Usually the product of blunt trauma, a hyphema is bleeding from the vessels of the iris into the anterior chamber.*

11. Assessment findings associated with hyphema include:
    0   A. Aching pain in the affected eye
    0   B. Blood at the top of the anterior chamber
    0   C. Blindness from the blood in the anterior chamber
    0   D. No change in visual acuity in the affected eye

12. An appropriate nursing diagnosis for Mr. Gordon would be:
    0   A. Social isolation
    0   B. Alteration in comfort, pain
    0   C. Fluid volume deficit, high risk for
    0   D. Ineffective airway clearance

13. Interventions for Mr. Gordon include proper patient positioning once his cervical spine has been cleared. Mr. Gordon should:
    0   A. Lay flat on his abdomen to decrease intraocular pressure
    0   B. Sit with his head elevated to decrease intraocular pressure
    0   C. Sit with head of bed at 45° angle, turned on the affected side
    0   D. Sit with head of bed at 45° angle, turned on the unaffected side

14. Nursing interventions are also aimed at protecting the eye from further injury while in the emergency department. This can be accomplished by:
    0   A. Administering antibiotic eyedrops into the affected eye to prevent infection
    0   B. Administering anesthetic eyedrops into the unaffected eye to decrease pain
    0   C. Covering both eyes with a shield or patch to decrease movement
    0   D. Covering only the affected eye with a shield or a patch to decrease movement

*Mr. Thomas, a 66-year-old, presents to the emergency department with complaints of a severe headache located along the left eyebrow. He states that he can barely see out of his left eye and when he looks toward the lights, he sees halos around them. Mr. Thomas denies head trauma and states this all began approximately 1 hour ago.*

15. You suspect Mr. Thomas has:
    0   A. Corneal abrasion
    0   B. Retinal detachment
    0   C. Central retinal artery occlusion
    0   D. Acute, narrow-angle glaucoma

16. As the triage nurse, you would classify Mr. Thomas as:
    0   A. Urgent
    0   B. Emergent
    0   C. Nonurgent
    0   D. Delayed care

17. Several classic assessment findings will assist the emergency medical team in their diagnosis of acute, narrow-angle glaucoma. The affected eye's pupil will be:
    0   A. Normal in size and reaction
    0   B. Dilated, yet reactive
    0   C. Constricted, nonreactive
    0   D. Semidilated, nonreactive

18. Upon palpation, the affected eye will feel:
    0   A. Normal texture
    0   B. Rock hard
    0   C. Like rubber
    0   D. Soft and mushy

19. The physician may use a tonometer to measure Mr. Thomas's intraocular pressure. The normal reading is 11 to 22 mm. You expect Mr. Thomas's to be:
    0   A. Lower than normal
    0   B. Higher than normal
    0   C. Within normal limits
    0   D. Unable to be determined

20. Mr. Thomas is given an analgesic for pain. Anticipatory care would also dictate that Mr. Thomas be given:
    0   A. An antibiotic
    0   B. An antiemetic
    0   C. An antiinflammatory
    0   D. An anticoagulant

21. You also anticipate a medical order for:
    0   A. Miotic eyedrops
    0   B. Mydriatic eyedrops
    0   C. Cycloplegic eyedrops
    0   D. Sublingual nitroglycerin

22. Mr. Thomas is also given 4% pilocarpine. What criteria should the nurse use to evaluate the effectiveness of this drug?
    0   A. An increase in intraocular pressure
    0   B. An increase in visual acuity
    0   C. An increase in blurred vision
    0   D. An increase in halos seen around lights

23. Mr. Thomas is given an osmotic diuretic. The rationale for this therapy for the patient with acute, narrow-angle glaucoma is that the diuretic will:
    0   A. Lower intraocular pressure
    0   B. Prevent cerebral edema
    0   C. Raise mean arterial pressure
    0   D. Improve cardiac output

24. Mr. Thomas's "attack" is broken. His vital signs are stable, visual acuity has improved, and pain has substantially subsided. He is given discharge instructions and has an appointment to see the ophthalmologist the next day. Mrs. Thomas begins to cry and expresses fear that her husband

has lost his vision forever. An appropriate reply would be:

- 0 A. Mr. Thomas's sight can return to normal with appropriate treatment and compliance with his healthcare providers' instructions.
- 0 B. Mr. Thomas will probably go blind in the future but many social programs can help him adjust to this change.
- 0 C. Mr. Thomas will probably go blind in the affected eye only, which means only minimal changes in his daily routine.
- 0 D. Mrs. Thomas should address these concerns with the ophthalmologist tomorrow when her husband's appointment is scheduled.

25. Central retinal artery occlusion (CRAO) is differentiated from acute angle-closure glaucoma by:
- 0 A. Painless onset of visual changes
- 0 B. History of contact lens use
- 0 C. Visual acuity unaffected by the disease
- 0 D. Gradual unilateral loss of vision

26. Mrs. Rug is a 78-year-old female brought to the emergency department for an eye problem. She states that she tripped on the rug and fell, striking the right anterior-lateral side of her face on the floor. There was no loss of consciousness. Her vision has reportedly progressively decreased in the right eye since the fall. Upon admission to the emergency department, Mrs. Rug states she can see only flashes of light but mainly sees a curtain effect in her right visual field. You suspect:
- 0 A. Acute angle-closure glaucoma
- 0 B. Corneal abrasion
- 0 C. Retinal detachment
- 0 D. Central retinal artery occlusion

27. Your primary interventions for Mrs. Rug are:
- 0 A. Bed rest and patches applied to both eyes
- 0 B. Measures to increase intraocular pressure
- 0 C. Head of bed elevated and patched right eye
- 0 D. Application of cold compresses and sublingual nitroglycerin

*Mr. Roberts, a 24-year-old carpenter, presents to the emergency department with complaints of pieces of wood in his left eye. Several large foreign bodies are visible. The eye is reddened, tearing, and painful. Visual acuity is normal.*

28. Your first nursing intervention for Mr. Roberts would be:
- 0 A. To vigorously irrigate the injured eye with dextrose in water
- 0 B. Manually remove the larger pieces of wood to prevent blindness
- 0 C. Anesthetize the eye with the appropriate eye drops for comfort
- 0 D. To test Mr. Robert's intraocular pressure with a tonometer

*It is determined that Mr. Roberts has sustained a corneal abrasion secondary to the foreign bodies. The affected eye is patched, and Mr. Roberts is provided with antibiotic ointment, as well as instructions on how to apply the ointment.*

29. Mr. Roberts should also be instructed that his eye pain will return. The pain can be relieved by:
- 0 A. Application of warm compresses and a metal shield over the injured eye
- 0 B. Application of an eye patch and application of a cool pack to the injured eye
- 0 C. Continuous instillation of topical anesthetics to the injured eye
- 0 D. Application of over-the-counter eye drops to decrease the pain to the injured eye

30. The legal definition of blindness is a visual acuity of:
- 0 A. 20/80 or less
- 0 B. 20/100 or less
- 0 C. 20/160 or less
- 0 D. 20/200 or less

31. A life-threatening complication of periorbital cellulitis is:
- 0 A. Decreased visual acuity on the affected side
- 0 B. Development of a brain abscess
- 0 C. Paralysis of extraocular muscles
- 0 D. Development of conjunctivitis

32. A 32-year-old unrestrained driver was involved in a head-on motor vehicle crash. The airbag was deployed. He is now complaining of pain in both eyes. The initial treatment of his eyes should include:
- 0 A. Administration of antibiotic ointment to decrease the risk of infection
- 0 B. Patching both eyes to decrease movement and allow them to rest

O    C. Liberal irrigation with large quantities of normal saline solution

O    D. Administration of cycloplegic and antibiotic eye drops

**33.** When removing a patient's contact lens, the emergency nurse should:

O    A. Use as much force as necessary to remove the lens from the eye

O    B. Instill all eye medications while the contact lens is still in place

O    C. Use only saline solutions with preservatives when removing contact lens

O    D. Look for lost lenses in the upper cul-de-sac of the eye

**34.** Complications related to eye irrigation include:

O    A. Corneal abrasions

O    B. Periorbital edema

O    C. Fine punctate keratitis

O    D. All of the above

**35.** Discharge instructions related to the instillation of eye drops should include:

O    A. Look down toward the floor when instilling the eye drops

O    B. Close or blink the eyes gently to spread the medication in the eye

O    C. Squirt a large amount of solution into the eye to save time

O    D. Gently pull the lower lid up when instilling the eye drops

## ANSWERS

1. **C. Assessment.**[1]
2. **B. Assessment.**[1]
3. **D. Assessment.**[1]
4. **A. Assessment.**[1]
5. **C. Assessment.** The patient with conjunctivitis usually has no change in visual acuity.[4]
6. **C. Analysis.**[4]
7. **B. Intervention.** Warm compresses will provide comfort to the patient with conjunctivitis.[4]
8. **B. Intervention.** Conjunctivitis is contagious, not only to other people but also to the patient's unaffected eye.[1,2]
9. **B. Assessment.**[3]
10. **C. Assessment.**[4]
11. **A. Assessment.** The patient with a hyphema will have pain and a decrease in visual acuity in the affected eye.[5]
12. **B. Analysis.**[5]

13. **B. Intervention.** The patient with a hyphema should assume an upright position.[5]
14. **C. Intervention.** Both eyes should be covered with either a patch or a shield to decrease movement and allow the eyes to rest.[2]
15. **D. Assessment.** Mr. Thomas has classic symptoms of acute narrow-angle glaucoma.[3]
16. **B. Assessment.** Mr. Thomas needs emergent therapy and interventions to preserve his eyesight.[3-5]
17. **D. Assessment.**[4]
18. **B. Assessment.** Narrow-angle glaucoma will produce a rock-hard globe on palpation.[4]
19. **A. Assessment.** A tonometer reading reflects the amount of plunger indentation on the eye. Patients with high intraocular pressure produce a low reading because the plunger cannot indent the eyeball very much. Patients with low intraocular pressure will produce a high reading because the plunger can indent the eyeball more.[3]
20. **B. Intervention.** Patients with acute narrow-angle glaucoma frequently experience nausea and vomiting. Anticipatory care would dictate the use of an antiemetic to decrease nausea and prevent vomiting.[5]
21. **A. Intervention.** Miotic eyedrops will constrict and decrease the size of the pupil to allow for aqueous humor drainage.[3]
22. **B. Evaluation.** The effectiveness of 4% pilocarpine eyedrops can be evaluated by an increase or improvement in visual acuity. Pilocarpine constricts the pupil, pulling the iris away from the cornea and out of the angle, allowing for the free flow of aqueous humor from the posterior to the anterior chamber.[4]
23. **A. Intervention.** The use of an osmotic diuretic for the patient with acute, narrow angle glaucoma serves to decrease intraocular pressure. Because diuretics "dehydrate" the body, the amount of aqueous humor produced will also hopefully be decreased, lowering intraocular pressure.[4]
24. **A. Intervention.**[4,5]
25. **A. Assessment.** CRAO is painless, and can be sudden or gradual in onset. Acute angle-closure glaucoma is usually very painful with a sudden onset. Both conditions are usually monocular and neither condition is necessarily binocular.[2]
26. **C. Assessment.**[3]
27. **A. Intervention.** Bedrest, bilateral eye patches, and occasionally, the need for a tranquilizer, are primary interventions for the patient with retinal detachment. You may also need to prepare the patient for surgery.[3]

28. **C. Intervention.** Providing anesthetic drops is a nursing intervention with the appropriate standing orders. This should be a priority of care as the patient will then be able to cooperate with all other procedures.[4]

29. **B. Intervention.** To alleviate his recurrent pain, Mr. Roberts should be instructed to apply the antibiotic ointment as directed, double patch the eye to achieve a tight eye patch, apply an ice pack, and use over-the-counter analgesics. The purpose of an eye patch is to protect the eye, absorb secretions, and promote comfort. A tight eye patch will act as a pressure dressing and will relieve pain as well as promote healing. Patients should never be given a bottle of topical anesthetics as it impairs corneal healing and promotes the development of corneal ulcers. Patients may also reinjure the eye without knowing it if they consistently use a topical anesthetic.[5]

30. **D. Assessment.**[6]

31. **B. Assessment.** The most serious complication of a periorbital cellulitis is the development of a brain abscess.[3]

32. **C. Intervention.** The gases in an airbag contain sodium hydroxide. Alkali solutions penetrate the eyes more easily than acids and require liberal irrigation with copious amounts of normal saline solution to ensure that the chemical has been removed.[6]

33. **D. Intervention.** When removing a contact lens from a patient's eye the emergency nurse should never use force to remove it; instill eye drops while the lens is still in place; use saline solutions with preservatives since it can damage the lens; and look for the lens in the cul-de-sac if its location is not obvious.[7]

34. **D. Assessment.** All of these are potential complications of eye irrigation.[8]

35. **B. Intervention.** Instillation of eye drops includes:
- Instruct the patient to look up
- Gently pull the eyelid down for drop instillation
- Instill a small amount of solution to decrease tearing
- Close or blink the eyes to spread the medication[9]

## REFERENCES

1. Egging D: Ocular emergencies. In Newberry L, editor: *Sheehy's emergency nursing principles and practice,* ed 4, St Louis, 1998, Mosby.
2. Barak A, Belkin M: The eyes have it, *Emerg Med Serv* 23(5):50-55, 1994.
3. Epifanio P: Ocular emergencies. In Jordan K, editor: *Emergency nursing core curriculum,* Philadelphia, 2000, WB Saunders.
4. Kitt S, Kaiser J: *Emergency nursing: a physiologic and clinical perspective,* Philadelphia, 1990, WB Saunders.
5. Jacobs BB, Hoyt S: *Eye trauma. Trauma nursing core course.* Des Plaines, IL, 2000, Emergency Nurses Association.
6. Watts D, Kokiko J: Air bags and eye injuries: assessment and treatment for ED patients, *J Emerg Nurs* 25(6):572-574, 1999.
7. Layman M: Contact lens removal. In Proehl J, editor: *Emergency nursing procedures,* ed 2, Philadelphia, 1999, WB Saunders.
8. Smallwood M: Eye irrigation. In Proehl J, editor: *Emergency nursing procedures,* ed 2, Philadelphia, 1999, WB Saunders,
9. Novonty-Dinsdale V: Instillation of eye medications. In Proehl J, editor: *Emergency nursing procedures,* ed 2, Philadelphia, 1999, WB Saunders.

## Chapter 14

# Organ and Tissue Donation and Posttransplant Emergencies

### REVIEW OUTLINE

I. Types of organ donors[1,2]
   A. Nonheartbeating donors: patients who have suffered cardiopulmonary arrest and have been declared dead.
   B. Heartbeating donors: patients who have been declared brain dead and whose organs have maintained viability by mechanical ventilation, fluids, and limited and selected medications.

II. Organs that may be transplanted
   A. Cornea
   B. Kidney
   C. Skin
   D. Liver
   E. Heart
   F. Lung
   G. Pancreas
   H. Bone
   I. Heart for valves
   J. Bone, ligament
   K. Middle ear

III. Physiological systems review
   A. Fluid and electrolytic balance
   B. Cardiac system
   C. Respiratory system
   D. Renal system
   E. Hepatic system
   F. Pancreatic system
   G. Neurological system
   H. Skeletal system
   I. Integumentary system
   J. Immunosuppression

IV. Assessment
   A. History related to the cause of death
   B. In-depth head-to-toe physical assessment
   C. Medical history
      1. Risk factors
      2. Current medications
      3. Previous illnesses and injuries

V. Issues related to organ donation
   A. Legislative issues
      1. Consolidated Omnibus Budget Reconciliation Act (COBRA), 1986
      2. Organ Donation Request Act, 1987
      3. Uniform Anatomical Gift Act
      4. State laws
         a. Routine referral
         b. Required request
      5. Hospital policy
      6. Emergency department policy
   B. Brain death
      1. Definition
      2. Criteria
      3. Brain death status
         a. State
         b. Federal
         c. Hospital policy
      4. Coroner's cases
   C. Nonheartbeating donors

VI. Identification of potential organ and tissue donors
   A. Respiratory (artificially maintained) and circulatory functions
   B. Tissue donation: either respiratory- and circulatory-maintained brain-dead patients or patients who have died of cardiorespiratory arrest (nonheartbeating donors)
   C. Identification of potential donor
      1. Medical history
      2. History of presenting injury or condition
      3. Present physiological condition
      4. Contraindications
      5. Brain death
   D. Organ procurement organization
      1. Protocols
      2. Role of coordinators
         a. With emergency department
         b. With families
         c. With donors

E. Brain death
   1. Definition
      a. Generally accepted (Harvard Brain Death Criteria)
      b. State
      c. Hospital policy
   2. Role of ethics committee
F. Criteria for organ donor suitability
   1. Vary according to organ and/or tissue involved
   2. Time frames for retrievability
G. Exclusionary criteria for donor identification
   1. Untreated septicemia
   2. Human immunodeficiency virus (HIV)
   3. Viral hepatitis
   4. Active tuberculosis
   5. Malignancy, except primary brain tumor
   6. Disease of the donated organ and/or tissue
   7. Chronic systemic disease

VII. Donor maintenance management
A. Goal: ensure organ viability
   1. Maintain optimal hydration
   2. Maintain adequate oxygenation
   3. Maintain hemodynamic stability
      a. Maintain adequate fluid hydration (central venous pressure [CVP] 8 to 12 cm)
      b. Maintain urine output ($>$100 ml/h)
      c. Maintain systolic blood pressure stability at $>$100 mm Hg
      d. Maintain electrolyte balance and blood glucose level
      e. Maintain normal body temperature
      f. Prevent and treat infection
B. Basic principles of donor management
   1. Resuscitation
   2. Organ perfusion
   3. Hydration
   4. Diuretics
   5. Avoidance of infection

VIII. Approaching families of potential donors
A. Establishing legal next of kin
   1. Spouse
   2. Adult brother or sister
   3. Guardian
   4. Any other person who is responsible for the disposal of the patient's body
B. Approach to family, intervention
   1. Obligations to approach
   2. Dignified, professional manner
   3. Positive attitude
   4. Knowledgeable
   5. Offer emotional support
   6. Answer questions, allow expression of feelings
   7. Accept and support decision of family
C. Involvement of others
   1. Physician
   2. Social worker
   3. Clergy
   4. Medical examiner and/or coroner
   5. Organ procurement coordinator
D. Answers to most commonly asked questions
   1. No cost
   2. No disfigurement
   3. No disruption of funeral arrangements
   4. Confidentiality maintained
   5. Donated organs always given to those in great need
   6. Religious leaders support organ donations
   7. Family can visit patient's body

IX. Specific emergency nursing considerations
A. Completing physical assessment
B. Obtaining a history
C. Awareness of organ and tissue donation inclusion and exclusion criteria
D. Knowledge of appropriate ways to approach families
E. Knowledge of brain death criteria
F. Awareness of role of organ procurement coordinator
G. Awareness of other support services personnel and referral agencies
H. Knowledge about donor management protocols
I. Awareness of legal next of kin
J. Coordination with intensive care unit
   1. Donor maintenance
   2. Documenting, reporting
   3. Following policy and/or procedures
K. Legal issues
   1. Legal next of kin
   2. Obligation by law to ask
   3. Telephone consent (witnessed)
   4. Documentation

X. Related nursing diagnoses
A. Breathing pattern, effective
B. Cardiac output, decreased
C. Coping, family, high risk for growth
D. Coping, ineffective, family
E. Fluid volume deficit, high risk for
F. Gas exchange, impaired
G. Grieving, anticipatory
H. Infection, high risk for

I. Skin integrity, impaired

J. Spiritual distress (distress of the human spirit)

K. Tissue perfusion, altered

L. Urinary elimination, altered patterns

XI. Posttransplant emergencies

A. Patient assessment

1. Location of the transplanted organ

2. Differences in symptoms: chest pain is different in the heart transplant patient because of denervation of the donated heart; there may be two P waves on the ECG because parts of both the donor's and recipient's hearts are kept

B. Immunosuppression

1. Drug reaction

a. Bone marrow suppression

b. Hepatic dysfunction

c. Leukopenia

C. Infection

D. Rejection

1. Fever

2. Fatigue

3. Irregular cardiac rhythm

4. Jaundice

5. Edema

6. Decreased appetite

E. Diagnostic tests

1. CBC with differential

2. Culture and sensitivity

3. Cardiac enzymes

4. Liver enzymes

5. Electrolytes

6. BUN and creatinine

There have been many advances in technology, surgical techniques, and immunosuppression to make transplantation successful. Organ donation has taken on both a national and international focus over the past 10 years. The supply of organs for transplant, however, remains a major factor limiting organ transplantation, and thousands of people await transplants each year. Many continue to die each year while waiting.[2] Two specific pieces of legislation mandate that hospitals and medical personnel inform all families of their option of organ and tissue donation. A brief overview of these laws is presented here. A discussion of the vital role emergency nurses play in identifying and maintaining potential donors follows.[3]

The first legislation, the Consolidated Omnibus Budget Reconciliation Act (COBRA), was passed in 1986. This became effective on Oct. 1, 1987, and made provisions requiring all hospitals receiving Medicaid or Medicare reimbursement to do the following:

1. Have written protocols for donor identification

2. Inform families of their option of organ and tissue donation

3. Observe discretion and sensitivity

4. Notify organ procurement organizations of potential organ or tissue donors[1,4]

The federal government also enacted a second piece of legislation, the Organ Donation Request Act (the "required request" act), in January 1987, because health care professionals had demonstrated reluctance in asking families for organ and tissue donation. This act outlined the following provisions:

1. The next of kin must be asked for consent

2. Consent may be secured by the attending physician

3. Deference should be paid to the donor's religious beliefs

4. Notification must be made to the organ procurement organization

5. No sanctions for hospital noncompliance, but funding may be withheld[3]

These legislative acts make it clear that hospitals must comply with the provisions outlined, or Medicare and Medicaid reimbursement may be withheld. "Required request" laws now exist in all states and require hospitals to notify the nearest organ procurement agency when brain death is diagnosed and also require request for organ and tissue donation when the deceased meet specified criteria.

Local procurement agencies play a large role in assisting the emergency department nurse in complying with these laws. The local organ procurement agency (OPA) is linked with the United Network for Organ Sharing System (UNOS) and, by way of a national computer system, connects with current information on all potential recipients and organs available. This system ensures that those with the greatest need receive organs and/or tissues first. The organ procurement agency serves a vital role in providing information and guidance to the emergency department nurse.

Since emergency department nurses are frequently the first health care professionals to identify a potential donor, they must be diligent in their efforts to identify and manage potential donors to help meet the increasing demand for organs and tissues. Although organ donors are usually transferred to the critical care unit for care until brain death has been declared and consent obtained from the family, the emergency department nurse provides emotional support for the family and provides proper nursing management of the patient prior to transport. Tissue donors may be identified and maintained in the emergency department, because no ventilatory or cardiovascular support is necessary. After the patient is determined to meet the criteria for organ and/or tissue donation, the emergency department nurse should follow the established protocol quickly and notify the local organ procurement organization.[5]

Nurses can facilitate the decision making of families who are considering donation, and they can work with the health care team to provide the concept of organ donation to families who have not considered it at all. This is important because, although many families would be willing to donate organs for transplantation, most families will not think of donation unless someone cares enough to let them know about this opportunity. The family's willingness to donate organs can be enhanced by allowing them to participate as much as possible in the end-of-life decision making and identifying ways to help the family cope with their feelings of helplessness and powerlessness.[6,7]

It is crucial that emergency department nurses know their state laws and hospital/departmental policies in relation to organ and tissue donation. They must be able to identify potential donors, know the role of the organ procurement agency, know the interventions to be used in the care of donor management, know how to approach families, and know the nursing diagnoses related to the care of these patients. Efforts to increase the number of available donor organs and tissues are underway to meet the steadily increasing demand. In addition, the emergency department nurse must become comfortable with approaching families and making a request. Increasing public awareness through education regarding the need to consider donation remains a role of the emergency department nurse.

With the advent of more effective immunosuppressive agents and an increase in the number of hospitals that perform organ and tissue transplantation, patients are living longer and more active lives than those in the past.[4] Because of this, emergency nurses may find themselves faced with the challenge of caring for a patient who is having a posttransplant complication. One of the most common complaints that brings posttransplant patients to the emergency department is fever, which may be a sign of infection or potential organ rejection.

The emergency nurse needs to be aware of the anatomical, physiological, and psychological impact that organ and tissue transplantation makes on patients' lives. The transplanted organ may be in a different anatomical location, such as the transplanted kidney that is placed lower in the pelvic cavity. Because of physiological differences in the transplanted heart, the patient will

not experience chest pain, or may have cardiac arrhythmia considered normal for that patient.[1,2]

Finally, the drugs that are used to prevent rejection may contribute multiple problems, including hepatic, renal, and infectious complications.[1,2,4]

## REVIEW QUESTIONS

*The rescue squad brings a 56-year-old man to the emergency department. He was on a construction site and fell from a bridge into a river. He has suffered severe head injuries and has fixed, dilated pupils. Cardiopulmonary resuscitation (CPR) was begun at the scene. The patient is brought to the emergency department under full CPR. After a brief period of additional resuscitation efforts, the patient is pronounced dead by the trauma team.*

1. How would the emergency nurse determine whether this patient is a potential organ donor?
   - A. Completing a physical examination and obtaining a detailed history
   - B. Calling the organ procurement agency with a potential referral
   - C. Asking the family's consent for potential organ and tissue donation
   - D. Notifying the coroner that the patient is a potential organ or tissue donor

2. Current federal and state laws require that:
   - A. Families of all potential donors must be asked about donation
   - B. Only families of medically suitable donors be asked about donation
   - C. Catholic families should not be approached about organ donation
   - D. Families should never be asked about donation while they are still in the ED

3. The emergency department nurse finds the deceased patient's driver's license among his belongings. The patient had signed the donor card. When the family is approached about organ donation, the patient's relatives vehemently oppose the idea of donation. The Uniform Anatomical Gift Act allows for:
   - A. The individual's decision to override the wishes of relatives
   - B. Hospitals to create their own policies about organ/tissue donation
   - C. The family's decision to override the patient's request
   - D. The need to contact a judge before any decision can be made

4. When the family is told that CPR was ineffective and that the patient has died, the family members begin to yell and scream. One of them attempts to hit the emergency physician and states, "he did not do enough!" The nursing diagnosis on which the emergency nurse would base care is:
   0   A. Coping, ineffective family, related to the suddenness of the patient's death
   0   B. Family processes, altered, related to the patient's sudden death
   0   C. Grieving, anticipatory, related to the suddenness of the patient's death
   0   D. Injury, high risk for, related to the family attempting to strike the emergency physician

5. Based on the family's reaction to the news of the loss of their family member, the best approach for the emergency nurse to use concerning organ/tissue donation would be to:
   0   A. Refrain from asking about organ donation because they are too upset to make a decision at this time
   0   B. Ask the family, and if they do not agree, try to convince them that they should donate because it is what the patient wanted
   0   C. Provide emotional support, such as from a chaplain, and when the family is calmer, offer them the option of donation
   0   D. Tell the family it is the nurse's job to ask them about organ donation, and they have to sign a paper saying the nurse did ask them

6. The major goal of organ donation management is to:
   0   A. Reassure family members that the organs of the deceased are donated to the person of their choice
   0   B. Ensure organ viability so that the organs can be used effectively in the patient who is to receive them
   0   C. To make sure the religious beliefs of the family are explored and respected by the organ procurement team
   0   D. Notify the appropriate agencies so that the organs can be transported by either air or ground to the receiving facility

7. A recommended method of maintaining fluid volume in the patient who is a potential organ donor is to:
   0   A. Slowly infuse dextrose 5% in water ($D_5W$) with 20 Meqs of potassium to maintain adequate organ perfusion
   0   B. Perform vigorous fluid resuscitation with crystalloids, colloids, and blood products to maintain organ perfusion
   0   C. Transfuse the patient with packed red blood cells only to maintain adequate organ perfusion
   0   D. Begin a dopamine drip to maintain a systolic pressure of 150 mm Hg to maintain adequate organ perfusion

8. If adequate fluid replacement therapy has been attempted and is unsuccessful, the best choice of vasopressors to be used to maintain a systolic blood pressure of greater than 100 mm Hg is:
   0   A. Dopamine
   0   B. Norepinephrine
   0   C. Dobutamine
   0   D. Azathioprine

9. A patient may be declared brain dead when which of the following criteria has been met?
   0   A. The patient exhibits conjugate eye movements in response to a caloric test
   0   B. The pupillary light reflex is intact and the patient has dilated pupils bilaterally
   0   C. Irreversible cessation of all functions of the brain, including the brain stem
   0   D. Cerebral angiogram that shows filling above the level of carotid bifurcation

10. A 35-year-old single woman has been deemed an appropriate candidate for organ donation. The nurse approaches the waiting room and finds twelve of the patient's relatives there. The sister of the patient has become the spokesperson for the family. The emergency department nurse needs to determine who is the legal next of kin. Of the following, the nurse should obtain consent from the:
    0   A. Patient's sister, since she is the spokesperson for the family
    0   B. Patient's boyfriend, since he was the last to speak to her
    0   C. Mother of the patient
    0   D. Woman who states she is the patient's closest friend

**11.** Which of the following is not an exclusionary criterion for organ donation?
- 0   A. Known positive HIV
- 0   B. Hepatitis B
- 0   C. Obesity
- 0   D. Active tuberculosis

**12.** Candidates for organ donation who are victims of a drowning or, in the case of severe burns, who require prolonged ventilatory support, have been thought to be less suitable for organ donation because of which of the following nursing diagnoses?
- 0   A. Fluid volume deficit, high risk for, related to prolonged ventilatory support
- 0   B. Infection, high risk for, related to prolonged ventilatory support
- 0   C. Poisoning, high risk for, related to prolonged ventilatory support
- 0   D. Breathing pattern, ineffective, related to ventilatory support

**13.** A 5-year-old child who had a heart transplant 6 months earlier is brought to the emergency department by her parents. They state that the child has had a fever of 102° F and has been nauseated and vomiting. The child was recently exposed to chickenpox by one of her cousins. Her parents state that she has received the human varicella-zoster immune globulin, but now has lesions on her abdomen. Which medication will the child need to receive on an emergent basis?
- 0   A. Tacrolimus
- 0   B. Ceftriaxone
- 0   C. Acyclovir
- 0   D. Gentamicin

**14.** A serious side effect of cyclosporine (Sandimmune) is:
- 0   A. Vomiting
- 0   B. Hepatotoxicity
- 0   C. Tremors
- 0   D. Oral candida

**15.** Patients who have received a heart transplant generally do not:
- 0   A. Develop congestive failure
- 0   B. Develop cardiac dysrhythmia
- 0   C. Develop immunosuppression reactions
- 0   D. Experience angina

## ANSWERS

1. **A. Assessment.** A thorough history and physical examination are essential to the initial assessment of donor suitability. A number of underlying conditions immediately exclude the potential donor from further consideration.[1,4,5]

2. **A. Intervention.** The law requires that all potential donors (or their families) be approached. Families may wish to have their relative's body donated for research if it is not suitable for organ/tissue donation. Sometimes, as in the case of cancer patients, middle ears may be suitable for donation. The patient may be mistakenly considered "medically unsuitable" for donation.[1,2,5]

3. **A. Assessment.** If the patient had properly complied with the provisions of the Uniform Anatomical Gift Act of the state in which he or she was a resident, the request of the patient to be an organ donor would take precedence over the wishes of the patient's family. The gift takes effect immediately on death and is, therefore, binding on relatives. Thus, technically, the decision of an individual to donate an organ is legally binding on the family. In practical terms, and as a matter of policy, however, few hospitals go against the wishes of family members if they choose not to proceed with donation. A common practice is to obtain consent for organ and tissue donation from the donor's next of kin.[1,2,4-6]

4. **A. Analysis.** The family is exhibiting an inability to cope with the tragic news of their family member's death. Although individuals react differently to a family member's death, violent and threatening behavior is not acceptable behavior. This family needs a lot of support, and a referral should be made to a member of the clergy or to a social worker.

5. **C. Intervention.** The timing of when organ/tissue donation is requested, and the way a family is approached, are key issues in obtaining consent for organ donation. Physicians and nurses may be reluctant to discuss organ donation with potential donor families, fearing that this will cause the families more distress. However, it has been found that organ donation may actually bring consolation to a grieving family.[5,6]

6. **B. Evaluation.** Ensuring organ viability is the primary goal in organ donor management. This is accomplished by maintaining optimal hydration, oxygenation, and hemodynamic stability.[1,3,5]

7. **B. Intervention.** Maintaining hemodynamic stability is mandatory in order to maintain adequate tissue perfusion. Fluid resuscitation with crystal-

loid, colloid, and blood products should be employed to maintain the patient's blood pressure. Dopamine may be used once adequate fluid resuscitation has been achieved.[8]

8. **A. Intervention.** Dopamine is the vasopressor of choice for restoring autoregulatory control. The use of norepinephrine should be avoided because it raises the body's oxygen demands and can constrict the vessels supplying major organs. Large doses of vasopressors should be avoided whenever possible to prevent vasoconstriction, which can also produce decreased organ perfusion.[8]

9. **C. Analysis.** Brain death may be declared when a person has sustained either irreversible cessation of circulatory and respiratory function or irreversible cessation of all functions of the brain, including the brain stem.[8]

10. **C. Intervention.** The legal priority of individuals from whom consent can be obtained for a patient's organ/tissue donation are (in this order): the patient's spouse, an adult son or daughter, either parent, an adult brother or sister, a guardian, or any other person authorized or under obligation to dispose of the body.[1-3,5,7]

11. **C. Assessment.** Obesity in an otherwise healthy individual is not an exclusionary criterion for organ donation.[1,3]

12. **B. Analysis.** Exposure to foreign substances such as soot, a chemical, or water, which may contain debris or bacteria, increases the patient's potential to develop infection.

13. **C. Intervention.** If the child has received the human varicella-zoster immune globulin and still develops chicken pox, she needs to be treated with intravenous acyclovir. The drug will need to be continued for 7 to 10 days.[4]

14. **B. Assessment.** A serious side effect of cyclosporine therapy is hepatotoxicity. Other side effects include nausea and vomiting, diarrhea, oral candida, pancreatitis, rash, tremors, and headache.[9]

15. **D. Assessment.** When the patient's heart is removed for transplant of the donor's heart, the parasympathetic and sympathetic innervation is severed and the patient no longer experiences angina.[10]

## REFERENCES

1. Cosby C: In Jordank, editor: *Emergency nursing core curriculum,* ed 5, Philadelphia, 2000, WB Saunders.

2. Lewis D, Valerius W: Organs from non-heart-beating donors: an answer to the organ shortage, *Crit Care Nurs* 19(2):70-74, 1999.

3. Rowland DJ: Organ and tissue donation in the emergency department. In Kitt S and others, editors: *Emergency nursing: a physiologic and clinical approach,* Philadelphia, 1995, WB Saunders.

4. Bernardo LM, Bove M: Care of the pediatric organ transplant recipient. In Kelley S, editor: *Pediatric emergency nursing,* Norwalk, 1994, Appleton & Lange.

5. Pedersen M: Tissue and organ donation. In Newberry L, editor, *Sheehy's emergency nursing principles and practice,* ed 4, St Louis, 1998, Mosby.

6. Riley L, Collican M: Needs of families of organ donors: facing death and life, *Crit Care Nurs* 19(2):53-59, 1999.

7. Roark D: The need for increasing organ donation among African Americans and Hispanic Americans: an overview, *J Emerg Nurs* 25(1):21-27, 1999.

8. Holmquist M, Chabalewski F, Blount T, and others: A critical pathway: guiding care for organ donors, *Crit Care Nurs* 19(2):84-100, 1999.

9. Sullivan J, Seem, Chabalewski F: Determining brain death, *Crit Care Nurs* 19(2):37-46, 1999.

10. Bush WW: Overview of transplantation immunology and the pharmacotherapy of adult solid organ transplant recipients: focus on immunosuppression, *AACN Clin Iss* 10(2):253-269, 1999.

11. Rourke T, Droogan M, Ohler L: Heart transplantation: state of the art, *AACN Clin Iss* 10(2):185-201, 1999.

# Chapter 15

# Orthopedic Emergencies

**REVIEW OUTLINE**

I. Anatomy and physiology[1,2]
  A. Function of the musculoskeletal system
    1. Support
    2. Protection
    3. Movement and leverage
    4. Storage of mineral salts and fats
    5. Red blood cell production
  B. Components of musculoskeletal system
    1. Bones
    2. Nerves
    3. Vessels
    4. Muscles
    5. Tendons
    6. Ligaments
    7. Joints
  C. Range of motion
  D. Neurovascular status affected by orthopedic injuries
    1. Circulation
    2. Sensory perception
    3. Motor function

II. Orthopedic assessment
  A. History
    1. Chief complaint
      a. Mechanism of injury
      b. Position of limb when injured
      c. Ability to use body part since injury
      d. Time of injury or onset
      e. Swelling, deformity
      f. First aid or treatment since onset
      g. Associated injuries
    2. Significant medical status
      a. Previous injury to same site
      b. Current medications
        (1) Steroids
        (2) Anticoagulants
        (3) Chemotherapy
      c. Allergies
      d. Immunization status
      e. Chronic diseases
        (1) Osteoporosis
        (2) Cancer
        (3) Diabetes
        (4) Cardiovascular disease
  B. Physical examination
    1. Overview
      a. Position of the injured limb(s)
      b. Degree of distress
      c. Skin color, moisture, and temperature
      d. Vital signs
    2. Affected part
      a. Deformity
      b. Swelling
      c. Ecchymosis
      d. Loss of function
      e. Abnormal position or mobility
      f. Point tenderness
      g. Lack of skin integrity
      h. Five Ps
        (1) Pain
        (2) Pulse
        (3) Paresthesia
        (4) Paralysis
        (5) Pallor
      i. Range of motion
  C. Neurological assessment (motor and sensory)
    1. Median nerve
    2. Ulnar nerve
    3. Radial nerve
    4. Tibial nerve
    5. Peroneal nerve
  D. Reflexes
    1. Biceps
    2. Brachioradialis
    3. Triceps
    4. Patellar
    5. Ankle reflexes
  E. Age-related characteristics[2,3]
    1. Pediatric
      a. Presence of the epiphyseal, or growth plate, until maturity
      b. Bones more porous, more susceptible to injury
      c. Periosteum is thicker and more vascular, healing occurs more quickly

d. During adolescence, growth occurs, legs elongate, hips and chests widen, and shoulders broaden

e. Fractures may indicate intentional abuse and injury

2. Geriatric

a. Loss of height with aging

b. Development of kyphosis with aging

c. Decrease in muscular strength and range of motion

d. Chronic disease states such as osteoporosis may also contribute to changes in aging

F. Diagnostic studies or procedures

1. Skeletal x-ray studies

2. CT scan

3. Technetium bone scans

4. Arteriograms

5. Magnetic resonance imaging (MRI)

6. Complete blood cell count (CBC) with differential

7. Electrolytes

8. Type and crossmatch

9. Coagulation studies

10. Urinalysis

11. Uric acid level

12. Wound cultures

13. Compartment pressure measurement

III. Related nursing diagnoses

A. Activity intolerance

B. Anxiety

C. Body image disturbance

D. Fear

E. Fluid volume deficit, high risk for

F. Infection, high risk for

G. Injury, high risk for

H. Knowledge deficit

I. Mobility, impaired physical

J. Pain

K. Posttrauma response

L. Powerlessness

M. Self-care deficit

N. Skin integrity, impaired, high risk for

O. Tissue perfusion, altered (peripheral)

IV. Collaborative care of the patient with an orthopedic emergency[4]

A. Airway maintenance

B. Bleeding/hemorrhage control

C. Blood and fluid replacement

D. Cardiac status monitoring

E. Amputated part preservation

F. Pharmacological interventions

1. Analgesics

2. Antibiotics

3. Antiinflammatory

a. Steroidal

b. Nonsteroidal

4. Muscle relaxants

5. Local/regional anesthesia

G. Immobilization

1. Splinting

2. Casting

3. Traction

a. Skin

b. Skeletal

4. Serial reassessment

5. Local comfort measures

a. Positioning

b. Cold

c. Heat

6. Wound care

7. Compartment pressure monitoring

8. Emotional support

9. Patient/family teaching

V. Specific orthopedic emergencies

A. Sprains, strains

B. Fractures

C. Dislocations, subluxations

D. Inflammatory conditions

1. Bursitis

2. Tendinitis

3. Joint effusion

E. Carpal tunnel syndrome

F. Amputations

G. Complications

1. Hemorrhage

2. Compartment syndrome

3. Fat embolus

Orthopedic emergencies are responsible for a considerable number of patient visits to emergency departments. Most are related to recent injuries incurred in our fast-moving society. Motor vehicle and bicycle crashes, falls, industrial equipment accidents, and sports activities are all contributors to bone, joint, tendon, and muscle problems.[5]

The musculoskeletal system is made up of 206 bones and skeletal muscle equaling 40% to 50% of body weight.[2] It has two major functions, the first of which is to provide a framework for the body. In doing so, the musculoskeletal system provides support and protection for the vital organs. The second purpose is to provide for leverage and movement of the various body parts and for the body as a whole. In considering the anatomy and physiology of this system, it is important to note that veins, arteries, and nerves follow the course of long bones and that damage to the bone may include and/or cause injury to any of these structures.

The musculoskeletal system undergoes changes from birth until death. Pediatric musculoskeletal differences include the presence of the epiphyseal or growth area, bones that are more porous, and a thicker periosteum. During adolescence, there are growth changes leading to adult development.

The geriatric patient's musculoskeletal changes include shortening of bones, ligaments, and tendons, decline in muscular strength, and a decrease in range of motion.

Musculoskeletal injuries may also be a sign of intentional injury. Because both children and some elderly persons may be in dependent situations, abuse may manifest itself in fractures. The mechanism of injury should match the type of injury being treated.

The most important nursing measure in the initial phase of caring for the patient who has an orthopedic emergency is to immediately assess the whole patient. Compound fractures, dislocations, and severe deformities have a dramatic appearance but are not life threatening. Stabilization of airway, breathing, and circulation (the ABCs) is essential and should not be overlooked or delayed. An important axiom to remember is that the most obvious may not be the most severe.

In obtaining a history of the chief complaint, careful scrutiny is given to the mechanism of injury. Factors such as force involved, trajectory, position of the limb when injured, time elapsed since the incident, activity or ability to use the body part since injury, and any first aid prior to seeking care all contribute to understanding the presenting problem. In addition, this information assists in discovering associated injuries of which the patient may be unaware. A history of any previous similar injury, as well as a review of current medications, use of alcohol or other drugs, and any significant medical history will be helpful. Special considerations of the elderly, infants, and children include the possibility of abuse and complications such as hypothermia and dehydration.

An objective assessment of the patient with an orthopedic emergency includes observing the affected area for abnormalities such as deformity, swelling, discoloration, loss of function, and abnormal position or movement. Palpation may reveal point tenderness or crepitus. Neurovascular status distal to the site is assessed initially and serially.

Interventions appropriate to the management of the emergency orthopedic patient include stabilizing the injured part as soon as possible. Open wounds are covered with sterile saline dressings. Splinting is performed using whatever device will immobilize the part and still allow access for circulatory checks. It is important to remember to pad the splint well and to immobilize the joint above and below the injury.

Pain control is an important facet of care. Local comfort measures of ice and elevation decrease venous congestion and reduce swelling, a major factor contributing to pain. In addition, pharmacological agents are indicated. Concurrent skin defects are cleansed and dressed as indicated. The potential for infection can be significant and requires administration of antibiotics.

An orthopedic emergency of life-threatening proportion is a fractured pelvis. Significant pelvic fractures are incurred in incidents involving severe, direct force. Tears in pelvic and lumbar vessels can result in rapid, massive blood loss. With pelvic fractures it is common to have injuries in other systems as well, especially the genitourinary and gastrointestinal systems. Interventions in this instance include aggressive fluid resuscitation, application of the pneumatic antishock garment (PASG) for stabilization and tamponade effect, and rapid identification and management of associated injuries.

## REVIEW QUESTIONS

1. A 34-year-old woman comes to the emergency department (ED) complaining of right wrist pain of 1 week's duration that is gradually becoming worse. She has no history of direct trauma to the extremity. Vital signs are B/P 116/82, HR 84, RR 16, and Temp 97.8° F. Pertinent subjective assessment obtained by the nurse includes:

    0   A. Family history of arm pain
    0   B. Activity prior to the onset of pain
    0   C. Current use of contraceptives
    0   D. Allergies to food or animals

2. Based on this patient's history, an examination of this patient's right arm may reveal:

    0   A. Discoloration at or distal to the wrist
    0   B. Abnormal mobility with movement
    0   C. Increased pain with motion
    0   D. Sensory deficit in the fingers

3. The appropriate nursing diagnosis on which to base care for this patient is:

    0   A. Mobility, impaired physical, due to pain with movement
    0   B. Infection, high risk for, related to the presence of pain
    0   C. Skin integrity, impaired, high risk for related to the presence of pain
    0   D. Tissue perfusion, altered (peripheral), related to limited movement due to pain

4. The physician prescribes ibuprofen for this patient. The nurse recognizes this drug as a:
   - 0  A. Synthetic narcotic
   - 0  B. Salicylate derivative
   - 0  C. Tricyclic antidepressant
   - 0  D. Nonsteroidal antiinflammatory agent

5. When discharging this patient, the emergency nurse instructs her to be rechecked by her physician in 1 week if she is not better. What specific instructions should the nurse give this patient for taking her medication?
   - 0  A. Take medication before meals
   - 0  B. Take medication with food or milk
   - 0  C. Double the dose if the medication is not effective
   - 0  D. Evenly space doses over a 24-hour period

6. An evaluative criteria to determine whether this patient's treatment is working is:
   - 0  A. The patient develops gastritis from taking the ibuprofen
   - 0  B. The patient regains full range of motion
   - 0  C. The patient continues to complain of pain
   - 0  D. The patient requires physical therapy for the rest of her life

*The rescue squad brings a 32-year-old man to the ED after being involved in a head-on motor vehicle crash. He was a restrained front seat passenger who required some extrication. He arrives on a long backboard awake, alert, and complaining of pain in both legs. He has some minor abrasions of the face, the left knee has a deep laceration with crepitus, and the right ankle is obviously deformed. Vital signs are B/P 122/72, HR 106, RR 24, and Temp 98.4° F.*

7. The emergency nurse's initial intervention upon receiving this patient should be to:
   - 0  A. Immobilize the cervical spine with a soft collar
   - 0  B. Apply a splint to the right ankle for comfort
   - 0  C. Assess and manage the patient's airway
   - 0  D. Inquire if others injured in the accident will be brought to this facility

8. While performing an objective assessment, the nurse notes that pulses are absent in the right foot. An appropriate intervention for this problem would be to:
   - 0  A. Splint the extremity above the knee so that no further harm may be done
   - 0  B. Expedite portable films of the right lower extremity to identify injury

   - 0  C. Attempt to straighten the deformity and apply a hare traction for comfort
   - 0  D. Notify the physician at once about this significant physical finding

9. The appropriate initial x-ray films to be obtained on this patient are:
   - 0  A. Cross-table cervical spine, chest, pelvis
   - 0  B. Cross-table cervical spine, pelvis, left knee
   - 0  C. Chest, pelvis, right ankle, and CT scan of the head
   - 0  D. Pelvis, left knee, right ankle, and MRI of the head

10. The mechanism of injury and the presence of left knee injury alerts the nurse to what possible associated injury?
    - 0  A. Left hip and/or acetabular injury
    - 0  B. Lumbar spine injury
    - 0  C. Left os calcis fracture
    - 0  D. Left lower tendon rupture

11. The physician orders ceftriaxone, 1 g, and gentamicin, 160 mg IV. Which nursing diagnosis is reflected in this order?
    - 0  A. Pain related to multiple fractures
    - 0  B. Infection, high risk for, related to an open fracture
    - 0  C. Tissue perfusion, altered (peripheral), related to an open fracture
    - 0  D. Anxiety related to the patient's immobility

12. A 4-year-old girl fell down the steps before arrival in the ED. Her only complaint is that she cannot move her right forearm. An x-ray film shows a right ulnar fracture involving only one side of the bone. This type of fracture is described as a:
    - 0  A. Barton fracture
    - 0  B. Galeazzi fracture
    - 0  C. Colles fracture
    - 0  D. Greenstick fracture

*A 55-year-old male who was a restrained driver struck a telephone pole at 60 miles per hour. The patient was entrapped for over 45 minutes. Upon arrival in the ED, the patient is alert and oriented, B/P 80/40, HR 140, RR 30, and Temp 94° F (rectal). The only obvious sign of trauma is a swollen left thigh and a large laceration on the inner aspect of his left thigh. The patient has on a C-collar and is fully immobilized on a backboard.*

13. The pelvic x-ray film shows an avulsion of the ischial spine and a total disruption of the soft

tissues on the left side of his pelvis. The patient is to be transferred to a level I trauma center by ground. What may the emergency nurse do to stabilize the patient's pelvis for transport?

0   A. Apply PASG to provide tamponade and bone immobilization during the transport process

0   B. Take the patient off the backboard and place on a soft mattress to decrease the pain that may occur with transport

0   C. Place pillows between the patient's legs and use cravats to stabilize the patient's legs

0   D. Place bilateral hare traction splints on both of the patient's femurs to stabilize the patient's pelvis

14. Based on the patient's injury and current vital signs, what nursing diagnosis should the emergency nurse use to plan his care?

0   A. Injury, high risk for, related to the movement required to evaluate the patient and transfer him for further care

0   B. Infection, high risk for, related to the wound on his left thigh and the need to transfer the patient for further care

0   C. Fluid volume deficit related to active loss of body fluid secondary to bleeding from his pelvic injury

0   D. Mobility, impaired, related to the patient's ability to assist in moving him from the emergency department stretcher to the transport stretcher

15. Signs and symptoms of an open pelvic fracture include all of the following except:

0   A. Paresis of the lower extremities

0   B. Blood from the urethra or vagina

0   C. Ecchymosis in the flank area

0   D. Low-riding prostate

16. The major complication of an open pelvic fracture is:

0   A. Coagulopathy

0   B. Exsanguination

0   C. Paraplegia

0   D. Sepsis

17. The patient has been given 9 L of crystalloid and 5 L of packed red blood cells. Which of the following lab values should the emergency nurse monitor during aggressive fluid resuscitation to avert any further complications?

0   A. Cardiac enzymes

0   B. BUN and creatinine

0   C. Coagulation studies

0   D. Liver function tests

18. The expected outcome for the patient being medicated for pain from a fractured ankle is:

0   A. Absence of pain after the administration of the medication

0   B. Decrease in the amount of swelling after the administration of the medication

0   C. Tolerance of the pain after administration of the medication

0   D. No change in pain after administration of the medication

19. A 26-year-old man is brought to the ED by the rescue squad. He is complaining of a sudden onset of shortness of breath, and he is restless and somewhat cyanotic. Vital signs are B/P 102/60, HR 138, RR 44, and Temp 102.8° F. The nurse's first intervention in caring for this patient is to:

0   A. Start high-flow oxygen by means of a nonrebreathing mask

0   B. Draw arterial blood gases from the patient's radial artery

0   C. Attach a cardiac monitor and obtain a 12-lead ECG

0   D. Establish an IV access and give a fluid bolus of normal saline

20. Further assessment reveals that the patient sustained fractures of his right tibia and fibula 2 days earlier in a soccer game. He was hospitalized until this morning and then discharged with a long leg cast in place. The nurse recognizes that this puts the patient at risk for:

0   A. Embolus secondary to deep venous thrombosis

0   B. Adult respiratory distress syndrome from his injury

0   C. Air embolus from an open fracture

0   D. Fat embolus from the lower extremity fracture

21. The initial blood gases on this patient reveal a pH of 7.21, $PCO_2$ of 66, $PO_2$ of 60, and bicarbonate level of 26. The nurse recognizes these values as:

0   A. Respiratory alkalosis

0   B. Metabolic acidosis

0   C. Respiratory acidosis

0   D. Metabolic alkalosis

22. Based on the initial evaluation, the most appropriate nursing diagnosis is:
    0   A. Airway clearance, ineffective, related to his shortness of breath
    0   B. Cardiac output, decreased, related to his change in blood pressure and pulse
    0   C. Anxiety related to returning to the emergency department
    0   D. Gas exchange, impaired, related to a fat embolus

23. The physician orders a heparin infusion. He orders 25,000 units of heparin in 500 ml of dextrose 5% in water ($D_5W$) to infuse at the rate of 1,000 units/h. The flow rate in milliliters per hour is:
    0   A. 12 ml per hour
    0   B. 24 ml per hour
    0   C. 20 ml per hour
    0   D. 6 ml per hour

*A 17-year-old youth comes to the ED complaining of left leg pain after being struck by an automobile and pinned against a wall. His lower left leg is deformed and markedly contused. He has no other apparent injury. Vital signs are B/P 128/86, HR 98, RR 20, and Temp 98.4° F.*

24. The nature of this patient's injury alerts the emergency nurse to the possibility of his developing:
    0   A. Osteomyelitis
    0   B. Deep venous thrombosis
    0   C. Compartment syndrome
    0   D. Secondary skin infection

25. An external cause of compartment syndrome is:
    0   A. Black widow spider bite of the hand
    0   B. Prolonged application of PASG
    0   C. Electrical burn of a lower extremity
    0   D. Open fracture of the lower extremity

26. Nursing assessment of this patient's lower leg includes:
    0   A. Observation for skin discontinuity
    0   B. Palpation of the posterior popliteal pulse
    0   C. Palpation of the dorsalis pedis and posterior tibial pulses
    0   D. Check for movement, sensation, and capillary refill of the toes

27. This patient is given fentanyl, 150 μg IV, for pain, and a long leg splint is applied. Thirty minutes after medication administration, he continues to complain of severe pain in his left leg, which increases with movement of his toes. Sensation and capillary refill remain intact. An appropriate nursing intervention at this time would be to:
    0   A. Notify the physician immediately
    0   B. Adjust the splint till the patient says he is more comfortable
    0   C. Reposition the patient's leg on some soft pillows
    0   D. Administer one half the first fentanyl dose

28. Measurement of compartment pressures is accomplished using a(n):
    0   A. Pulse oximeter
    0   B. Manometer
    0   C. Sphygmomanometer
    0   D. Air splint

29. Evidence of compartment syndrome may be reflected in which other system?
    0   A. Pulmonary
    0   B. Cardiac
    0   C. Renal
    0   D. Gastrointestinal

30. The nursing diagnosis that best reflects the problems of compartment syndrome is:
    0   A. Pain (acute) related to decreased blood flow to the extremity
    0   B. Gas exchange, impaired related to decreased blood flow to the extremity
    0   C. Skin integrity, impaired, high risk for related to decreased blood flow
    0   D. Tissue perfusion, altered, peripheral related to decreased blood flow

31. A 12-year-old male caught his right hand in a corn-picker while attempting to clean it. He has suffered an amputation of the first four digits. The life squad transports the patient and his digits to the emergency department. Detriments to the possibility of reimplantation of his digits include:
    0   A. Length of time of less than 12 hours since the amputation
    0   B. Availability of a qualified reimplantation team at the receiving facility
    0   C. Crush/avulsion type injuries to the amputated extremities
    0   D. Upper-extremity amputations such as fingers and forearms

**32.** A 17-year-old male with a severe ankle sprain has been given crutches for ambulation. Appropriate fitting of these crutches includes:

0   A. Each hand piece should be fitted so that the elbow is flexed at 60 degrees

0   B. Crutches should fit so that each arm piece is two finger widths below the axilla

0   C. Crutches should fit so that all the weight of the upper body is on the axilla

0   D. Tips of the crutches should be placed 12 inches to the front of the patient

**33.** Initial emergency nursing interventions for the management of a joint dislocation include:

0   A. Apply firm traction to reduce an abnormally deformed joint dislocation

0   B. Leave any distal constricting jewelry in place for patient comfort

0   C. Immobilize the joint below the level of injury only for patient comfort

0   D. Immobilize the joint and extremity in position of comfort

**34.** A 23-year-old male patient presented to the ED complaining of swelling, redness, tenderness, and excessive warmth to his left elbow. The patient states he has no history of medical problems. He is diagnosed with a septic joint. The most common pathogen that causes a septic joint is:

0   A. *Streptococcus*

0   B. *Gonococcus*

0   C. *Clostridium*

0   D. *Staphylococcus*

**35.** An ankle radiograph should be obtained when:

0   A. The patient is able to bear weight on the ankle upon admission to the ED

0   B. The patient does not have bone tenderness over the posterior edge or tip of the lateral malleolus

0   C. The patient does not have bone tenderness over the posterior edge or tip of the medial malleolus

0   D. The patient is unable to bear weight on the injured extremity immediately after injury and in the ED

## ANSWERS

1. **B. Assessment.** The most beneficial information concerning this patient's problem can be derived from learning what the patient was doing before the pain began. Most often the nurse will discover some repetitive activity involving the affected joint, in this case the wrist.[4]

2. **C. Assessment.** Excessive, continued stress on an area produces inflammation of the involved tendons. Movement exacerbates the pain.[4]

3. **A. Analysis.** The goal in treatment of tendinitis is to reduce irritation by immobilizing the affected area. In addition, local application of heat may be beneficial.[6]

4. **D. Intervention.** Ibuprofen and the other nonsteroidal antiinflammatory medications are first-line agents for inflammatory conditions such as tendinitis. The action of these drugs is related to inhibition of prostaglandin synthesis; however, the exact method of action is not known.[7]

5. **B. Intervention.** A common side effect of the nonsteroidal antiinflammatory drug is gastrointestinal upset. Taking the medication with food or milk helps protect the stomach from irritation.

6. **B. Evaluation.** The relief of pain and the ability to use the extremity as before would indicate that the treatment is working.

7. **C. Intervention.** Evaluating the status of airway, breathing, and circulation (ABCs) should be the automatic first response to every patient. The appearance of deformed limbs should never divert the nurse from a basic primary assessment.[4]

8. **D. Intervention.** Initial and serial reevaluation of circulation distal to the injury is a nursing responsibility. A pulseless extremity is a serious emergency and should be brought to the physician's attention at once so appropriate collaborative interventions can be initiated.[4]

9. **A. Intervention.** Initial x-ray films are taken on a patient with multiple trauma immediately after stabilizing the ABCs to rule out life-threatening injuries. A cross-table cervical spine film helps identify serious neck injury. A chest film is taken to look for pneumothorax or hemothorax and for any mediastinal shift. A pelvis film will reveal fractures that could cause massive blood loss. These x-ray studies can be done quickly by portable machine and create minimal disruption of patient care.[8]

10. **A. Assessment.** In a front-end collision, the patient sustains a blow to the knee while in the flexed position. This energy is transmitted up the femur to the flexed hip joint, causing hip fracture, acetabular fracture, or posterior hip dislocation. Careful evaluation of this patient's left hip and pelvis is indicated.[8]

11. **B. Analysis.** Compound fractures, such as this patient's left knee injury, are prime targets for serious

infection. Vigorous prevention of this complication is begun early in the patient's stay.[6]

12. **D. Assessment.** A greenstick fracture is a longitudinal fracture that involves only one side of the cortex of the bone. Because the periosteum is thicker in children, the fracture may not go completely through the bone. A Barton fracture is a radial fracture associated with dislocation of the carpal bones and the hand. A Galeazzi fracture involves the middle to distal third of the radius associated with radioulnar subluxation. A Colles fracture involves a fracture of the distal radius with volar angulation, along with a Salter type II epiphyseal fracture of the ulnar styloid.[4]

13. **A. Intervention.** Even though the use of PASG remains controversial, one indication of their use that still remains is for the management of pelvic fractures, particularly during transport. PASG can immobilize the pelvic bones and provide a tamponade effect that may prevent retroperitoneal bleeding.[8]

14. **C. Analysis.** Blood loss from a pelvic fracture has been found to range between 750 to 6,000 ml. The emergency care should be directed to replacing the patient's lost volume and monitoring the effects of the resuscitation.[6,8]

15. **D. Assessment.** An open pelvic fracture results in a direct communication between the fracture and the vagina, perineum, groin, rectum, or laceration. Signs and symptoms of an open pelvic fracture include paresis, ecchymosis of the perineum, groin, flanks, blood from the urethra and vagina, and a high-riding prostate.[9]

16. **B. Assessment.** Because of the large vessels located in the pelvis, the most serious complication of an open pelvic fracture is exsanguination.[9]

17. **C. Evaluation.** Open pelvic fractures have a high mortality of between 40% and 60%. The major cause of early death is exsanguination. Late death from open pelvic fractures is associated with multiple organ failure and sepsis.[9]

18. **C. Evaluation.** Pain medication will only help the patient tolerate pain. Until the ankle is appropriately treated and healing begins, the pain will not be gone.

19. **A. Intervention.** All of the interventions listed are indicated in the early care of this patient; however, the first priority is to provide supplemental oxygen. Tachypnea, restlessness, and cyanosis are clear-cut signs of respiratory distress and must be addressed immediately.[8]

20. **D. Assessment.** A serious complication in patients who have sustained long bone fractures is fat embolus. This phenomenon is characteristically seen 12 to 48 hours after injury. The remobilization is thought to be a result of fat and marrow break-off directly related to the fracture, as well as a result of changes in circulating lipids secondary to stress.[8]

21. **C. Assessment.** Interpretation of the ABCs should begin with the pH. Normal pH is 7.35 to 7.45. Because this patient's pH is reported at 7.21, he is in a state of acidosis. Next, note the $PCO_2$. This reflects the respiratory side of the acid-base equation. Normally the value should be 35 to 45 mm Hg. A value of 66 mm Hg indicates retained carbon dioxide. A normal bicarbonate level is 22 to 26 MEq and represents the metabolic or buffer system component. The patient's value of 26 falls within the normal range. This patient's blood gases demonstrate a respiratory acidosis.[10]

22. **D. Analysis.** The respiratory compromise this patient is experiencing is at the alveolar-capillary level, where carbon dioxide–oxygen exchange occurs. Because emboli have obstructed vessels in the lungs, there is a decreased area in which gas exchange can take place.[6]

23. **C. Intervention.** 25,000 U in 500 ml is 50 U/ml. To determine the number of milliliters per hour, divide what is desired (1,000 U) by what you have (50 U) to arrive at the correct amount of 20 ml/h.[7]

24. **C. Assessment.** Compartment syndrome is a real possibility in orthopedic injuries whose mechanism of injury is a crushing force. The most common site of development is the anterior compartment of the lower leg.[8] The forearm may also be affected.

25. **B. Assessment.** There are both external and internal causes of compartment syndrome. Internal causes include crushing injuries, burns, spider and snakebites, and prolonged hypotension and ischemia. External causes of compartment syndrome include prolonged application of PASG, skeletal traction, or lying in the same position for an extended period of time.[8]

26. **D. Assessment.** Compartment syndrome develops when tissue pressures within a limited space, the muscle compartment, exceed the intraarterial hydrostatic pressure, causing collapse of capillaries and venules, and subsequent tissue necrosis. Loss of a pulse distal to the affected area is a late sign. Initial and frequent checks for motion, sensation, and capillary refill are most valuable in detecting this complication early.[5]

27. **A. Intervention.** A hallmark sign of developing compartment syndrome is severe pain, not relieved by narcotics, that increases with muscle stretching.

This finding needs to be reported immediately, so that proper medical intervention may ensue.[5]

28. **B. Intervention.** The quick and easy way of obtaining compartment pressures is with a setup using a three-way stopcock, IV tubing, a syringe of saline, and a mercury manometer. Normal compartment pressures should be less than 20 mm Hg.[11]

29. **C. Evaluation.** When this complication advances to the stage of muscle death, myoglobinuria and subsequent renal complications may develop.[8]

30. **D. Analysis.** This diagnosis is defined as a decrease in oxygenation and nutrition at the cellular level due to a deficit in capillary blood supply.[6] This is an accurate physiological description of what happens in compartment syndrome.

31. **C. Assessment.** The possibility of reimplantation decreases with amount of damage done to the amputated parts; availability of an experienced reimplantation team; and the amount of time that has elapsed since the injury. Generally greater than 24 hours decreases the changes of a successful reimplantation.[10]

32. **B. Intervention.** When fitting patients with crutches the arm piece should be 2 inches or two finger widths from the axilla; no weight should be placed on the axilla because nerve damage may occur; the tips of the crutches should be placed 6 inches to the side and to the front; and the elbows flexed at 30 degrees.[10]

33. **D. Intervention.** The joint and extremity should be immobilized in position of comfort initially unless there is neurovascular compromise. If there is neurovascular compromise, only gentle traction should be applied until the pulse returns. Constricting jewelry should be removed to prevent further damage.[12]

34. **B. Assessment.** The most common pathogen to cause a septic joint, particularly in a young person, is the gonococcal organism.[13]

35. **D. Assessment.** Evidence-based research has demonstrated that ankle radiographs are not always necessary to rule out a fracture. The Ottawa Ankle Rules state that a radiograph should be obtained when:
- The patient is unable to bear weight on their ankle immediately after injury or in the emergency department
- The patient has bone tenderness at the posterior edge or tip of the lateral malleolus
- The patient has bone tenderness at the posterior edge or tip of the medial malleolus[13]

## REFERENCES

1. Walker J: Orthopedic emergencies. In Jordan K, editor: *Emergency nursing core curriculum,* ed 5, Philadelphia, 2000, WB Saunders.
2. Bickley LS: *Bate's guide to physical examination and history taking,* Philadelphia, 1999, Lippincott.
3. Engel J: *Pediatric assessment,* St Louis, 1993, Mosby.
4. Phelan A: Musculoskeletal trauma. In Kelley S, editor: *Pediatric emergency nursing,* Norwalk, 1994, Appleton & Lange.
5. Jagmin MG: Musculoskeletal emergencies. In Kitt S and others, editors: *Emergency nursing: a physiologic and clinical perspective,* Philadelphia, 1995, WB Saunders.
6. Kim MJ, McFarland GK, McLane AM: *Pocket guide to nursing diagnoses,* St Louis, 1993, Mosby.
7. McKenry L, Salerno E: *Pharmacology in nursing,* St Louis, 1998, Mosby.
8. Strange JM, Kelly PM: Musculoskeletal injuries. In Cardona V, and others, editors: *Trauma nursing: from resuscitation through rehabilitation,* Philadelphia, 1994, WB Saunders.
9. Ziglar M, Parrish R: An 18-year-old male patient with multiple trauma including an open pelvic fracture, *J Emerg Nurs* 20:265-270, 1994.
10. James C: Orthopedic and neurovascular trauma. In Newberry L, editor: *Sheehy's emergency nursing principles and practice,* ed 4, St Louis, 1998, Mosby.
11. Proehl J: Compression syndrome, *J Emerg Nurs* 14:283-290, 1988.
12. Campbell J: Extremity trauma. In Campbell J, editor: *Basic trauma life support,* ed 4, Upper Saddle River, NJ, 2000, Brady/Prentice Hall Health.
13. Selfridge-Thomas J: *Emergency nursing an essential guide for patient care,* Philadelphia, 1997, WB Saunders.

# Chapter 16

# Pain Management

## REVIEW OUTLINE

I. Definition of pain
  A. From the Greek word *poine,* which means penalty or punishment
  B. Pain[1]: is a sensory experience associated with actual or potential tissue damage as well as physiological and psychological responses. Pain is a personal experience and may be whatever the patient says it is. Pain is manifested in both verbal and nonverbal behaviors, physiological responses, and emotional and spiritual responses.
  C. Acute pain
  D. Chronic pain

II. Sources of pain in the prehospital, transport, and emergency department environments
  A. Pain from the illness of injury
  B. Pain from procedures
    1. Intravenous insertion
    2. Gastric tube insertion
    3. Blood draws
    4. Chest tube insertion
    5. Cardiopulmonary resuscitation (CPR)
  C. Environment
    1. Noise
    2. Light
    3. Excessive heat or cold

III. Perception and response to pain
  A. Patient's previous experience with pain
  B. Source of the pain
    1. Physical
    2. Emotional
    3. Spiritual
  C. Caregiver reactions to the patient's pain
  D. Response to pain learned and influenced by
    1. Age
    2. Socioeconomic status
    3. Gender
    4. Ethnicity
    5. Cultural beliefs
    6. Values

IV. Barriers to pain management in the prehospital, transport, and emergency department environment
  A. Lack of knowledge about pain management
  B. Lack of knowledge about pharmacology of pain medications
  C. Fear of addiction
  D. Respiratory depression and hypotension
  E. Concentrating on life-threatening illness and injury

V. Physiology of pain
  A. Nociceptors
  B. A-fibers
  C. C-fibers
  D. Spinal cord
  E. Neurons
    1. Medial
    2. Lateral
  F. Afferent pathways
  G. Efferent pathways

VI. Theories of pain
  A. Gate theory of pain
  B. Pattern theory
  C. Neurotransmitters

VII. Pain assessment
  A. Identify the source of the pain
  B. Determine the level of the pain (pain rating)
    1. FACES pain rating scale
    2. Numeric pain scales
    3. Visual analog scales
  C. Determine the patient's response to the pain
    1. Physiological
    2. Emotional
    3. Spiritual
  D. Related nursing diagnoses
    1. Pain
    2. Pain, chronic

VIII. Pain management
  A. Patient's past experiences
  B. Conscious sedation

C. Pain management pharmacology
   1. Opioids
   2. Dissociative agents
   3. Benzodiazepines
   4. Non-opioid agents
   5. Sedative, hypnotics
   6. Local anesthetics
IX. Patient assessment and management
   A. Monitoring of airway, breathing, circulation (ABCs)
      1. Respiratory rate
      2. Pulse oximeter
      3. $CO_2$ monitoring
   B. Circulation
      1. Cardiac monitor
      2. Blood pressure
      3. Pulse
   C. Neurological status
      1. Protect patient from injury
      2. Orient patient
      3. Decrease outside stimulation
   D. Patient's response is dosage related
   E. Availability of appropriate antagonists
   F. Sedation scale
   G. Additional methods to manage pain and enhance pharmacological management
      1. Cutaneous stimulation
         a. Hot
         b. Cold
      2. Distraction
      3. Relaxation
      4. Proper positioning
      5. Soaking
      6. Comfort measures
      7. Therapeutic presence
      8. Therapeutic touch
      9. Music
      10. Therapeutic listening
      11. Accupressure
      12. Acupuncture

## REVIEW QUESTIONS

1. Acute pain is:
   O   A. Persistent over a period of time, usually 6 months or greater
   O   B. May be the result of an unknown source causing suffering
   O   C. Makes one feel hopeless, depressed, and powerlessness
   O   D. Is a significant sign of a physical or emotional injury

2. Reasons why pain management is not always given high priority in patient care in the prehospital setting include:
   O   A. Prehospital providers are well-versed about the pharmacology of pain management
   O   B. Administration of a dissociative agent in the prehospital environment may cause significant respiratory depression
   O   C. Prehospital providers are not concerned about the patient becoming addicted to narcotics
   O   D. Prehospital providers are more focused on the patient's illness or injury, and pain management is not a primary concern

3. A 3-month-old infant is brought to the emergency department by his parents. The parents state that he has not stopped crying. He has a firm, distended abdomen. The diagnosis of peritonitis and sepsis is made. An example of inappropriate information related to the management of pain in the pediatric patient is:
   O   A. Children respond the same as an adult to most pain medications
   O   B. Children's nervous systems are immature, and they perceive pain differently
   O   C. It is easier to hold small children down (brutaine) then to medicate them
   O   D. Children will experience respiratory depression more quickly than the adult patient

4. Reliable indicators of pain in the neonate include all of the following *except:*
   O   A. Squeezing their eyes shut
   O   B. Palmar sweating
   O   C. No change in heart rate
   O   D. Nasolabial furrow

5. Stimulation of the nociceptors causes the release of:
   O   A. Histamines
   O   B. Endorphins
   O   C. Enkephalins
   O   D. GABA

6. Pain medications used in the prehospital and emergency department environment should:
   O   A. Possess multiple side effects
   O   B. Have a long duration of action
   O   C. Produce multiple complications
   O   D. Provide sedation as well as analgesia

7. The medication ketamine is classified as a:
   - O  A. Sedative-hypnotic
   - O  B. Dissociative agent
   - O  C. Local anesthetic
   - O  D. Non-opioid analgesic

8. A 42-year-old male was given fentanyl and midazolam intravenously for conscious sedation to reduce his fractured ankle. A splint has been applied and he is to be referred to his orthopedic physician for follow-up. The emergency nurse may determine that the patient is ready to be discharged when:
   - O  A. His family is ready to take him home by car
   - O  B. He easily falls back to sleep when not stimulated
   - O  C. He can ambulate using his crutches
   - O  D. When his oxygen saturation ranges between 85% and 90%

9. The transport team is called to a referring facility to transport a patient who has been involved in an all-terrain vehicle (ATV) rollover. He is awake and alert, but in acute respiratory distress because of a severe pulmonary contusion and multiple rib fractures. His oxygen saturation is 90% on high flow oxygen. Because of the length of the transport, the patient is intubated using RSI for oxygenation. He is given vecuronium to facilitate his oxygenation. During the 3-hour transport, which medications will the patient require for comfort?
   - O  A. Midazolam and vecuronium for sedation and amnesia during the length of the transport from the referring to the receiving facility
   - O  B. Fentanyl and vecuronium for sedation and analgesia during the length of the transport from the receiving to the referring facility
   - O  C. Morphine sulfate and vecuronium for analgesia and to facilitate oxygenation during the length of the transport from the referring to the receiving facility
   - O  D. Fentanyl, midazolam and vecuronium for sedation, amnesia, analgesia and to facilitate ventilation and oxygenation

10. Massage may be effective in relieving pain in selected situations because:
   - O  A. It decreases the blood flow to the injured area
   - O  B. Causes retention of the toxins to only the injured area

- O  C. It releases the patient's endorphins through relaxation
- O  D. The patient wants it to no matter what others may say

## ANSWERS

1. **D. Assessment.** Acute pain is a significant sign of a physical or emotional injury. It is sudden in onset and works as a protective mechanism. Patients experiencing acute pain are hopeful that it will be relieved soon.[1]

2. **D. Intervention.** Explanations for not providing pain management in the prehospital and emergency care environment include:
   a. Lack of knowledge about pain management and pain medications
   b. Fear of causing addiction (both the patient and the care provider)
   c. Respiratory depression and hypotension may occur with the administration of some pain medications
   d. Focus on the patient's illness or injury.[2] The risk of adverse effects in the pediatric patient being treated with pain medications are directly related to the rate of drug administration, total dose, and combination with other medications.[4]

3. **B. Assessment.** Myths about children and pain management include:
   a. Children perceive pain differently than adults because they have immature nervous systems
   b. Children are more sensitive to pain medication than adults and may suffer a respiratory arrest if given pain medication
   c. It is easier to hold a small child down (brutaine) than to administer pain medication[3,4]

4. **C. Assessment.** Indicators of pain in the neonate include:
   a. Changes in heart and respiratory rates, including both bradycardia and tachycardia
   b. Palmar sweating
   c. Vagal tone
   d. Nasolabial furrow
   e. Crying[4]

5. **A. Assessment.** Stimulation of the nociceptors causes the release of histamines, serotonin, bradykinins, prostaglandins, potassium, and acetylcholine.[5]

6. **D. Intervention.** Pain medications that are used in the prehospital and emergency department environments should:
   a. Cause minimal side effects.
   b. Possess uniform efficacy.

c. Have a short and controllable duration of action.

d. Possess few contraindications.

e. Produce both a sedative and analgesic affect. In order to do this most effectively, combinations of medications generally need to be administered.

7. **B. Assessment.** Ketamine is a dissociative agent that causes dissociation between the thalamoneocortical and limbic systems, preventing higher centers from perceiving visual, auditory, and painful stimuli.[6]

8. **C. Evaluation.** The patient who has undergone a procedure that required conscious sedation should be awake, able to ambulate (this patient would need to demonstrate this with crutches); drink and swallow.[1]

9. **D. Intervention.** The patient will require medications that will provide sedation, amnesia, analgesia and assist in facilitating ventilation and oxygenation.[7,8]

10. **C. Intervention.** Research has demonstrated that massage therapy may be useful in decreasing patient pain in selected situations because:

a. It causes the release of endorphins through relaxation

b. It releases toxins from the injured area

c. Touch has been demonstrated to assist in pain management

d. It increases blood flow to the injured area[9]

## REFERENCES

1. Albrecht S, Bernardo L: Pain management. In Jordan K, editor: *Emergency nursing core curriculum,* ed 5, Philadelphia, 2000, WB Saunders.

2. Selbst M, Clark M: Analgesic use in the emergency department, *Ann Emerg Med* 19(9):1010-1013, 1990.

3. Woolard D, Terndrup T: Sedative-analgesic agent administration in children: Analysis of use and complications in the emergency department, *J Emerg Med* 12(4):453-461, 1994.

4. American Academy of Pediatrics: Prevention and management of pain and stress in the neonate, *AAP Policy Statement* 105(2):454-461, 2000.

5. Trautman D: Pain management. In Newberry L, editor: *Sheehy's emergency nursing principles and practice,* ed 4, St Louis, 1998, Mosby.

6. Barsan W, Jastremski M, Syverud S: *Emergency drug therapy,* Philadelphia, 1991, WB Saunders.

7. Semonin-Holleran R, editor: *Flight nursing principles and practice.* St Louis, 1996, Mosby.

8. Krupa D, editor: *Flight nursing core curriculum,* Park Ridge, IL, 1997, Road Runner Press.

9. Morse J: The science of comforting, *Reflections* 22(4):6-10, 1996.

# Chapter 17 _____

# Respiratory Emergencies

**REVIEW OUTLINE**

I. Anatomy and physiology[1]
   A. Anatomy
      1. Nasal cavity
      2. Oropharynx
      3. Mucous membrane
      4. Larynx
      5. Epiglottis
      6. Vocal cords
      7. Cricothyroid membrane
      8. Trachea
      9. Bronchi
     10. Bronchiole
     11. Alveoli
     12. Lung parenchyma (right three lobes; left two lobes)
     13. Pleura
     14. Mediastinum
     15. Sternum
     16. Manubrium
     17. Xiphoid process
     18. Sternal angle
     19. Scapulae
     20. Clavicle
     21. Ribs
     22. Thoracic vertebrae
     23. Esophagus
     24. Heart
     25. Diaphragm
     26. Intercostal muscles
     27. Accessory muscles
     28. Expiratory muscles
     29. Aorta
     30. Nerves associated with respirations
   B. Physiology
      1. Oxygen transport, gas exchange
      2. Ventilation: inspiration, expiration
      3. Tidal volume
      4. Nervous system innervations
      5. Positive-negative pressure flow system

II. Assessment[1-3]
   A. Inspection
      1. Airway patency
      2. Work of breathing
        a. Use of accessory muscles
        b. Level of consciousness
        c. Respiratory rate and depth
        d. Skin color
        e. Cyanosis
        f. Flaring of nares
        g. Sternal retraction
        h. Patient's posture
      3. Tachypnea
      4. Bradypnea
      5. Apnea
      6. Splinting
      7. Audible wheezing
      8. Inspiratory stridor
      9. Productive cough, sputum
     10. Presence of wounds, scars, impaled objects
   B. Palpation
      1. Pain, tenderness
      2. Crepitus
      3. Skin temperature
   C. Assessment landmarks
      1. Anterior chest
        a. Midsternal line
        b. Anterior axillary line
        c. Midaxillary line
      2. Posterior chest
        a. Posterior axillary line
        b. Scapular line
        c. Vertebral line
   D. Percussion
      1. Flatness
      2. Dullness
      3. Resonance
      4. Hyperresonance
      5. Tympany
   E. Auscultation
      1. Evaluate all lung fields
      2. Inspiration, expiration
      3. Normal breath sounds
        a. Vesicular
        b. Bronchovesicular

c. Bronchial

d. Tracheal

4. Adventitious breath sounds

   a. Wheezes

   b. Rhonchi

   c. Crackles

5. Absence of breath sounds

F. Age-related characteristics[1-3]

1. Pediatric

   a. Pediatric airway smaller and shorter than adult

   b. Tongue is large and may easily block the airway

   c. Cricothyroid membrane narrow, forming an anatomical cuff

   d. Chest is rounded in children under 6 years of age

   e. Infant's sternum is pliable and may appear to be "caving" in with inspiration

   f. Children less than 7 years of age use their diaphragm for breathing

   g. Chest wall is thinner in younger children

   h. Ribs and sternum more cartilaginous and flexible in younger children

   i. Respiratory rates faster in infants and young children

2. Geriatric

   a. Vital capacity decreases

   b. Skeletal changes of aging may result in kyphosis or "barrel chest"

   c. Gag reflex diminishes, leaving elderly adult at greater risk for aspiration

G. History

1. Onset of symptoms

2. History of trauma, mechanism of injury

3. Pain on inspiration or expiration

4. Cough

   a. Onset

   b. Sputum

   c. Related symptoms

   d. Time of the day

5. Fever, chills

6. Smoking history

7. Medical history

8. Productive cough, sputum

9. Work history (e.g., "black lung")

10. Environmental history

11. Date of last tuberculosis (TB) test, chest radiograph

12. HIV status

13. Recent international travel

14. Recent travel in southwestern United States or hiking and staying in an enclosed space where rodents may live

15. Associated diseases (e.g., heart disease, emphysema, asthma, allergies)

H. Diagnostic studies or procedures

1. Chest radiograph studies

2. Blood gases

   a. pH

   b. $pCO_2$

   c. $pO_2$

   d. $HCO_3$

   e. Arterial

   f. Capillary

   g. Venous

3. Pulse oximetry

4. End-tidal $CO_2$ monitoring

5. ECG

6. Sputum evaluation

7. Laboratory tests

   a. CBC with differential

   b. Electrolytes

   c. Amylase

   d. Liver function tests

8. CT/MRI/ultrasound of the chest

9. Esophagogram

10. Lung scan (VQ scan)

III. Related nursing diagnoses

A. Airway clearance, ineffective

B. Anxiety

C. Aspiration, high risk for

D. Breathing pattern, ineffective

E. Fatigue

F. Fear

G. Gas exchange, impaired

H. Infection, high risk for

I. Knowledge deficit

J. Pain

IV. Collaborative care of the patient with a respiratory emergency

A. Airway management

1. Airway adjuncts

2. Delivery of oxygen

3. Intubation

B. Ventilation

1. Bronchodilators

2. Humidification

C. Cardiac monitor

D. Antibiotics

E. Thoracentesis

F. Autotransfusion

G. Chest tube insertion

H. Thoracotomy (open and closed)

V. Specific respiratory emergencies
   A. Chest pain differentiation
   B. Chronic obstructive pulmonary disease
   C. Pneumonia
   D. Acute respiratory distress syndrome (ARDS)
   E. Pulmonary embolus
   F. Hyperventilation syndrome
   G. Epiglottitis
   H. Croup
   I. Bronchiolitis
   J. Foreign body aspiration
   K. Rib fractures
   L. Flail chest
   M. Pneumothorax
   N. Tension pneumothorax
   O. Hemothorax
   P. Pulmonary contusion
   Q. Ruptured diaphragm
   R. Tracheal trauma

No matter what the origin of the respiratory emergency, the emergency nursing assessment of the patient must begin with an evaluation of the patient's airway and its patency, effort and effectiveness of ventilation, and the level of oxygenation. Many triage areas now have a pulse oximeter available to obtain a "spot" check on the status of the patient in respiratory distress and provide the emergency nurse with additional noninvasive information about the patient.

The amount of data that is collected in relation to the patient's respiratory distress will depend on the patient's history and ability to provide information. Many patients and their families with chronic respiratory problems who develop distress are quite well versed in the treatment of their disease and can be a good source of information concerning what they need.

Shortness of breath (dyspnea), chest pain, cough, and cyanosis may be difficult symptoms to quickly classify their cause. Chest pain may be pulmonary, cardiac, or of an abdominal origin. Cyanosis may be the result of poor perfusion or a toxicological emergency.[4] Just as with other body systems, the respiratory system may be the source of the disease or injury or simply where the disease or injuries' symptoms manifest themselves.

## Chest Pain

The assessment of the patient with chest pain can cause some difficult problems for the emergency nurse. There are numerous causes of chest pain, including those that require emergent interventions and those that may require little, if any, nursing and/or medical care.

The origins of chest pain may include asthma, acute bronchitis, chronic obstructive pulmonary disease (COPD), pneumonia, pulmonary embolus, and/or a traumatic injury to the chest that may result in rib fractures, pulmonary contusion, pneumothorax, or hemothorax.

## Asthma

Asthma is a response of the lung to various stimuli that cause narrowing of the airway. These stimuli may include specific allergens, such as dust and molds, stress, or intoxicants.[4] Even though asthma can be successfully treated in the emergency department, the death rate from acute asthma has been increasing. Reasons that have been suggested for this increase in death include the lack of access to care and the increased use of bronchodilators that may mask a worsening respiratory status. The National Heart, Lung, and Blood Institute have issued Guidelines for the Diagnosis and Management of Asthma. These guidelines act as an algorithm for the treatment of asthmatics in the emergency department and offer one of the few ways patients may receive evidence based care.[5]

## Chest Trauma

Chest trauma accounts for approximately 25% of deaths related to trauma.[6] The patient with chest trauma requires a rapid and organized emergency nursing assessment so that injuries and potential threats to life, such as a tension pneumothorax, can be rapidly identified and appropriate interventions provided.

It is important to keep in mind that trauma to the chest may not result in injury to the chest alone. Contained in the thoracic cavity are the heart, great vessels, and some abdominal organs. Injuries to any of these vessels or organs can be life threatening.

## Pediatric Respiratory Emergencies

The most common cause of cardiopulmonary arrest in the pediatric patient is interference with the child's airway and ventilation.[3,7,8] The child's airway is different from the adult airway. It is smaller in diameter and shorter in length. The tongue is larger and may easily obstruct the airway. The narrowest part of the pediatric airway is the cricothyroid ring, which forms a physiologic cuff. These differences require that the emergency nurse be familiar not only with the impact of these differences but also with how the pediatric airway should be appropriately managed.

Signs and symptoms of pediatric respiratory distress include the following: increased respiratory rate, decreased respiratory rate, apnea, fatigue, head bobbing, stridor, prolonged expiration, grunting, retractions, nasal flaring, altered mental status, and cyanosis.[3,7,8]

## Pulmonary Diseases

Over the past 10 years, emergency departments (EDs) have seen an increase in various pulmonary diseases that may be entities in and of themselves or symptoms of other disease states. For example, the patient who is HIV positive may also have a viral or fungal type of pneumonia. Pneumonia that may be seen in the HIV-infected patient include PCP, histoplasmosis, cryptococcosis, Legionella, and Nocardia.[10]

There has been a significant increase in the number of patients with tuberculosis in recent years in the United States. Many of these patients seek care in the emergency department, which poses particular challenges to emergency nursing practice.[11] Some of these challenges include early identification of the disease, appropriate triage and isolation of infected patients, and provision of methods to decrease the emergency department staff's risk of infection.

Finally, because of the emergence of unfamiliar diseases, such as the hantavirus, or the reemergence of diseases thought conquered, such as pertussis, the emergency nurse needs to continuously keep up-to-date on information that protects not only their patients but also themselves.[12]

## REVIEW QUESTIONS

### Asthma

*A 30-year-old man comes to the ED complaining of shortness of breath. The patient states that he has been treated for asthma in the past and has not taken any medication for over a month. He is alert, oriented, and barely able to speak. His color is pale and his skin is diaphoretic.*

1. What specific physical signs may indicate acute respiratory distress in the adult asthmatic patient?
   O   A. Paroxysmal coughing
   O   B. Sternocleidomastoid retractions
   O   C. Audible wheezing
   O   D. Nausea and vomiting

2. This patient has a PEF of 85 L/min. This is an indication of:
   O   A. Moderate obstruction
   O   B. No obstruction
   O   C. Severe obstruction
   O   D. Minor obstruction

3. After assessment of this patient's lung function, what intervention should the emergency nurse initiate?
   O   A. Administration of a corticosteroid
   O   B. Administration of theophylline
   O   C. Administration of a bronchodilator
   O   D. Administration of an antibiotic

4. An initial nursing diagnosis for the patient having an acute asthmatic attack may be:
   O   A. Health maintenance, altered related to his diagnosis of asthma
   O   B. Fluid volume excess related to his fluid intake
   O   C. Activity intolerance related to his diagnosis of asthma
   O   D. Anxiety related to his inability to breathe

5. The emergency physician orders a dose of methylprednisone for the patient. The most effective way to administer the drug to this patient is?
   O   A. Orally
   O   B. Inhaler
   O   C. Intramuscularly
   O   D. Intravenously

6. An indication that the asthmatic patient may need to be intubated would include all of the following *except:*
   O   A. A change in mental status, such as confusion, agitation, or unresponsiveness
   O   B. Respiratory arrest from work of breathing and fatigue
   O   C. Blood gas results of pH, 7.35; $Po_2$, 100; and $Pco_2$, 40
   O   D. Inability of the patient to talk and provide an adequate history

7. A trigger of pediatric asthma in an urban setting is:
   O   A. Soy bean pollen
   O   B. Cockroaches
   O   C. Pigeon feathers
   O   D. Horse dandruff

8. An ominous sign that indicates marked airflow obstruction in the asthmatic is:
   O   A. Expiratory wheezing
   O   B. Expiratory stridor
   O   C. Paroxysmal coughing
   O   D. "Silent chest"

9. The most effective method of administering a bronchodilator to a patient in severe distress is:
   - O  A. Administering the medications every hour
   - O  B. Continuous nebulization of the medication
   - O  C. Two to three puffs every 3 to 4 hours
   - O  D. Allow the patient to chose which method is most comfortable

10. When teaching the patient with asthma how to use a metered dose inhaler (MDI), the emergency nurse should instruct him or her to:
    - O  A. Clean the mouthpiece daily with soap and water
    - O  B. Soak the mouthpiece for 20 minutes daily in Clorox
    - O  C. Store the canister in the freezer to keep the drug potent
    - O  D. Use the MDI as often as the patient thinks that he or she needs it

## Pneumonia

*The paramedics bring a 52-year-old man to the ED. He generally lives outside, but the weather has been cold and he was forced to live in the local shelter. Today, he presents with fever, chills, and a productive cough of blood-tinged yellow sputum. A chest radiograph reveals a right lower lobe pneumonia. He states that he has smoked 1 to 2 packs per day for 40 years and has not received any preventive health care for 5 years.*

11. Pneumonia, an acute infection of the lung parenchyma, may be caused by all of the following *except*:
    - O  A. *Mycoplasma pneumoniae*
    - O  B. *Legionella pneumophila*
    - O  C. Human immunodeficiency virus
    - O  D. *Streptococcus pneumoniae*

12. An important emergency nursing intervention for the patient being treated for pneumonia is:
    - O  A. Ordering the appropriate antibiotic to treat the infection
    - O  B. Providing the patient with fluids and obtaining a sputum
    - O  C. Deciding when the patient should be intubated
    - O  D. Ordering a blood gas analysis to evaluate oxygenation

13. One method that can measure the ventilatory status of this patient is:
    - O  A. Placing him on a pulse oximeter with a disposable probe
    - O  B. Placing the patient on a cardiac and apnea monitor
    - O  C. Placing the patient on a $CO_2$ monitor
    - O  D. Placing the patient on a noninvasive blood pressure monitor

14. Factors that may limit the usefulness of a pulse oximeter include:
    - O  A. Limited ambient light
    - O  B. Carbon monoxide poisoning
    - O  C. Normovolemia
    - O  D. Limited patient movement

15. Atypical infiltrates are also noted on this patient's chest radiograph. Active tuberculosis is diagnosed in addition to his pneumonia. This patient:
    - O  A. Should remain in the treatment room he is currently in
    - O  B. Be discharged back to the homeless shelter for care
    - O  C. Be admitted to an open ward on the floor
    - O  D. Be moved to a controlled air flow room for isolation

## Chest Pain

*A 30-year-old woman comes to the ED with severe chest pain, shortness of breath, and diaphoresis. She states that the pain began suddenly and is crushing. Her B/P (palpable) is 80, her monitor shows a sinus tachycardia, and her RR is 48.*

16. When obtaining a history from this patient specific to the complaint of chest pain, the emergency nurse should ask about:
    - O  A. Any history of recent surgery or long bone fractures
    - O  B. The date of the patient's last chest radiograph
    - O  C. The patient's previous occupation
    - O  D. Any history of hyperventilation

17. The patient states she recently had an abdominal hysterectomy. A fluid bolus of 500 ml normal saline brings the patient's blood pressure to 100/60. An emergent lung scan is performed and demonstrates a pulmonary embolus. What medication should be started in the emergency department to treat this patient?
    - O  A. Heparin calcium
    - O  B. Dicumarol
    - O  C. Dipyridamole
    - O  D. Vitamin K

18. Based on the patient's presenting blood pressure, which nursing diagnosis is appropriate to mange her care?
    - O  A. Injury, high risk for, related to her recent surgery
    - O  B. Tissue perfusion, altered (cardiopulmonary), manifested by her hypotension
    - O  C. Thought processes, altered, related to her hypotension
    - O  D. Skin integrity, impaired, related to her hypotension

19. The patient is given a bolus of 10,000 units of heparin, and a drip is begun at the rate of 1,000 U/h. Potential complications with the use of heparin include:
    - O  A. Intracerebral hemorrhage
    - O  B. Chills, fever, and urticaria
    - O  C. Oral and rectal bleeding
    - O  D. All of the above

*A 17-year-old man presents to triage complaining of shortness of breath, severe chest pain, and difficulty swallowing. The triage nurse notes that the patient's voice is hoarse and he is sitting forward in order to breathe.*

20. What important piece of history should the triage nurse obtain?
    - O  A. The date of the patient's last immunization
    - O  B. Recent use of illicit drugs
    - O  C. Presence of breath sounds bilaterally
    - O  D. Presence of ST elevation in lead II

21. The patient is taken emergently into the treatment area. A physical finding that may indicate a pneumomediastinum is:
    - O  A. Hamman's crunch
    - O  B. Kernig's sign
    - O  C. Kerr's sign
    - O  D. Homans' sign

22. A complication of pneumomediastinum includes:
    - O  A. Neck pain
    - O  B. Sore throat
    - O  C. Pneumothorax
    - O  D. Pericardial tamponade

*The rescue squad brings a 53-year-old man to the ED. The patient was found camping outside and states he is from out of town and has yet to find a new home. He states that he has a history of alcohol abuse and has not eaten for 2 days.*

*The patient is complaining of shortness of breath, a cough, and fatigue.*

23. All of the following place this patient at risk for tuberculosis *except:*
    - O  A. Alcohol abuse
    - O  B. Homelessness
    - O  C. Proper diet
    - O  D. His age

24. A primary screening tool for tuberculosis is:
    - O  A. Chest radiograph
    - O  B. Acid-fast bacteria (AFB) sputum smears
    - O  C. Blood cultures
    - O  D. Purified protein derivatives (PPD)

**Pediatric Respiratory Emergencies**

25. A rare cause of chest pain in the pediatric patient is:
    - O  A. Asthma
    - O  B. Pneumonia
    - O  C. Kawasaki's disease
    - O  D. Rib fracture

26. A 5-year-old girl is brought to the ED by her family. Her parents state that she has been febrile, lethargic, and unable to lie down and has been drooling. During the initial assessment of this patient, the emergency nurse should do all of the following *except:*
    - O  A. Assess the child's level of consciousness
    - O  B. Look down the child's throat
    - O  C. Assess the child's respiratory status
    - O  D. Assess the child's circulatory status

27. The initial care for the child who is suffering respiratory distress from acute epiglottitis would include:
    - O  A. Administration of chloramphenicol
    - O  B. Administration of racemic epinephrine
    - O  C. Obtaining x-ray films of the child's neck
    - O  D. Preparing the child for intubation

28. The most common cause of epiglottitis is:
    - O  A. Streptococcus
    - O  B. *Haemophilus influenzae*
    - O  C. Staphylococcus
    - O  D. Pneumococcus

29. A mother comes to the ED carrying her 18-month-old child, who has stridor and is cyanotic. The mother states that the child was eating a hot dog before her symptoms began.

The emergency nurse's initial interventions should include:

0  A. Opening the child's mouth and trying to remove the food
0  B. Delivering four back blows and four chest thrusts
0  C. Grabbing the child by the legs and turning her upside down
0  D. Performing a needle cricothyrotomy with a 14-gauge needle

30. The emergency nurse performs the appropriate sequence of foreign body airway obstruction (FBAO) management for the conscious infant. An indication that the maneuvers are not being effective is:

0  A. Expulsion of the object
0  B. The child begins to cry
0  C. The child becomes unconscious
0  D. The child's color improves

31. The most common item aspirated by children less than 3 years of age is:

0  A. A toy
0  B. A hot dog
0  C. A peanut
0  D. Hard candy

32. Foreign-body aspiration should be suspected in the pediatric patient when:

0  A. The child does not respond to conventional treatment for respiratory distress
0  B. The child's chest x-ray film does not show any infiltrates or pneumothoraces
0  C. The child's respiratory rate returns to normal after conventional interventions
0  D. The child is found to be afebrile after emergency department hydration

33. The initial management of the child experiencing an acute asthma attack is:

0  A. Administration of bronchodilators
0  B. Hydration with 20 ml/kg of normal saline
0  C. Administration of high-flow oxygen by nasal cannula
0  D. Administration of prophylactic antibiotics

34. A 3-month-old infant is brought to the ED by his parents because of a "stuffy" nose and difficulty breathing. When teaching the parents how to care for the sick infant, the emergency nurse should be sure that the parents understand all of the following except:

0  A. Infants lose fluids through rapid breathing
0  B. Infants are obligate nose breathers
0  C. Infants cry when sick and may never be consoled
0  D. Infants need to be kept warm but not made excessively warm

35. Respiratory syncytial virus (RSV) is not transmitted by:

0  A. Large droplet aerosols
0  B. Sneezing
0  C. Visitors
0  D. Hand washing

## Thoracic Trauma
### Pneumothorax

*A 30-year-old man has attempted suicide by shooting himself in the left upper chest. On arrival in the ED, the patient is alert, complaining of shortness of breath, and is pale and diaphoretic. His vital signs are B/P (palpable) 80, HR 140, RR 32.*

36. The emergency nurse needs to assess quickly for the presence of:

0  A. Breath sounds
0  B. Peripheral edema
0  C. Capillary refill
0  D. Altered mental status

37. No breath sounds are auscultated on the left side. The patient respiratory distress increases and he becomes agitated. Until a physician is available, a critical intervention the emergency nurse may perform is:

0  A. Obtain central line access
0  B. Perform needle thoracostomy
0  C. Place the patient on a pulse oximeter
0  D. Obtain an emergent chest radiograph

38. Based on the emergency nurse's initial assessment of this patient, the primary nursing diagnosis would be:

0  A. Injury, high risk for related to a gunshot wound to the chest
0  B. Fluid volume deficit related to a gunshot wound to the chest
0  C. Activity intolerance related to the gunshot wound to the chest
0  D. Gas exchange, impaired related to the gunshot wound to the chest

39. After the emergency nurse performs the needle thoracostomy, evaluation of the effectiveness of this procedure would include all of the following except:
    - O A. A rush of air after insertion of the needle
    - O B. Improvement in the patient's blood pressure
    - O C. A dramatic increase in the patient's shortness of breath
    - O D. Decrease in the patient's shortness of breath

40. The classic signs and symptoms of a tension pneumothorax include all of the following except:
    - O A. Equal breath sounds bilaterally
    - O B. Tracheal deviation away from the affected side
    - O C. Distended neck veins
    - O D. Cyanosis and diaphoresis

41. A flail segment may be stabilized by:
    - O A. Placing sandbags on the injured segment
    - O B. Strapping the patient to a backboard
    - O C. Positioning the patient on the injured side
    - O D. Applying skin traction to the injured chest wall

### Myocardial Contusion

*A 19-year-old man was riding his bicycle and hit a hole in the road at a high rate of speed. He struck his chest on the ground. On arrival in the ED, the patient is alert and complaining of chest pain. His vital signs are stable, but the rescue squad reports that the patient's pulse is irregular.*

42. Because of the mechanism of injury, the initial assessment of this patient should include assessment for the presence of:
    - O A. Chest wall ecchymosis
    - O B. Periorbital ecchymosis
    - O C. Scrotal ecchymosis
    - O D. Abdominal ecchymosis

43. An important intervention in the care of this patient would be:
    - O A. Monitoring and treating cardiac dysrhythmia
    - O B. Performing and documenting a Glasgow Coma Scale
    - O C. Preparing the patient for hospitalization
    - O D. Administering prescribed medications for pain

44. Because of the possibility of cardiac dysrhythmia in this patient, the nursing diagnosis the emergency nurse may base interventions on is:
    - O A. Fluid volume deficit, high risk for related to the mechanism of injury
    - O B. Infection, high risk for related to the skin abrasions on his chest
    - O C. Skin integrity, impaired related to the skin abrasions on his chest
    - O D. Cardiac output, decreased related to a myocardial contusion

45. The patient continues to have frequent premature ventricular contractions (PVCs) and is given lidocaine, 50 mg, as an IV bolus. A continuous drip is maintained at the rate of 2 mg/min. The emergency nurse evaluates the patient for the presence of lidocaine toxicity by observing for:
    - O A. The onset of seizures
    - O B. The absence of ventricular dysrhythmia
    - O C. Redness at the IV site
    - O D. The presence of chest pains

### Pulmonary Contusion

*An 18-year-old woman was an unrestrained back seat passenger in an automobile involved in a collision. The patient was thrown against the backseat. On arrival in the ED, she is awake and complaining of chest pain. Her vital signs are B/P 110/70, HR 90 and regular, and RR 32.*

46. All of the following signs and symptoms indicate a possible pulmonary contusion in this patient except:
    - O A. A sucking chest wound
    - O B. Shortness of breath
    - O C. Restlessness and agitation
    - O D. The presence of severe chest injuries

47. Because of the mechanism of injury and bruising on the patient's chest, a pulmonary contusion is suspected and confirmed with a chest radiograph. During the initial management of this patient, the emergency nurse should:
    - O A. Give the patient a fluid bolus to keep her blood pressure above 120/80
    - O B. Prepare the patient for elective intubation to maintain an oxygen saturation of 98%
    - O C. Limit fluids unless the patient develops hypovolemia from an associated injury
    - O D. Administer 3 L of oxygen by a nonrebreather face mask

**48.** Based on the medical diagnosis given to this patient, the emergency nurse would base care on which of the following nursing diagnoses?

0   A. Thought processes, altered, related to the patient's being admitted to the emergency department

0   B. Gas exchange, impaired, related to the injury of the lung parenchyma from the pulmonary contusion

0   C. Thermoregulation, ineffective, related to the patient's 30-minute entrapment

0   D. Activity intolerance, related to the patient's chest injury

**49.** A 16-year-old man is brought to the ED after having been thrown 25 feet from his car. He is complaining of severe chest pain and shortness of breath. During the primary assessment, bowel sounds are auscultated over the right chest. What injury is suspected?

0   A. Pneumothorax

0   B. Hemothorax

0   C. Aortic dissection

0   D. Ruptured diaphragm

**50.** A 3-year-old girl arrives in the ED in severe respiratory distress. The emergency physician has decided the child needs to be intubated. What size and type of tube should the emergency nurse prepare?

0   A. A 4.5 uncuffed endotracheal tube

0   B. A 4.5 cuffed endotracheal tube

0   C. A 3.0 uncuffed endotracheal tube

0   D. A 3.0 cuffed endotracheal tube

## ANSWERS

1. **B. Assessment.** Retractions of the sternocleidomastoid muscle usually indicate severe asthma. This occurs because of increased air trapping, which forces the patient to use accessory muscles to lift the rib cage in order to generate higher negative pleural pressures.[4,13]

2. **C. Assessment.** Obtaining a peak expiratory airflow (PEF) from the patient having an asthma attack will provide the emergency nurse with important information about the patient's pulmonary status. A PEF of less than 100 L/min indicates severe obstruction; a PEF of 100 to 200 L/min indicates moderate obstruction. The PEF can also be used to assess the effectiveness of the prescribed medical treatment the patient receives while in the emergency department. The PEF should improve >10% over baseline after treatment, or reach a minimum of 300 L/min.[5,13]

3. **C. Intervention.** A beta-agonist, which will cause bronchodilation, is used as the initial treatment of the asthmatic patient.[4,5] Frequently used beta-agonists include metaproterenol sulfate and albuterol.

4. **D. Analysis.** The inability to breathe, no matter what the cause, will generate anxiety. The emergency nurse will need to include interventions that will help decrease the patient's anxiety, as well as provide medication and physical comfort. A useful intervention would be structuring the environment so that the patient is not left alone. This can be done by placing the patient in a visible area of the department.[14]

5. **A. Intervention.** The use of steroids in the management of acute asthma in the emergency department has become a common treatment. However, the method of administration remains controversial. Research has demonstrated that IM or IV administration is not more effective than oral administration. Inhaled corticosteroids continue to be evaluated in the acute setting, but are currently not recommended.[5,13,15]

6. **C. Evaluation.** All of the above, except the blood gas results, would indicate that the asthmatic patient may need to be intubated. If the patient were unable to verbalize or cough, this would be an indication of severe distress that may need to be treated with intubation.[4]

7. **B. Assessment.** It has been found that 23% to 60% of children living in an urban environment who have asthma have a sensitivity to cockroaches.[16]

8. **D. Assessment.** A "silent chest" is an indication of marked airflow obstruction in an asthmatic patient. Wheezes indicate that air is getting in and out even though there is obstruction. No sound means no air movement and is a premoribund sign that requires immediate intervention.[5,16]

9. **B. Intervention.** Continuous nebulization has been found to be most effective in the initial acute care of the patient with asthma.[5,13]

10. **A. Intervention.** The patient should clean the mouthpiece daily by removing the medication canister and cleaning with mild soap and water twice a week. The MDI should be protected from freezing and overheating. The patient should only use the MDI as instructed and either contact his or her physician or return to the emergency department if the symptoms do not improve.[17]

11. **C. Assessment.** Bacteria that have been found to cause pneumonia include *Legionella*, *Mycoplasma*,

and *Streptococcus pneumoniae.* HIV infection can contribute to the patient's being at risk for developing pneumonia, but does not cause it.[17]

12. **B. Intervention.** The patient with pneumonia is at risk of becoming dehydrated. Providing fluids for these patients is an important nursing intervention.[17]

13. **C. Evaluation.** The pulse oximeter does not provide information about the ventilatory status of the patient. In order to monitor the ventilatory status of this patient, the emergency nurse should place the patient on a $CO_2$ monitor. Ventilatory status is measured by $CO_2$ tension and acid base balance (pH).[18]

14. **B. Assessment.** Factors that limit the usefulness of pulse oximetry include carboxyhemoglobin, methemoglobin, hypovolemia, excess ambient light, patient motion, and nail polish.[18]

15. **D. Intervention.** Active tuberculosis provides a risk for transmission to other patients and the people caring for the patient. The patient needs to be moved and admitted to a controlled air flow room.[19]

16. **A. Assessment.** When obtaining a history from a patient who is experiencing chest pain, the emergency nurse obtains information about the possible causes of the chest pain. A part of this history is identification of risk factors. Recent surgery, immobility, trauma, use of oral contraceptives, pregnancy, and obesity are risk factors for pulmonary embolus.[4]

17. **A. Intervention.** Since the patient has suffered an acute pulmonary embolus, the initial treatment would include the administration of a direct-acting anticoagulant. Heparin calcium is a direct-acting anticoagulant because it activates antithrombin III and factor $X^a$, which neutralize thrombin.[20]

18. **B. Analysis.** Tissue perfusion, altered (cardiopulmonary), would be an appropriate nursing diagnosis. This condition is a result of the pulmonary emboli. Included in the signs and symptoms of this nursing diagnosis is the patient's low blood pressure. The initial care of this patient by the emergency nurse will be based on interventions to improve tissue perfusion.[14]

19. **D. Evaluation.** Heparin can cause all of the above complications, including, in rare instances, the actual formation of more clots, which may cause chest pain, neurological deficits, and diminished pulses in extremities.[20]

20. **B. Assessment.** When obtaining historical information from a patient with this type of symptomatology, the triage nurse should elicit whether the patient has been smoking crack or inhaling co-

caine. Answers C and D are physical assessment parameters, not historical parameters.[16]

21. **A. Assessment.** Hamman's crunch is an indication of a pneumomediastinum. Hamman's crunch is a crunching sound that is heard during systole.[21,22]

22. **C. Evaluation.** Pneumomediastinum results from air in the mediastinal tissues. This is the result of barotrauma (smoking crack, inhaling cocaine), which causes increased pressure and alveoli rupture. Signs and symptoms include chest and neck pain, sore throat, difficulty swallowing, and subcutaneous emphysema. Complications of pneumomediastinum include the development of a pneumothorax.[21,22]

23. **C. Assessment.** Risk factors for the development of tuberculosis include close contacts with people with TB, foreign-born people in countries with high incidence of TB, old and young, malnutrition, homeless people and migrants, alcohol and drug abuse, HIV, chronic renal failure and certain malignancies.[19]

24. **D. Assessment.** In the emergency department, tuberculosis is generally a suspected diagnosis since definitive diagnosis usually takes several days. Tuberculosis should be suspected if the patient complains of a "constellation" of signs and symptoms including fatigue, night sweats, cough, and low-grade fever. A chest x-ray film may show cavitations or diffuse infiltrates. The primary screen for TB is the PPD. This test requires 2 to 3 days before it can be appropriately evaluated.[19]

25. **C. Assessment.** Kawasaki's disease is a rare cause of chest pain in the pediatric patient. It causes cardiac ischemia.[13]

26. **B. Assessment.** The history and physical presentation of this child are strongly suggestive of epiglottitis. Because of the possibility of obstruction, the child's throat should not be examined until the child is in a safe environment that includes personnel capable of emergency airway management. The potential dangers of evaluating the child's throat include precipitating laryngospasm and complete obstruction leading to respiratory arrest.[7,8]

27. **D. Intervention.** When the child is suffering acute respiratory distress from epiglottitis, the first intervention is to prepare the child for intubation. Administration of antibiotics would come after airway stabilization. Administration of racemic epinephrine is not recommended for the child with epiglottitis because of the potential of laryngospasm.[7,8]

28. **B. Assessment.** The most common cause of epiglottitis is *Haemophilus influenzae.*[7,8]

29. **B. Intervention.** According to the Basic Life Support Guidelines for Infant FBAO Management (conscious) of the American Heart Association, the emergency nurse should determine airway obstruction, place the infant face down and deliver four back blows, and then turn the infant over on the back and deliver four thrusts in the midsternal region. This is repeated until the object is expelled or the infant becomes unconscious.[3]

30. **C. Evaluation.** As noted in the previous answer, an indication that these maneuvers are not effective would be the child's becoming unconscious.[3]

31. **B. Assessment.** The most common item that is aspirated by the child under age 3 years is the hot dog.[3,7,8]

32. **A. Evaluation.** If the child does not respond to conventional therapy for respiratory distress, the emergency nurse should suspect the potential for foreign body aspiration, particularly if there is an unclear patient history.[8]

33. **A. Intervention.** The management of the child with asthma is based on obtaining bronchodilation. It has been shown that this can be done well with the use of a beta-agonist such as albuterol, terbutaline, or metaproterenol.[8]

34. **C. Evaluation.** An early indication of hypoxia in the infant is irritability. It is important for the emergency nurse to teach parents the signs and symptoms of early hypoxia so that there may be early intervention in the management of pediatric respiratory emergencies.[8]

35. **D. Assessment.** RSV is highly contagious. It is transmitted by direct contact from large-droplet aerosols, sneezing, and multiple visitors. The most effective way to decrease transmission is by hand washing and limiting visitors.[7,8]

36. **A. Assessment.** Following the formula of airway, breathing, and circulation, the emergency nurse would assess the patient's ability to maintain his airway. This patient is alert and able to speak but is complaining of shortness of breath. In assessing ventilation (breathing), the emergency nurse would auscultate for the presence or absence of breath sounds. Because one of the major interventions in the management of chest trauma is ensuring adequate ventilation, the absence of breath sounds and the complaint of shortness of breath indicate the need for interventions to return adequate airflow.[6]

37. **B. Intervention.** Until a chest tube can be inserted to improve the patient's ventilation, the emergency nurse should prepare for and perform a needle thoracostomy. Two areas can be used for a needle thoracostomy: the second intercostal space in the midclavicular line or the fifth intercostal space in the midaxillary line. A large-bore needle is used (14 gauge), and the area should be prepared with antiseptic solution; the needle is inserted on the injured side.[22]

38. **D. Analysis.** Once again, based on the ABCs, the initial nursing diagnosis on which to establish nursing interventions would be impaired gas exchange. The emergency nurse's interventions would initially be directed at providing interventions to correct the injuries that are impairing the patient's gas exchange.

39. **C. Evaluation.** The purpose of a needle thoracostomy is to improve the symptoms of tension pneumothorax, which include shortness of breath and hypotension. If there is no improvement or the patient's shortness of breath increases, another needle may need to be placed. The needle may not have completely entered the chest cavity, or it may have become kinked.

40. **A. Assessment.** The signs and symptoms of a tension pneumothorax include tracheal deviation, respiratory distress, unilateral absence of breath sounds, distended neck veins, and cyanosis.[21,22]

41. **C. Intervention.** Positioning the patient on the injured side is one method that may be used to stabilize a flail segment and improve oxygenation. However, the patient's cervical spine needs to be appropriately immobilized until cervical spine injury is ruled out.[6]

42. **A. Assessment.** Because the mechanism of injury involves the patient striking his chest and the patient is complaining of chest pain, the emergency nurse should assess the patient for the presence of chest wall injury. This would include the presence of abrasions or contusions on the chest wall.[21]

43. **A. Intervention.** Cardiac contusions leave the patient at risk for the development of life-threatening injuries related to cardiac damage. The most important initial intervention based on the presence of an irregular pulse would be the monitoring and treatment of cardiac dysrhythmia.

44. **D. Analysis.** The patient with myocardial contusion may suffer decreased cardiac output for several reasons. First, damage to the myocardium may result in pericardial tamponade, valvular disruption, and coronary artery occlusion. In addition, the patient may also suffer cardiac dysrhythmia, such as premature ventricular contractions and tachycardia, and conduction abnormalities.[14]

45. **A. Evaluation.** There are many indications of lidocaine toxicity, including hypotension, bradycardia, drowsiness, dizziness, and seizures.[20]

46. **A. Assessment.** The signs and symptoms of pulmonary contusion include a high index of suspicion based on the mechanism of injury, dyspnea, and ineffective cough, restlessness and agitation, and the presence of other severe chest injuries.[21,22]

47. **C. Intervention.** If the patient does not have hypotension from another related injury, such as an abdominal injury, fluids should be restricted for the patient with a pulmonary contusion. Because of the injury to the patient's lungs, the patient is at risk for developing complications from fluid overload, such as ARDS and hypoxia. Diuretics and steroids may be considered for the treatment of these patients.[6]

48. **B. Analysis.** Because of the injury to the patient's lungs and the possibility of a pulmonary contusion, the patient's care should be based on keeping her oxygenated. Defining characteristics of this nursing diagnosis include confusion, somnolence, restlessness, irritability, and inability to move secretions, hypoxia, and hypercapnia.[14]

49. **D. Assessment.** Based on mechanism of injury and the presence of bowel sounds in the patient's chest cavity, a ruptured diaphragm would be suspected.[22]

50. **A. Intervention.** The formula for calculating the tube size is 16 + the age of the child divided by 4. The approximate size is 4.5. The tube should be uncuffed for a 3-year-old child.[3]

## REFERENCES

1. Bates B: *Guide to physical examination and history taking,* Philadelphia, 1995, JB Lippincott.
2. Engel J: *Pediatric assessment,* St Louis, 1993, Mosby.
3. Chameides L, Hazinski F: *Pediatric advanced life support,* Dallas, 1997-1999, The American Heart Association.
4. Mackey D: Pulmonary emergencies. In Kitt S and others, editors: *Emergency nursing: a physiologic perspective,* Philadelphia, 1995, WB Saunders.
5. Bonner S, Holleran R, editors: Overhauled asthma guidelines: the way you care for patients will be revamped. In *ED Nursing,* 1999, American Health Consultants.
6. Hurn P, Hartsock R: Thoracic injuries. In Cardona V and others, editors: *Trauma nursing: from resuscitation through rehabilitation,* Philadelphia, 1994, WB Saunders.
7. Phelan A: Respiratory emergencies. In Kelley S, editor: *Pediatric emergency nursing,* Norwalk, 1994, Appleton & Lange.
8. Haley K, Eckles N, Baker B, editors: *Emergency nursing core course,* Park Ridge, IL, 1999, Emergency Nurses Association.
9. James C: Respiratory emergencies. In Jordan KS, editor, *Emergency nursing core curriculum,* ed 5, Philadelphia, 2000, WB Saunders.
10. Varghese G, Crane L: Evaluation and treatment of HIV-related illnesses in the emergency department, *Ann Emerg Med* 24:503-511, 1994.
11. Curry J: Identifying the patient with tuberculosis and protecting the emergency department staff, *J Emerg Nurs* 20:293-304, 1994.
12. Brillman J and others: Hantavirus: Emergency department response to a disaster from an emerging pathogen, Ann Emerg Med 24:429-436, 1994.
13. Candioty V: Shortness of breath. In Davis M, editor: *Signs and symptoms in emergency medicine,* St Louis, 1999, Mosby.
14. Kim MJ, McFarland GK, McLane AM: *Pocket guide to nursing diagnoses,* St Louis, 1993, Mosby.
15. Afilalo M, Guttman A, Colacone A, and others: Efficiency of inhaled steroids (beclomethasone dipropionate) for treatment of mild to moderately severe asthma in the emergency department: a randomized clinical trial, *Ann Emerg Med* 33(3):304-309, 1999.
16. Mattera CJ: Crashing asthmatics, *JEMS* 24(10):30-33, 1999.
17. Koran Z, Howard PK, Baxter CS: Respiratory emergencies. In Newberry L, editor: *Sheehy's emergency nursing principles and practice,* ed 4, St Louis, 1998, Mosby.
18. Durren M: Getting the most from pulse oximetry, *J Emerg Nurs* 18:340-342, 1992.
19. Almeida S: Infectious and communicable diseases. In Newberry L, editor, *Sheehy's emergency nursing principles and practice,* ed 4, St Louis, 1998, Mosby.
20. McKenry L, Salerno E: *Pharmacology in nursing,* St Louis, 1998, Mosby.
21. Kearney K: Thoracic trauma. In Newberry L, editor: *Sheehy's emergency nursing principles and practice,* ed 4, St Louis, 1998, Mosby.
22. Jacobs BB, Baker P, editors: *Trauma nursing core course,* Park Ridge, IL, 1995, Emergency Nurses Association.

# Chapter 18

# Shock Emergencies

## REVIEW OUTLINE

I. Definition of shock: no matter what the clinical insult, there is inadequate cellular metabolism

II. Etiologies of shock
   A. Alterations in circulating volume
   B. Alterations in pump function
   C. Alteration in peripheral vascular resistance

III. Pathophysiology of shock
   A. Amount of oxygen available for tissue consumption
   B. Amount of oxygen extracted from tissue
   C. Oxygen consumption dependent upon
      1. Cardiac output
      2. Hemoglobin concentration
      3. Arterial oxygen saturation
      4. Venous oxygen saturation
   D. Oxygen debt is the difference between tissue oxygen demand and oxygen consumption. Patient's preexisting condition will have an impact on how the body responds to a clinical insult that interferes with oxygen demand and consumption i.e., chronic obstructive pulmonary disease (COPD), sickle cell anemia, cardiovascular diseases
   E. Heat shock proteins: accumulate after a wide variety of clinical insults, associated with stress tolerance, potential biomarkers of early tissue injury, and resistance to subsequent insult
   F. Apoptosis: Physiological process of cell deletion that occurs during embryogenesis, metamorphosis, tissue atrophy and tumor regression. It is an active process that is energy dependent and requires a cascade of signal-transducing events.

IV. The body's response
   A. Cellular response
      1. Cell destruction
   B. Immune system response
      1. Activation of complement cascade system
      2. Macrophage response
      3. Neutrophils
      4. Slow-reacting substance of anaphylaxis
   C. Neurologic system response
      1. Alteration in cerebral perfusion pressure
   D. Cardiac system response
      1. Decrease in cardiac output
      2. Development of dysrhythmia
      3. Myocardial depressant factor (MDF)
   E. Pulmonary system response
      1. Acute lung injury
      2. Acute respiratory distress
   F. Renal system response
      1. Decrease in urinary output
      2. Decrease in detoxification
   G. Gastrointestinal system response
      1. Priming beds for circulating neutrophils
      2. Provoke multiple organ failure
   H. Integumentary system response
      1. Pale, cooler, fragile skin
      2. Less protection
      3. Hypothermia

V. Compensatory mechanisms
   A. Neural response
      1. Triggering of baroreceptors
      2. Release of catecholamines
      3. Vasoconstriction
   B. Hormonal response
      1. Production of angiotensin II-vasoconstriction
      2. Aldosterone
      3. Pituitary gland
      4. Fall in thyroid hormone
      5. Production of glucagons
   C. Fluid shifts
      1. Into the general circulation
      2. Fluid resuscitation–third spacing
   D. Skeletal muscle
      1. Major reservoir of amino acids
      2. Proteolysis

VI. Classification of shock
   A. Systemic inflammatory response syndrome (SIRS)
   B. Classification of sepsis

C. Multiple organ dysfunction syndrome

D. Multiple organ failure

E. Compensated

F. Uncompensated

G. Irreversible

VII. Patient assessment

    A. History of a clinical insult

        1. Trauma: blood and fluid loss

        2. Infection

        3. Myocardial infarction

        4. Tension pneumothorax

        5. Pericardial tamponade

        6. Allergic reaction

        7. Medical illness: GI bleeding, hepatic, pancreatitis

        8. Vaginal bleeding

        9. Trauma in pregnancy, rupture ectopic pregnancy

      10. Immunocompromised conditions

    B. Source of the clinical insult

    C. Airway

    D. Breathing

    E. Circulation

        1. Skin color

        2. Skin temperature

        3. Level of consciousness

        4. Urinary output

    F. Neurological

    G. Diagnostic procedures

        1. CBC with differential

        2. Serum electrolytes

        3. Creatinine and BUN

        4. Coagulation studies

        5. Arterial blood gas

        6. Drug screen

        7. Cardiac enzymes

        8. Cultures

        9. Type and crossmatch

      10. ECG

    H. Radiology

        1. Chest radiograph

        2. CT

        3. MRI

VIII. Related nursing diagnosis

    A. Impaired gas exchange

    B. Fluid volume deficit

    C. Decreased cardiac output

    D. Altered tissue perfusion

    E. Spiritual distress

    F. Grieving, anticipatory

IX. Collaborative care of the patient in shock

    A. Airway management

    B. Ventilation management

        1. Intubation for oxygenation

        2. Chemical paralysis

        3. Sedation

    C. Circulatory management

        1. Fluid resuscitation

        2. Operative management

        3. Antibiotics

        4. Steroids

        5. Vasoactive drugs

    D. Prevention

        1. Vaccinations

        2. Injury prevention

        3. Age-related interventions

X. Age-related considerations

    A. Pediatric patient[1]

        1. Pediatric myocardial fibers are shorter and less compliant. In order to increase cardiac output, the child's heart rate will increase.

        2. Infants have a higher cardiac output and less oxygen reserve.

        3. Infant circulating blood volume 90 ml/kg and 80 ml/kg in the child, small blood loss can be significant.

        4. Hypotension is a late sign of circulatory compromise in the infant and child.

        5. Because a greater percentage of the child's body weight is water, children at greater risk of becoming dehydrated with fluid loss.

    B. Geriatric patient[2]

        1. Preexisting cardiovascular disease may limit the geriatric patient's ability to respond to the initial clinical insult that causes SIRS.

        2. Cardiac output and stroke volume decrease with aging, leaving the patient at risk of rapidly developing hypoxemia and hypoxia with blood and fluid loss.

        3. Renal changes due to aging affect the kidneys' ability to reabsorb and to concentrate urine, which may result in fluid and electrolytes imbalances.

---

*S*hock has been described as the "rude unhinging of the machinery of life." It is a syndrome that results from inadequate perfusion of tissues.[2] Shock was initially described based on changes in the patient's vital signs. For example, a systolic blood pressure of 90 mm Hg or less. Today, shock has been recognized as a systemic response to a clinical insult that results in decreased oxygen to the cells.[3] The syndrome of shock has begun to be described as systemic inflammatory response syndrome (SIRS) to encompass all of the physiological responses that the body goes through.[4] Examples of clinical insults include trauma, infection, and anaphylaxis.

When the patient is in shock, all of the body systems will respond. Many of these responses produce familiar signs and symptoms such as altered mental status, skin pallor, diaphoresis, hypotension, and decreased urinary output.

The management of the patient in shock begins with recognition of its cause. If the patient has lost volume or is acutely infected, the source of the systemic response must be identified and dealt with. Airway, breathing, and circulation are assured so that adequate oxygen is available to the cells.[5]

However, the most effective treatment for shock remains prevention. Assuring that people are properly vaccinated, wear seat belts, understand fire safety, and stay healthy and injury free are but a few examples of how to prevent shock and its devastating consequences.

## REVIEW QUESTIONS

1. A 34-year-old African American male is brought to the emergency department (ED). He was the restrained driver in a car that was "T-boned" on his side. He was entrapped for 45 minutes. Upon arrival in the emergency department, he has an altered mental status with a calculated Glasgow Coma Scale of 8. His skin is diaphoretic. His vital signs are BP 80/52; HR 144R; and RR 36. Which of the following is the most critical intervention?
   O  A. Insertion of two large-bore intravenous catheters
   O  B. Preparation for emergent intubation and oxygenation
   O  C. Insertion of a urinary catheter for circulatory monitoring
   O  D. Preparation for an emergent CT of the head and abdomen.

2. Fluid resuscitation has been initiated. A positive end-point for fluid resuscitation in the ED is:
   O  A. Decrease in the patient's peripheral pulses
   O  B. Decrease in the patient's level of consciousness
   O  C. Maintenance of adequate peripheral perfusion
   O  D. Maintenance of the patient's hypertension

3. The patient's history of sickle cell anemia will affect his:
   O  A. Oxygen delivery
   O  B. Oxygen use

   O  C. Oxygen demand
   O  D. Oxygen debt

4. Oxygen consumption is dependent upon all the following **except:**
   O  A. Cardiac output (CO)
   O  B. Hemoglobin concentration (Hb)
   O  C. Arterial carbon dioxide ($PCO_2$)
   O  D. Oxygen saturation ($SaO_2$)

5. A unit of O-negative packed red blood cells is to be administered because of persistent hypotension. The emergency nurse administers the blood through a blood filter because:
   O  A. The filter will prevent the hypothermia that may develop with the administration of blood
   O  B. The filter will prevent the debris that is found in banked blood from being infused and causing potential complications
   O  C. The filter will prevent the development of the clotting problems that are associated with the infusion of banked blood
   O  D. The filter will prevent the development of the hypokalemia that is associated with the infusion of banked blood

6. An example of a neural compensatory mechanism that is triggered in the shock state is:
   O  A. Vasodilation to increase the cardiac output
   O  B. Production of angiotensin-II to increase systolic blood pressure
   O  C. Proteolysis of muscle tissue to produce adenosine triphosphate (ATP)
   O  D. Increase in heart rate to increase cardiac output

7. An 18-year-old male was riding a bicycle when he struck a rock and flew over the handlebars, landing on his head. He now complains of "numbness all over." His vital signs are BP 88/48; HR 48R, and RR 12. He is probably in:
   O  A. Cardiogenic shock
   O  B. Neurogenic shock
   O  C. Hemorrhagic shock
   O  D. Anaphylactic shock

8. Once the patient's primary interventions have been managed, which nursing diagnosis would be most appropriate on which to base the patient's care:
   O  A. Hyperthermia related to the patient's inability to maintain his body temperature

O  B. Infection, high risk for, related to the abrasions he sustained in the fall

O  C. Hypothermia related to his inability to maintain his body temperature

O  D. Noncompliance related to his refusal to wear a helmet when riding his bike

9. The neurosurgeon has ordered high-dose steroid administration. The patient weighs 155 lbs. His initial loading dose should be:

O  A. 2035 mg of methylprednisone over 15 minutes

O  B. 1150 mg of methylprednisone over 25 minutes

O  C. 1860 mg of methylprednisone over 15 minutes

O  D. 4650 mg of methylprednisone over 20 minutes

10. In anaphylaxis, chemical mediators target:

O  A. Smooth muscle of the bronchopulmonary tree

O  B. Smooth muscle of the abdominal cavity

O  C. Striated muscles in the lower extremities

O  D. Myocardial muscle to decrease cardiac output

11. A 10-year-old female presents to the ED with severe shortness of breath, wheezing, and facial edema. Her mother says she was just stung by a yellow jacket. The initial dose of epinephrine for this child is (she weighs 30 kg):

O  A. 0.3 mg epinephrine 1:1000 SQ

O  B. 0.3 mg epinephrine 1:10000 SQ

O  C. 0.3 mg epinephrine 1:1000 IM

O  D. 0.3 mg epinephrine 1:1000 IV

12. A 20-year-old male fell 20 feet from a tree, striking his chest. He presents with severe shortness of breath. No breath sounds are auscultated on the right side, and crepitus is palpated on the right side of his chest. His heart rate is 138R, and there is no palpable blood pressure. He is experiencing:

O  A. Hemorrhagic shock

O  B. Distributive shock

O  C. Obstructive shock

O  D. Vasogenic shock

13. The initial critical intervention for this patient is:

O  A. Insertion of a 14-gauge needle into his left second intercostal space, mid-clavicular line followed by chest tube insertion

O  B. Insertion of a 14-gauge needle into his right second intercostal space, mid-clavicular line followed by chest tube insertion

O  C. Administration of high-flow oxygen with a 10 L binasal cannula

O  D. Turning the patient on his affected side to increase his ability to ventilate more effectively

14. The mother of a 4-month-old infant has brought the infant to the triage desk. Her mother states that she has been vomiting and has had loose stools for the past 24 hours. She is lethargic, pale, cool, and clammy. No peripheral pulses can be palpated, and she has weak central pulses. Her capillary refill is greater than 5 seconds. This child is in:

O  A. Compensated hypovolemic shock

O  B. Stable hypovolemic shock

O  C. Uncompensated hypovolemic shock

O  D. Partially compensated hypovolemic shock

15. The child is placed on a high-flow oxygen mask, and an intraosseous needle is inserted in her right tibia. An initial fluid bolus is ordered. The child weighs 15 lbs. How much fluid bolus should be administered to this baby?

O  A. 120 ml of normal saline

O  B. 240 ml of normal saline

O  C. 120 ml of dextrose in water

O  D. 150 ml of normal saline

16. An indication that the child is improving is:

O  A. A decrease in her level of consciousness

O  B. A palpable radial pulse or pedal pulse

O  C. A decrease in her body temperature

O  D. A capillary refill time of greater than 6 seconds

17. The parents of a 15-month-old male bring him to the emergency department. They state that he has had a high fever and vomiting and is now very irritable. His mother states that he has "bruises" on his leg but has no history of recent trauma. The child's vital signs are HR 160R, RR 38, and rectal temperature of 103° F. There are pupura on both lower extremities. The most probable cause of this child's illness is:

O  A. *Neisseria meningitidis*

O  B. *Haemophilus influenzae*

O  C. *Streptococcus pneumoniae*

O  D. All of the above

18. The initial systemic response that occurs in septic shock is caused by:
   - O A. The loss of volume that occurs in sepsis due to fever
   - O B. The endotoxins of the infecting bacteria, virus, or fungus
   - O C. The immune system's response to the invading organism
   - O D. The cardiovascular system's response to the invading organism

19. A 62-year-old patient in septic shock has been started on a Levophed (norepinephrine) drip at 2 µg/min. A serious complication of the use of norepinephrine is:
   - O A. An increase in cardiac output
   - O B. Peripheral vasoconstriction
   - O C. Reduction of renal blood flow
   - O D. Increase in systolic blood pressure

20. An example of a preventive strategy that may be used in the emergency department to decrease the risk of sepsis in the elderly population is:
   - O A. Administration of the pneumococcal vaccine to patients over 65 years of age
   - O B. Provision of information related to recognition of the signs and symptoms of sepsis
   - O C. Referral of the elderly patients to a healthcare provider to ensure that all their vaccinations are up-to-date
   - O D. Provision of written material that outlines when all vaccinations should be obtained

## ANSWERS

1. **B. Intervention.** The patient's respiratory rate, altered mental status, heart rate, and blood pressure indicate the need for emergent intubation and oxygenation.[5]

2. **C. Evaluation.** Fluid resuscitation end-points include maintaining the patient's level of consciousness; maintaining an adequate blood pressure, generally a systolic pressure between 90 and 100 mm Hg or even lower with uncontrolled hemorrhage; and maintenance of the patient's peripheral perfusion.[6]

3. **D. Assessment.** The oxygen debt is the difference between tissue oxygen demand and oxygen consumption. The effects of the patient's injury and current health status will affect the oxygen debt.

4. **C. Assessment.** Oxygen consumption is dependent upon the patient's cardiac output, hemoglobin concentration, and the oxygen saturation.[7]

5. **B. Intervention.** There is debris in banked blood that may cause additional injury to the patient. Blood should always be administered with a filter to prevent this potential complication.[5]

6. **D. Assessment.** The body's neural compensatory mechanisms include the triggering of baroreceptors, release of catecholamines, and vasoconstriction to increase cardiac output. Catecholamine release will cause tachycardia in an attempt to increase cardiac output.[7]

7. **B. Assessment.** Injuries to the spinal cord and brain will block the outflow of the sympathetic nervous system. This results in hypotension and bradycardia.[6]

8. **C. Analysis.** The loss of vasomotor tone leaves the patient at great risk of becoming hypothermic because he is unable to maintain his body temperature through vasoconstriction (poikilothermia).[8]

9. **C. Intervention.** The patient weighs 155 lbs., which is 62 kg. The initial loading dose of methylprednisone is 30 mg/kg over 15 minutes.[2]

10. **A. Assessment.** The SRSA targets specific organs, including the smooth muscle of the bronchopulmonary tree and tissue in the upper airway. This leads to bronchospasm and airway edema, compromising the patient's airway and ability to ventilate effectively.[8]

11. **A. Intervention.** The correct dosage calculation is 0.1 mg/kg epinephrine 1:1000 SQ. The child weighs 30 kg; therefore the dose is 0.3 mg of epinephrine 1:1000 SQ. The epinephrine may be given IV if the child's condition dictates, however, it would be 0.3 1:10000.[9]

12. **C. Assessment.** The patient is experiencing obstructive or mechanical shock. Causes of obstructive shock include tension pneumothorax, pericardial tamponade, and myocardial contusion. The injury causes obstruction of venous return and lowers cardiac output.[6]

13. **B. Intervention.** The patient's chest should be needled with a 14-gauge needle at the second intercostal space, MCL. Since his decreased breath sounds are on the right side, that is where the needle should be inserted. A chest tube will then need to be inserted.[2,6]

14. **C. Assessment.** This child is in uncompensated hypovolemic shock. Her level of consciousness, her skin color and temperature, a capillary refill greater than 5 seconds, and the absence of peripheral pulses indicate uncompensated shock.[10]

15. **A. Intervention.** The initial fluid bolus for this baby is 120 ml of normal saline. The baby weighs 15 lbs. (6 kg) $\times$ 20 ml = 120 ml.[10]

16. **B. Evaluation.** Return of peripheral pulses would be an indication that the fluid resuscitation is effective.[10]

17. **D. Assessment. All of the above.** The child has significant signs and symptoms of meningitis and/or meningococcemia. Any of these bacteria can cause these signs and symptoms, and it may be difficult to differentiate the cause in the ED. History of recent exposure to any of these diseases would assist in differentiation, but treatment should not be delayed. A key piece of history is whether the child has been exposed to an infected child or the presence of meningococcemia cases in the community.[1]

18. **B. Assessment.** The initial response of the body to the invading organism's endotoxins initiates a systemic response. For example, the immune system responds by releasing interleukins, tissue necrosis factor, and SRSA.[5,7]

19. **C. Evaluation.** The most serious complication of the use of norepinephrine is the reduction of blood flow to the kidneys. This can be very serious in shock states where hypovolemia has not been corrected, leading to acute renal failure. Norepinepherine has a high affinity for alpha receptors, causing peripheral arteriolar vasoconstriction and return of blood to the central circulation to increase cardiac output. It can also activate beta$_1$ receptors in the heart and increase the force of the myocardial contraction to result in an increase in cardiac output.[9]

20. **A. Intervention.** Research has demonstrated that written information and referral does not assure follow-up. Actual administration of vaccines in the emergency department provides the first step in preventive health care.[11,12]

## REFERENCES

1. Haley K, Eckles N, Baker P, editors: *Emergency nursing pediatric course,* Park Ridge, IL, 1999, Emergency Nurses Association.
2. Jacobs BB, Baker P, editors: *Trauma nursing core course,* Park Ridge, IL, 2000, Emergency Nurses Association.
3. Shoemaker WC: Diagnosis and treatment of shock and circulatory dysfunction. In Grenvik A, editor: *Textbook of critical care,* ed 4, Philadelphia, 2000, WB Saunders.
4. Bone R: Sepsis, sepsis syndrome, and the systemic inflammatory response syndrome (SIRS): Gulliver in Laputa, *JAMA* 273:155-156, 1992.
5. Chapman C: Shock emergencies. In Newberry L, editor: *Sheehy's emergency nursing principles and practice,* ed 4, St Louis, 1998, Mosby.
6. Fowler R, Pepe P, Lewis R: Shock evaluation and management. In Campbell JE, editor: *Basic trauma life support,* ed 4, Upper Saddle River, NJ, 2000, Brady/Prentice Hall Health.
7. Selfridge-Thomas J: Shock. In Kitt S, Selfridge-Thomas J, Proehl J, Kaiser J, editors: Philadelphia, 1995, WB Saunders.
8. Horvath C: Shock emergencies. In Jordan K, editor: *Emergency nursing core curriculum,* ed 5, Philadelphia, 2000, WB Saunders.
9. McKenry L, Salerno E: *Pharmacology in nursing,* ed 20, St Louis, 1998, Mosby.
10. Chameides L, Hazinski MF: *Pediatric advanced life support,* Dallas, 1997-1999, American Heart Association.
11. The Task Force on Community Preventative Services: Reviews of evidence regarding interventions to improve vaccination coverage in children, adolescents, and adults, *Am J Prevent Med* 18(1S):97-140, 2000.
12. Steffen S, Herringshaw M: Fulminate pneumococcal septicemia in the asplenic patient: a case study with urgent implications for recognition and prevention, *J Emerg Nurs* 25(2):102-106, 1999.

# Chapter 19

# Toxicological Emergencies

**REVIEW OUTLINE**

I. General management of the patient with a toxicological emergency
  A. Airway, breathing, circulation (ABCs)
    1. Assure a patent airway
    2. Monitor for respiratory changes
    3. Place the patient on a cardiac monitor
    4. Establish a large-bore intravenous line
    5. Insert a Foley catheter when indicated
  B. Termination of the toxicological exposure
    1. Remove the victim from the toxic environment
    2. Determine how the patient was exposed to the toxin (orally, intravenously, through the skin)
    3. Decontaminate the patient when indicated
    4. Induce vomiting when indicated (current research continues to demonstrate that this may become an obsolete practice)
    5. Perform gastric lavage when ordered
    6. Record the amount of emesis and a description of the emesis, saving a sample
    7. Administer a specific antidote when indicated
    8. Administer naloxone, dextrose 50% ($D_{50}$), thiamine, and oxygen
    9. Administer charcoal to neutralize the poison
    10. Administer a cathartic to enhance excretion of the toxin

II. History related to the toxicological emergency
  A. What was the patient exposed to or what did the patient take
  B. When was it taken
  C. What route (intravenous, intramuscular, oral, inhaled)
  D. What interventions have been done before admission to the emergency department (ED)
  E. Has the patient done this before (intentional or unintentional)
  F. Patient's medical history
  G. Allergies

  H. Medications
  I. History of mental health problems
  J. History of substance abuse

III. Identification of the toxin
  A. Presence of burns around or in the mouth
  B. Odor of the patient's breath
    1. Alcohol
    2. Garlic
    3. Oil of wintergreen
    4. Bitter almond
  C. Eyes
    1. Pinpoint pupils: narcotics, chloral hydrate, phenothiazine, insecticides
    2. Dilated pupils: alcohol, amphetamines, cocaine, tricyclics
    3. Nystagmus: vertical, horizontal
  D. Vital signs
    1. Bradycardia: beta-blockers, digitalis toxicity, organophosphate poisoning
    2. Tachycardia: tricyclics, cocaine and crack, amphetamines, hallucinogens
  E. Neurological assessment
    1. Mental depression
    2. Excitability
    3. Pupillary changes
    4. Extraocular eye movements
  F. Changes in respiratory patterns
    1. Tachypnea
      a. Amphetamines
      b. Alcohols
      c. Salicylates
      d. Cocaine
      e. Tricyclic antidepressants (TCAs)
  G. Changes in body temperature
    1. Hypothermia
      a. Ethanol
      b. Carbon monoxide
      c. TCAs
      d. Barbiturates
  H. Excessive salivation and lacrimation
    1. Organophosphates
  I. Carbomates

IV. Collaborative care of the patient with a toxicological emergency
  A. ABCs (primary interventions)
    1. Ensure a patent airway
    2. Arterial blood gases
    3. Cardiac monitor
    4. Large-bore intravenous line
    5. Specific antidote when available
    6. Neurological assessment
    7. Terminate toxic exposure
    8. Identify nature of the toxin
      a. Poisindex
      b. Poison Control Center
      c. Environmental Protection Agency (EPA)
      d. Local experts
    9. Gastric decontamination
      a. Syrup of Ipecac
      b. Activated charcoal
      c. Gastric lavage
    10. Other decontamination when indicated (i.e., clothing, skin, and so on)
    11. Urinary catheter for accurate measurement of intake and output
    12. Administration of dextrose 50% ($D_{50}$), naloxone, thiamine, oxygen
    13. Administration of charcoal
    14. Administration of a cathartic
    15. Family assessment and care
V. Related nursing diagnoses
  A. Airway clearance, ineffective, related to toxic exposure
  B. Aspiration, high risk for
  C. Breathing pattern, ineffective, related to toxic exposure
  D. Cardiac output, decreased, related to toxic exposure
  E. Coping, ineffective, related to a drug overdose
  F. Fluid volume deficit related to toxic exposure
  G. Gas exchange, impaired, related to toxic exposure
  H. Hyperthermia related to toxic exposure
  I. Injury, high risk for, related to toxic exposure
  J. Knowledge deficit
  K. Poisoning, high risk for
  L. Sensory/perceptual alterations related to toxic exposure
  M. Skin integrity, impaired, potential, related to toxic exposure
  N. Violence, high risk for: self-directed or directed at others, related to toxic exposure
VI. Specific toxicological emergencies
  A. Acetaminophen poisoning
  B. Salicylate poisoning
  C. Alcohol poisoning
    1. Ethanol
    2. Methanol
    3. Ethylene glycol
  D. Sedative-hypnotic poisoning
  E. Household products poisonings
    1. Hydrocarbons and petroleum distillates
    2. Caustic agents
  F. Cyanide
  G. Heavy metals
    1. Iron
    2. Lead
  H. Tricyclic antidepressants
  I. Toxic inhalants
  J. Cardiovascular medications
    1. Beta-blockers
    2. Calcium channel blockers
    3. Digitalis
  K. Food poisonings
  L. Plant poisoning
  M. Organophosphates
  N. Carbon monoxide
  O. Substance abuse
    1. Amphetamine
    2. Cocaine
    3. Heroin
    4. Hallucinogens

A person has been "poisoned" when they have suffered a chemical injury to one or more body systems. Each year millions of patients are cared for in the emergency department who have been intentionally or unitentially poisoned. Intentional poisoning still accounts for a significant number of deaths in the United States each year. Many times patients are poisoned by medications that were prescribed to help, not hurt the patient. The majority of poisonings still occur in children under the age of 6 years.[1,2] However, the majority of substance abuse or intentional exposure to poisons occurs in the 18- to 34-year-old age group.[3]

There are literally thousands of medications, plants, and chemicals that patients may be poisoned by. Very few antidotes are available, although research continues to be directed at affecting the most toxic substances.[5,6] The American Heart Association has issued specific guidelines for the resuscitation of a patient who has suffered a toxic exposure in order to aid in the management of these patients.[4]

The review questions presented in this chapter offer examples of some of the most frequent types of poisonings seen by the ED nurse. The assessment, analysis, intervention, and evaluation components in the care of the poisoned patient are addressed.

## MANAGEMENT OF THE POISONED PATIENT

Supportive care is the key to management of the poisoned patient. Airway, ventilation, and circulatory maintenance are the mainstays of care of the poisoned patient. Unfortunately, compared with the number of poisons contained in the human environment, there are few antidotes known.

In addition to meeting the physical and physiological needs of the poisoned patient, the emergency nurse needs to provide emotional care. Particular attention needs to be given to why or how the patient was poisoned. Was it an environmental problem, an unintentional poisoning, or an intentional poisoning? It is important to assess whether the poisoning may have been a form of abuse, particularly if a child or elderly adult is involved.

## ACETAMINOPHEN POISONING

Acetaminophen is contained in many over-the-counter drugs. Its most popular name is Tylenol. Poisoning by acetaminophen can be very lethal. The drug, if not properly eliminated, can cause hepatic, renal, and cardiac failure. Ingestions of 7.5 g or 150 mg/kg are considered potentially toxic.[7]

## SALICYLATE POISONING

Aspirin is the most common type of salicylate. It is one of the oldest nonprescription drugs used by humankind. As with acetaminophen, many over-the-counter drugs contain salicylates. There are three types of salicylate toxicity. Mild toxicity occurs with ingestions of less than 150 mg/kg, moderate toxicity occurs with ingestions of 150 to 300 mg/kg, and severe toxicity occurs with ingestions of 300 to 500 mg/kg.[8]

## TRICYCLIC ANTIDEPRESSANT POISONING

Antidepressants are used to treat depression in adults, and nocturnal enuresis and painful neuropathies in diabetic patients. In addition to tricyclic antidepressants, there are bicyclic and tetracyclic antidepressants. However, the most frequently prescribed antidepressants are tricyclic.[5]

The exact toxic level of poisoning cannot always be determined, because the drug accumulates in body tissues. The patient is treated according to the presenting symptoms. Tricyclic antidepressants in toxic amounts induce the release of norepinephrine and then inhibit its reuptake, directly block alpha action, exert a quinidinelike effect on myocardial tissue, and cause atropinelike anticholinergic effects.[2] The most common cause of death in cyclic poisoning is related to cardiac toxicity. Signs and symptoms of cardiac toxicity include depression of myocardial contractility, prolongation of the QT interval, heart block, atrial and ventricular dysrhythmia, and sudden cardiac death.[9] It is very important to remember that these drugs can be very toxic to the pediatric patient in what would appear to be small amounts to the adult patient.

## HYDROCARBON POISONING

Hydrocarbons are contained in many substances that may be ingested, inhaled, or spilled directly onto the skin. Examples of hydrocarbons include gasoline, kerosene, turpentine, and camphor. The most common types of hydrocarbon poisoning seen by the emergency department (ED) nurse include ingestion of gasoline and kerosene, and dermal exposure by these same substances.[5]

Hydrocarbon poisoning may cause pulmonary and cutaneous injuries. The major effects of ingestion of hydrocarbons are on the lungs, gastrointestinal tract, and central nervous system.[3]

## ORGANOPHOSPHATE POISONING

Organophosphates are contained in many commercial insecticides. Their mechanism of action is achieved by their ability to combine with acetylcholinesterase. This causes increased salivation, vomiting, bronchospasm, bradycardia, muscle fasciculations, paralysis, ataxia, confusion, seizures, and coma.[10]

## REVIEW QUESTIONS

*A 20-year-old woman is brought to the ED by the rescue squad. Her mother states that the patient has been anxious about her new job and has been taking lorazepam (2 mg), which was prescribed by the family physician. An empty pill bottle, along with a bottle of wine, was found by her bed. Currently the patient is responding only to deep, painful stimuli and she has vomited.*

1. The initial assessment of this patient would include which of the following?
   - 0  A. Consulting the toxicology file to determine a lethal dose of lorazepam
   - 0  B. Determining the patient's ability to protect her airway

O    C. Evaluating the patient's rhythm by performing a 12-lead ECG

O    D. Determining if the patient is truly suicidal or just anxious

2.  What would be the most appropriate intervention in the initial management of this patient?
    O    A. Prepare the patient for intubation to protect her airway
    O    B. Obtain intravenous access to administer flumazenil
    O    C. Place the patient on a cardiac monitor to assess her rhythm
    O    D. Administer ipecac as soon as possible to empty her stomach

3.  The emergency physician has decided to administer flumazenil to confirm the diagnosis of suspected benzodiazepine poisoning. Flumazenil should be administered:
    O    A. Slowly over 5 minutes
    O    B. Rapidly over 15 to 30 seconds
    O    C. Mixed with $NaHCO_3$
    O    D. Through a small vein

4.  A life-threatening side effect to flumazenil administration is:
    O    A. Agitation
    O    B. Sweating
    O    C. Seizures
    O    D. Dizziness

5.  What would be an appropriate nursing diagnosis for this patient?
    O    A. Coping, ineffective individual, related to use of drugs and alcohol to manage her anxiety
    O    B. Poisoning, potential for, related to ingestion of an unknown amount of lorazepam and alcohol
    O    C. Family processes, altered, related to attempted suicide by a family member who is having work problems
    O    D. Infection, potential for, related to poisoning and being immobile for several hours of treatment in the emergency department

6.  One of the parameters that must be monitored to evaluate the effectiveness of flumazenil is:
    O    A. The patient's level of consciousness
    O    B. The patient's urinary output
    O    C. The patient's peripheral pulses
    O    D. The patient's drug screen

7.  Benzodiazepines potentiate the activity of:
    O    A. Epinepherine
    O    B. Gamma-aminobutyric acid
    O    C. Acetylcholine
    O    D. Dopamine

8.  The purpose of charcoal in the care of the poisoned patient is to:
    O    A. Absorb toxins from the gastrointestinal tract
    O    B. Induce vomiting and remove all the remaining toxins
    O    C. Prevent cardiac dysrhythmia that may result from absorbed toxins
    O    D. Decrease the possibility of bleeding from absorbed toxins

9.  Charcoal adminstration is contraindicated when:
    O    A. The patient has ingested a toxic amount of salicylate
    O    B. The patient has ingested a toxic amount of a tricyclic
    O    C. The pediatric patient is less than 5 years of age
    O    D. The patient has ingested a caustic or corrosive substance

10. What is an important assessment parameter in the care of the patient who has ingested a toxic amount of acetaminophen?
    O    A. The serum acetaminophen level immediately following ingestion
    O    B. The serum acetaminophen level 24 hours after ingestion
    O    C. The serum acetaminophen level 4 hours after ingestion
    O    D. The serum acetaminophen level 48 hours after ingestion

11. A 3-year-old child was brought to the ED by her family after drinking approximately 120 ml of children's liquid acetaminophen. Four hours after ingestion, the child's acetaminophen level remains at a toxic level. Which medical interventions should the emergency nurse expect?
    O    A. An order for an additional dose of oral charcoal, 50 g
    O    B. Initiation of an intravenous solution containing sodium bicarbonate, 1 mEq/kg
    O    C. An order for Ipecac, 15 ml in a glass of orange juice followed by three glasses of water
    O    D. An order for N-acetylcysteine, 140 mg/kg in a glass of orange juice

12. N-acetylcysteine counteracts the effect of acetaminophen by:
    - 0   A. Stimulating the production of vitamin K to prevent bleeding
    - 0   B. Increasing hepatic production of glutathione, protecting the liver
    - 0   C. Stimulating the production of glucagon and absorbing the acetaminophen
    - 0   D. Decreasing the effects of liver enzymes stimulated by the acetaminophen

13. Which of the following assessment parameters may be used by the emergency department nurse to evaluate the toxicity of an acetaminophen poisoning?
    - 0   A. Liver function studies
    - 0   B. Serial arterial blood gases
    - 0   C. Coagulation studies
    - 0   D. Electrolytes

*A 23-year-old woman comes to the ED complaining of abdominal pain. She states that she took a bottle of aspirin after having a fight with her boyfriend. She is currently alert, and her skin is hot and dry. Her vital signs are B/P 90/50, P 130, and R 32. A set of blood gases are drawn, and the results are pH 7.40, $Po_2$ 100, $Pco_2$ 20, and $HCO_3$ 18.*

14. These gases reflect the patient's:
    - 0   A. Metabolic acidosis
    - 0   B. Respiratory alkalosis
    - 0   C. Respiratory acidosis
    - 0   D. Metabolic alkalosis

15. In addition to gastric emptying and charcoal administration for the patient who has suffered salicylate poisoning, which of the following interventions may be useful?
    - 0   A. Administering a specific antidote for salicylate poisoning
    - 0   B. Administering fresh frozen plasma to decrease coagulopathies
    - 0   C. Initiating forced diuresis and alkalinization
    - 0   D. Administering acetylcysteine either orally or intravenously

16. What nursing diagnosis would pertain to the patient who has a toxic level of salicylates?
    - 0   A. Swallowing, impaired, related to mental status changes caused by salicylates
    - 0   B. Fluid volume deficit, high risk for, related to fluid loss from nausea and vomiting

    - 0   C. Family processes, altered, related to the patient taking an intentional overdose
    - 0   D. Infection, high risk for, related to the skin injury that may occur with bleeding

17. Because of the bleeding complications that may occur with salicylate poisoning, what laboratory value should the emergency department nurse evaluate?
    - 0   A. Type and screen for packed red blood cells
    - 0   B. BUN and creatinine level
    - 0   C. Prothrombin time and partial thromboplastin time
    - 0   D. Arterial blood gases

18. An 18-month-old boy has ingested an unknown amount of his mother's amitriptyline. His sister gave the pills to him, believing they were candy. He is brought to the ED protecting his airway but only responding to deep, painful stimuli. Signs and symptoms of tricyclic toxicity include:
    - 0   A. Hypothermia
    - 0   B. Constricted pupils
    - 0   C. Urinary incontinence
    - 0   D. Sinus tachycardia

19. The first step in the management of this child is:
    - 0   A. Insert a nasogastric tube and begin lavage with room temperature water
    - 0   B. Insert a nasogastric tube and instill 50 g of charcoal along with a cathartic
    - 0   C. Secure the child's airway by intubation with a cuffed endotracheal tube
    - 0   D. Secure the child's airway by intubation with an uncuffed endotracheal tube

20. The method of gastric decontamination recommended for the person who has been poisoned by a toxic level of a tricyclic antidepressant is:
    - 0   A. Insertion of a nasogastric tube for gastric lavage and lavage with copious amount of normal saline
    - 0   B. Administration of 30 ml of syrup of Ipecac through a nasogastric tube with a large amount of normal saline
    - 0   C. Administration of activated charcoal mixed in 500 ml of orange juice or whatever fluid the patient will tolerate
    - 0   D. Administration of syrup of Ipecac orally, followed by eight glasses of warm distilled water

**21.** A pertinent nursing diagnosis for the patient who has been poisoned by cyclic antidepressants would be:

0    A. Noncompliance related to excessive ingestion of prescribed medications despite appropriate instructions

0    B. Social isolation related to depression and inability to express their need for counseling

0    C. Cardiac output, decreased, related to the quinidinelike effects of cyclic antidepressant toxicity

0    D. Injury, high risk for, related to the effects of cyclic antidepressant poisoning on the neurological and cardiovascular systems

**22.** Because of the capability of tricyclic antidepressants to block the reuptake of norepinephrine, what assessment parameter should be constantly evaluated by the emergency department nurse?

0    A. Temperature

0    B. Capillary refill

0    C. Blood pressure

0    D. Urinary output

**23.** A gastric tube is to be inserted for gastric lavage. The optimal position for this procedure would be:

0    A. Place the patient in the side-lying right lateral decubitis position

0    B. Place the patient in the side-lying left lateral decubitis position

0    C. Place the patient prone with the head of the bed lowered

0    D. Place the patient supine with pillow under the shoulders

**24.** Physostigmine should not be administered as an antidote for tricyclic toxicity because:

0    A. It can cause sinus tachycardia

0    B. It can cause atrial flutter

0    C. It can cause bradycardia

0    D. It can cause first-degree heart block

**25.** Tricyclic toxicity is very difficult to treat because:

0    A. They bind to the hemoglobin

0    B. They bind to the plasma proteins

0    C. They bind to white blood cells

0    D. They bind to muscle cells

*A 1-year-old child has ingested an unknown amount of gasoline from an open container. He is awake, alert, and crying appropriately with a respiratory rate of 40. He smells like gasoline.*

**26.** Because the patient has ingested a hydrocarbon, the initial assessment of this patient will be focused on his:

0    A. Cardiac rhythm

0    B. Respiratory system

0    C. Gastrointestinal system

0    D. Central nervous system

**27.** Initial interventions for the management of this child should include:

0    A. Placement of a temperature probe

0    B. Supplental oxygen as tolerated

0    C. Placement in an isolation room

0    D. Placement in a protective crib

**28.** The patient is placed on 100% oxygen by mask. His respiratory rate has decreased to 28 breaths per minute. However, he continues to smell of gasoline. In order to prevent any further injury to this child, the emergency nurse should:

0    A. Prepare the child for endotracheal intubation to secure his airway as a precaution because of gasoline absorption

0    B. Wash the child's skin with soap and water to prevent further absorption of the gasoline

0    C. Administer 50 g of charcoal to prevent further absorption of the gasoline into the child's internal system

0    D. Administer 15 ml of ipecac to prevent further absorption of the gasoline into the child's internal system

**29.** A relevant nursing diagnosis in the care of this child would be:

0    A. Injury, high risk for, related to his age and curiosity

0    B. Gas exchange, impaired, related to pulmonary injury

0    C. Cardiac output, decreased, related to hydrocarbon ingestion

0    D. Aspiration, high risk for, related to hydrocarbon ingestion

**30.** What additional information should be obtained by the ED nurse to evaluate the child's home environment?

0    A. The number of siblings in the house in which the child lives

0   B. The location of the gasoline and other possible toxins in the home

0   C. Who is responsible for the child's care on a day-to-day basis

0   D. The distance from the child's home to the ED

*An elderly man attempted to commit suicide by locking himself in a closet and spraying himself with insecticide. On arrival in the ED, the patient is comatose, and his ECG shows sinus bradycardia.*

**31.** In addition to the initial assessment of the patient's ABC status, the emergency nurse should also consider:

0   A. How the patient was exposed to the toxin

0   B. The age of the patient and the effects of the toxin

0   C. Whether the patient is depressed or has attempted suicide in the past

0   D. Whether the patient has any other medical or psychological problems

**32.** In addition to stabilizing this patient's ABCs, the emergency nurse should prepare to:

0   A. Administer epinephrine 1:1,000 intravenously

0   B. Administer 50 g of charcoal through a nasogastric tube

0   C. Decontaminate the patient with soap and water

0   D. Place the patient on a pulse oximeter

**33.** The initial drug of choice to reverse the toxic effects of organophosphate poisoning is:

0   A. Lidocaine, 1 mg/kg

0   B. Sodium bicarbonate, 1 mEq/kg

0   C. Atropine, 1 to 5 mg

0   D. Calcium chloride, 10 mg

**34.** Pralidoxime is used in the mangement of organophosphate posioning because it:

0   A. Blocks acetylcholinesterase

0   B. Regenerates acetylcholinesterase

0   C. Regenerates acetylcholine

0   D. Blocks epinepherine

**35.** An appropriate nursing diagnosis for this patient would be:

0   A. Knowledge deficit related to the inappropriate use of an insecticide

0   B. Coping, ineffective individual, related to depression

0   C. Thought processes, altered, related to organophosphate poisoning

0   D. Family processes, altered, related to age

**36.** What outcome in this patient would indicate the effectiveness of atropine in the treatment of organophosphate poisoning?

0   A. Decreased salivation

0   B. Increased bradycardia

0   C. Increased ataxia

0   D. Cardiopulmonary arrest

**37.** The antidote administered for iron toxicity is:

0   A. N-acetylcysteine

0   B. Vitamin K

0   C. Deferoxamine

0   D. There is no antidote

*A 2-year-old child is brought to the ED by her mother. The mother states that the child has chickenpox and has become confused and hyperactive and is having difficulty walking. She does not have a fever, and her other vital signs are also within a normal range. The only medication the mother has been using is Caladryl lotion to decrease the child's itching.*

**38.** What type of toxicity is this child suffering from?

0   A. Acetaminophen

0   B. Diphenhydramine

0   C. Salicylate

0   D. Calcium chloride

**39.** A 40-year-old woman has taken an overdose of atenolol. She presents to the ED awake, with B/P of 80/56 and HR 38. Which of the following medications will be administered to manage this patient's toxicity?

0   A. Atropine sulfate

0   B. Epinephrine 1:1,000

0   C. Calcium chloride

0   D. Glucagon hydrochloride

**40.** A 4-year-old boy took 10 tablets of his grandmother's Calan SR (verapamil). He presents to the ED with a B/P of 86/48, a HR 32 and a RR of 30. The drug of choice to reverse the effects of the Calan SR (verapamil) is:

0   A. Calcium chloride

0   B. Digitalis

0   C. Adenosine

0   D. Epinephrine

**ANSWERS**

1. **B. Assessment.** The most important component of the initial assessment of the poisoned patient is the patient's ability to use his or her airway. Many poisons alter the patient's mental status, and the patient could quickly be at risk for aspiration, hypoventilation, and apnea.[11]

2. **A. Intervention.** The initial management of the poisoned patient is based on supportive management of ABCs. Since this patient has an altered level of consciousness and has vomited, intubation is indicated. Ipecac should not be given to a patient who is not capable of protecting his or her airway.[11]

3. **B. Intervention.** Flumazenil should be administered rapidly over 15 to 30 seconds through a large vein. The drug should not be mixed with any other medications.[12]

4. **C. Assessment.** A serious and life-threatening side effect of flumazenil administration is the precipitation of seizures. Patients with a history of seizures and those with mixed overdoses, particularly tricyclics, should not be given this drug.[12]

5. **B. Analysis.** The most appropriate nursing diagnosis, and one on which the emergency nurse could develop this patient's plan of care, would be poisoning, potential for, related to ingestion of an unknown amount of lorazepam and alcohol. Because of the possible life-threatening complications that may occur with poisoning, and the nature of the episodic care provided by the ED nurse, this particular diagnosis would encompass many of the relevant nursing actions that would be required by this patient.[13]

6. **A. Evaluation.** The patient's level of consciousness should be closely monitored. One potential problem with flumazenil administration in the patient with benzodiazepine overdose is resedation.[12]

7. **B. Intervention.** Benzodiazepines potentiate the affects of gamma-aminobutyric acid (GABA), which is an inhibitory neurotransmitter. A positive side-effect is a decrease in anxiety and in some cases amnesia. However, an overdose of the drug can cause sedation and a depressed mental status.[14]

8. **A. Intervention.** Charcoal is a finely divided black powder with an extensive internal network of pores that absorb substances. For charcoal to be effective, it needs to be given as quickly as possible after ingestion of the toxic substance.[14] Research has suggested that in certain poisonings, charcoal alone, rather than combined with the use of ipecac, may be useful in the initial treatment of the alert poisoned patient. It has been found that many patients are unable to keep charcoal down until several hours after ipecac has been administered, thus being deprived of the charcoal's ability to absorb the poison.[15]

9. **D. Intervention.** Charcoal is contraindicated when the patient has ingested a caustic or corrosive substance. Pediatric doses of charcoal include infant 1 g/kg and children 25 to 50 g/kg.[5]

10. **C. Assessment.** All patients should have a serum acetaminophen level drawn 4 hours after ingestion. The serum level immediately following ingestion will offer little information about the potential toxic level the patient may have ingested.[7]

11. **D. Intervention.** N-acetylcysteine is indicated when the serum acetaminophen level remains at a toxic level after 4 hours or if an acetaminophen level cannot be obtained before 10 hours after ingestion. N-acetylcysteine is given orally. It may cause vomiting and may have to be given through a nasogastric tube. It is interesting to note that N-acetylcysteine is given intravenously in other countries, such as Australia. There are currently some centers giving it intravenously in this country, but this has not yet received FDA approval.[7]

12. **B. Intervention.** N-acetylcysteine stimulates an increase in the production of glutathione, which metabolizes the hepatotoxicity intermediately created by acetaminophen toxicity.[7]

13. **A. Evaluation.** Since acetaminophen poisoning is particularly toxic to the liver, baseline hepatic studies should be drawn. The peak hepatotoxicity occurs 72 to 96 hours after ingestion.[7]

14. **B. Assessment.** Salicylate poisoning initially will stimulate the respiratory center of the central nervous system. This manifests itself in an increased respiratory rate and causes respiratory alkalosis.[8]

15. **C. Intervention.** Salicylate poisoning is treated with gastric emptying, charcoal administration, and alkaline diuresis. Alkaline diuresis will increase the pH of the patient's urine and improve free salicylate excretion.[8,16]

16. **B. Analysis.** Salicylate poisoning may cause excessive fluid loss from nausea, vomiting, sweating, and hyperventilation, all of which can lead to dehydration.[13]

17. **C. Evaluation.** Bleeding problems may develop in severe salicylate poisoning. This occurs because of impaired platelet aggregation and decreased thrombin.[8,16]

18. **D. Assessment.** Because tricyclic toxicity stimulates anticholinergic activity and has quinidinelike effects on the cardiovascular system, the signs and symptoms of tricyclic toxicity include altered level

of consciousness, decreased respirations, seizures, urinary retention, sinus tachycardia with widened QRS, hyperpyrexia, and hypotension.[5,11,16]

19. **D. Intervention.** Since the child already has an altered mental status, his airway should initially be protected. The age of the child requires that the child needs to be intubated with an uncuffed endotracheal tube.[5]

20. **A. Intervention.** Tricyclic poisoning can cause rapid changes in mental status and will easily place the patient at risk of vomiting and aspiration if the patient is given anything orally. Tricyclic antidepressants exert an anticholinergic effect that may cause pills and pill fragments to remain in the stomach for a long period of time. Gastric lavage, and then administration of charcoal, will help ensure that the drug is removed from the patient's system.[5,11,16]

21. **C. Analysis.** The most appropriate nursing diagnosis would be C, because the toxic cardiac and neurological effects of cyclic antidepressants are lethal.[13]

22. **C. Evaluation.** Since the supply of norepinephrine is depleted by the body, and the tricyclic antidepressant is blocking the reuptake of norepinephrine, hypotension will result. It is important to recognize this toxic effect early so that appropriate intervention can be initiated.[5,8,16]

23. **B. Intervention.** The patient should be placed in the side-lying left lateral decubitis position to protect his airway (particularly if he is not intubated) and to facilitate drainage of the lavage fluid.[5]

24. **C. Intervention.** Physostigmine can cause bradycardia and asystole in a person poisoned by tricyclics.[9]

25. **B. Assessment.** Tricyclic antidepressants bind to the plasma proteins, which make them very diffiuclt to remove from the body.[11]

26. **B. Assessment.** Because hydrocarbon ingestion initially affects the respiratory system, the patient's respiratory system will need to be assessed. Included in this assessment should be the patient's normal respiratory rate and any indications of respiratory distress, including dyspnea, wheezes, stridor, hemoptysis, and cyanosis.[5,11]

27. **B. Intervention.** If the child has suffered pulmonary injury, supplemental oxygen will be needed.[5]

28. **B. Intervention.** Because some hydrocarbons (particularly gasoline) can be absorbed through the skin, and the emergency nurse is unsure of the amount of gasoline ingested, the child's skin should be decontaminated by washing it with soap and water. External gasoline can also cause burns.[5,11]

29. **D. Analysis.** One of the major complications with hydrocarbon ingestion is the potential for aspiration because of vomiting. The emergency nurse's plan of care needs to include interventions that will prevent any further injury to the pulmonary system from aspiration.[5,13]

30. **B. Evaluation.** An important role for the emergency nurse is teaching prevention. Obtaining information about the location of possible poisons, and then teaching the child's parents how to prevent any further accidents, could prevent a future tragedy.[5]

31. **A. Assessment.** The method of exposure needs to be considered, particularly in relation to insecticide poisoning. As noted in the history, the patient sprayed the insecticide all over himself in an enclosed place.[10,11]

32. **C. Intervention.** He suffered not only inhalation exposure but also dermal exposure. Therefore, he will need to have his clothes removed and his skin cleansed with soap and water to remove any remaining insecticide.[10,11]

33. **C. Intervention.** Atropine is administered in doses of 1 to 5 mg and repeated every 15 minutes.[10,11]

34. **B. Intervention.** Pralidoxime is an additional antidote for the treatment of organophosphate poisoning. It works by regenerating acetylcholinesterase.[10]

35. **B. Analysis.** A suicidal patient is displaying ineffective coping. The patient has chosen behavior that is detrimental, and suicide precautions will need to be instituted while he is in the emergency department.[13]

36. **A. Evaluation.** Atropine will reverse the muscarinic effects of organophosphate poisoning, which include salivation, lacrimation, urinary and fecal incontinence, vomiting, miosis, bronchospasm, and bradycardia.[10,11]

37. **C. Intervention.** Deferoxamine is the antidote for iron toxicity. This medication will turn the urine a vin rose color, which indicates that the iron is binding with the drug.[5]

38. **B. Assessment.** Caladryl lotion contains diphenhydramine to help decrease the amount of itching that accompanies some skin lesions such as those in chicken pox. If the lotion is applied in large amounts, to large areas of skin or to broken skin, it can be absorbed and cause toxic side effects. Diphenhydramine toxicity causes anticholinergic effects, including confusion, paradoxic hyperactivity, disorientation, and ataxia. The lotion needs to be removed to prevent any further absorption.[12]

39. **D. Intervention.** Glucagon hydrochloride has been found to be effective in the management of

propranolol toxicity. Glucagon may increase the intracellular level of calcium within the myocardium.[5]

40. **A. Intervention.** Calcium chloride is the drug that is used to manage the toxic side effects of calcium channel blocker intoxication. Unlike verapamil toxicity, which causes hypotension and bradycardia, nifedipine toxicity causes hypotension and tachycardia.[5]

## REFERENCES

1. Litovitz T, Kelin-Schwartz W, Dyer K, and others: 1997 annual report of the American Association of Poison Control Centers toxic surveillance system, *Am J Emerg Med* 16(5):443-497.
2. McCaig LF, Burt CW: Poisoning-related visits to emergency departments in the United States, 1993-1996, *J Toxicol Clin Toxicol* 77(7):817-826, 1999.
3. Department of Health and Human Services: *Mid-Year 1998 preliminary emergency department data from the drug abuse warning network,* Rockville, MD, July, 1999, SAMHSA.
4. International Liason Committee on Resuscitation: *ILCOR advisory statements: special resuscitation situations,* Dallas, 1999, American Heart Association.
5. Haley K, Eckles N, Baker P, editors. *Emergency nursing pediatric course,* Park Ridge, IL, 1999, Emergency Nurses Association.
6. Zimmerman HE, Burkhart KK, Donovan JW: Ethylene glycol ad methanol posioning: Diagnosis and treatment, *J Emerg Nurs* 25(2):116-120, 1999.
7. Perry H, Shannon M: Acetaminophen. In Haddad L, Shannon M, Winchester J, editors: *Poisoning and drug overdose,* ed 3, Philadelphia, 1998, WB Saunders.
8. Krenzelok E, Kerr F, Proudfoot AT: Salicylate toxicity. In Haddas L, Shannon M, Winchester J, editors: Poisoning and drug overdose, ed 3, Philadelphia, 1998, WB Saunders.
9. Pentel P, Keyler D, Haddad L: Tricyclic antidepressants and selective serotonin reuptake inhibitors. In Haddad L, Shannon M, Winchester J, editors: *Poisoning and drug overdose,* ed 3, Philadelphia, 1998, WB Saunders.
10. Diaz J, Lopez A: Voluntary ingestion of organophosphate insecticide by a young farmer, *J Emerg Nurs* 25(4):266-268, 1999.
11. McDeed-Breault C: Toxicological emergencies. In Jordan K, editor: *Emergency nursing core curriculum,* ed 5, Philadelphia, 2000, WB Saunders.
12. Deglin J, Vallerand A: *Davis' drug guide for nurses,* ed 6, Philadelphia, 1999, FA Davis.
13. Kim MJ, McFarland GK, McLane AM: *Pocket guide to nursing diagnoses,* St Louis, 1993, Mosby.
14. Dean BS: Ingestions and poisoning. In *Pediatric nursing,* Norwalk, 1994, Appleton & Lange.
15. Albertson TE and others: Superiority of activated charcoal in the treatment of acute toxic ingestions, *Ann Emerg Med* 18:56, 1989.
16. Criddle LM: Toxicologic emergencies. In Newberry L, editor: *Sheehy's emergency nursing principles and practice,* ed 4, St Louis, 1998, Mosby.

# Chapter 20

# Wound Management Emergencies

## REVIEW OUTLINE

I. Anatomy of the integumentary system[1]
  A. Largest organ system
  B. Epidermis
    1. Avascular
    2. Composed primarily of epithelial cells
    3. Responsible for regeneration of skin
  C. Dermis
    1. Composed of connective tissue, fibroblasts, microphages, and fat cells
    2. Vascular
    3. Has lymph channels and nerves
  D. Hypodermis
    1. Contains subcutaneous tissues
    2. Contains smooth muscle, the areolar bed, blood vessels, and nerves

II. Function of the skin
  A. Protection
  B. Temperature control
  C. Excretion of salt and water
  D. Preservation of body fluids
  E. Production of vitamin D

III. Process of wound healing
  A. Methods of wound healing
    1. Primary intention
    2. Secondary intention
    3. Tertiary intention
  B. Injury
  C. Inflammatory phase
    1. Homeostasis
    2. Phagocytosis
  D. Proliferation phase
    1. Granulation
    2. Epithelialization
  E. Maturation phase

IV. Assessment of the integumentary system[1]
  A. History
    1. Mechanism of injury
      a. Direction and amount of force
      b. Associated injuries
      c. What may have been responsible for the injury: weapon, fall, animals, insects, and so on

2. Time when injury occurred
3. Risk for contamination
4. Amount and type of bleeding
5. Level of pain
6. Amount of disability
7. Numbness or tingling distal to the injury
8. Previous interventions prior to arrival in the emergency department
  B. Medical history
    1. Chronic illness
      a. Diabetes
      b. Cancer
      c. Peripheral vascular disease
      d. Osteoporosis
      e. Arthritis
      f. Sickle cell anemia
      g. Immunosuppressive diseases
    2. History of recent surgery
    3. Medications
      a. Aspirin
      b. Immunosuppressants
      c. Steroids
      d. Anticoagulants
  C. Tetanus status
  D. Psychosocial history
    1. Intentional vs. nonintentional injury
  E. Age-related characteristics[1-3]
    1. Pediatric
      a. Growth/development
        (1) Younger children have thinner skin, more easily injured
        (2) Skin changes occur with adolescence
        (3) Immunization status
        (4) Intentional vs. nonintentional injury
    2. Geriatric
      a. Changes in skin texture and turgor, wrinkling, fragility
      b. Less elasticity
      c. Diminished temperature sensation
      d. Skin becomes dry, flaky

e. Skin discolorations
  (1) Liver spots
  (2) Seborrheic keratosis
  (3) Cherry angiomas

F. Inspection
  1. General appearance of the patient
  2. Edema
  3. Redness
  4. Presence of foreign bodies
  5. Extent of damage to the skin
  6. Presence of bite/fang marks

G. Neurovascular assessment
  1. Flexion
  2. Extension
  3. Palpation of distal pulses
  4. Palpation of skin temperature
  5. Capillary refill
  6. Sensation
  7. Two-point discrimination
  8. Neurological function
  9. Vascular status

V. Collaborative care of the patient with surface trauma[4,5]
  A. Airway, breathing, circulation (ABCs)
  B. Control of bleeding
  C. Assess for other life-threatening injuries
  D. Assess and manage patient's pain
  E. Goals of wound care
    1. Prevention of infection
    2. Promotion of rapid healing
    3. Prevention of scarring
  F. Forensic considerations
    1. Always keep in mind that the wound may be evidence or contain evidence
    2. Describe entrance and exit
    3. Preserve evidence in appropriate containers
    4. Label containers with patient's identification, location where evidence obtained, and date and time
  G. Wound care
    1. Assessment of the wound
    2. Assessment of the patient's neurovascular status
    3. Cleansing of the wound
    4. Irrigation of the wound
    5. Anesthesia
    6. Hair removal (never shave eyebrows)
    7. Closure
      a. Sutures
      b. Staples
      c. Adhesive tapes
      d. Tissue adhesives

8. Suture, staple, adhesive tape removal
9. Dressing application
10. Discharge instructions

H. Medications
  1. Tetanus/tetanus immune globulin
  2. Antibiotics
  3. Rabies prophylaxis

VI. Related nursing diagnoses
  A. Anxiety
  B. Infection, high risk for
  C. Fluid volume deficit
  D. Knowledge deficit
  E. Pain
  F. Skin integrity, impaired

VII. Selected wounds
  A. Abrasion
  B. Abscess
  C. Avulsion
  D. Amputation
  E. Contusion
  F. Lacerations
  G. Puncture wounds
  H. Wound-related infections

The skin, or integumentary system, is the largest organ system of the body. Its functions are protection, control of body temperature, primary sensation, excretion of water and salt, preservation of body fluids, and production of vitamin D. Injuries to the skin, or integumentary system, are a common reason for patients to come to the emergency department (ED). There are many sources of these injuries, including thermal or chemical sources, punctures (or penetrating trauma), lacerations, and abrasions.[4] This chapter focuses on some of the most common types of surface trauma seen in the ED.

The collaborative care of the patient who has suffered an injury to the integumentary system includes the prevention of infection, promotion of rapid healing, and prevention of scarring.[4] Proper cleansing of the wound is important in the prevention of infection.[4] There are many types of solutions that can be used to cleanse a wound. It is important to be familiar with the solution being used to prevent any further injury to the wound. Many solutions should be diluted.[5] In addition, irrigation of the wound with sterile water or normal saline helps to remove debris and contaminants.[5]

Whenever the skin has been penetrated, the tetanus status of the patient should be evaluated. Recommended tetanus prophylaxis is provided by the Centers for Disease Control and Prevention (CDC).

The type of wound determines specific interventions, such as suturing, stapling, or the use of tissue adhesives, the time when the wound occurred, and the extent of injury caused by the wound. Surface injuries older than 6 hours are generally considered contaminated and may not be closed in the same manner as a wound that occurred later.

Wounds may result from either intentional or non-intentional injury. Observing the pattern of injury will provide the emergency nurse with important information. Wound patterns may indicate the presence of other injuries; signs of defense or intentional injury that may require that the patient needs to be protected from himself or others; and finally, wounds may be evidence of a crime.[7] If photographs cannot be obtained, the wound should either be drawn or described on the patient's chart. Any evidence that is collected should be labeled and placed in a paper bag to prevent degradation.

Integumentary injuries are some of the most common problems that present to the emergency department. Early recognition of potential complications and high-quality wound management will prevent further injuries to the patient.[8]

## REVIEW QUESTIONS

1. Which of the following wounds has the greatest potential for infections?
   - 0   A. Shearing injury caused by a knife
   - 0   B. Shearing injury caused by glass
   - 0   C. Avulsion injury from a skin tear
   - 0   D. Compression injury to the hand

2. Wounds to which area of the body are at greatest risk for infection?
   - 0   A. The elbow
   - 0   B. The scalp
   - 0   C. The foot
   - 0   D. The face

3. The most common skin pathogen is:
   - 0   A. *Pasteurella multocida*
   - 0   B. *Staphylococcus aureus*
   - 0   C. *Vibrio vulnificus*
   - 0   D. *Pseudomonas aeruginosa*

4. A 21-year-old male cut his finger on a knife while at work. The wound is clean, but will require several stitches. The patient states that his last tetanus vaccination was 11 years ago. The most appropriate vaccination he should receive is:
   - 0   A. A tetanus-diphtheria toxoid
   - 0   B. A tetanus immune globulin
   - 0   C. A tetanus-diphtheria toxoid and a tetanus immune globulin
   - 0   D. No vaccination is necessary at this time

5. Which of the following is an indication for antibiotic therapy in wound management?
   - 0   A. A wound that is repaired within 2 hours of injury
   - 0   B. An uncomplicated wound without any drainage
   - 0   C. Wounds over a prosthetic joint
   - 0   D. A superficial abrasion to the scalp

6. An 18-year-old man comes to the emergency department complaining of abrasions to both his thighs. The patient states that he was riding his motorcycle and lost control, scraping his legs on the road. Physical examination reveals that the patient has large abrasions on the tops of both of his thighs. A wound complication common to abrasions is:
   - 0   A. A large loss of fluids from the skin
   - 0   B. Contamination of the wound by debris
   - 0   C. Open wounds to the bone
   - 0   D. Loss of sensation to the injured area

7. Contamination of an abrasion by asphalt may leave a patient at risk for:
   - 0   A. The development of a third-degree burn from the asphalt
   - 0   B. An anaphylactic reaction to the asphalt
   - 0   C. Tattooing from retained asphalt
   - 0   D. Development of tetanus from the asphalt

8. A 20-year-old woman comes to the triage nurse complaining of a severe laceration on her right wrist. The patient states that she tripped and put her hand through a plate glass door. The patient has a towel wrapped around the extremity. She is pale and diaphoretic. Her B/P is 90/60, and her P is 120. The initial care of this patient should be based on which of the following nursing diagnoses?
   - 0   A. Fluid volume deficit related to blood loss from the wrist laceration
   - 0   B. Skin integrity, impaired related to the wrist laceration
   - 0   C. Pain related to the wrist laceration
   - 0   D. Anxiety related to the potential for disfigurement from the wrist laceration

*A 32-year-old male painter presents to the emergency department complaining of pain in his left hand. The patient states that earlier that day he had injected his left index finger with his paint gun. Upon evaluation, his left index finger is found to be swollen, pale, and tender to the touch.*

9. The extent of this type of high-pressure injection injury (HPI) depends on all of the following *except*:
   - 0   A. The age of the patient who has been injured
   - 0   B. Site of the injury
   - 0   C. Characteristics of the substance injected
   - 0   D. Amount of the substance injected

10. The emergency nurse should prepare this patient for:
    - 0   A. Immediate debridement of the injured left finger to determine the extent of damage
    - 0   B. Immediate infiltration of the injured finger to manage the patient's pain during evaluation
    - 0   C. Immediate administration of the antidote to the paint substance that the patient may have injected in the wound
    - 0   D. Immediate evaluation and admission to the operating room for surgical evaluation of the wound

11. All of the following are factors that will delay wound healing *except:*
    - 0   A. Corticosteroid therapy
    - 0   B. Excessive body fat
    - 0   C. Adequate blood supply
    - 0   D. Diabetes mellitus

12. An injury where skin is peeled away from an extremity is:
    - 0   A. Contusion
    - 0   B. Laceration
    - 0   C. Abscess
    - 0   D. Avulsion

13. A 23-year-old male suffered a 15 cm deep laceration to his left forearm while digging a ditch when a chunk of rock struck it. The bleeding has been stopped. The initial nursing diagnosis upon which to base this patient's care would be:
    - 0   A. High risk for infection related to the size and depth of his left forearm laceration

    - 0   B. Knowledge deficit related to the safety regulations that prevent work injuries
    - 0   C. Risk for impaired skin integrity related to his left forearm laceration
    - 0   D. Impaired physical mobility related to his left forearm laceration

14. An example of a vegetative foreign body is:
    - 0   A. Metal splinter
    - 0   B. Straight pin
    - 0   C. Glass shard
    - 0   D. Wood splinter

15. A method that is effective in decreasing the pain of infiltration when administering a local anesthetic is:
    - 0   A. Injecting the local anesthetic directly into the wound
    - 0   B. Cooling the local anesthetic before injection
    - 0   C. Injecting the local anesthetic through the wound edges
    - 0   D. Buffering the anesthetic agent with epinephrine

16. A 2-year-old child suffered a 2.5 cm laceration to his right eyebrow after tripping on a rug and striking his head on a coffee table. There was no loss of consciousness. Preparation of this child's wound for closure should include:
    - 0   A. Shaving his eyebrow to remove hair follicles and decrease the risk of infection
    - 0   B. Directly scrubbing the wound with a hard sterile brush and undiluted povidone-iodine
    - 0   C. Allowing devitalized tissue to remain in the wound to enhance healing
    - 0   D. Irrigating the wound with normal saline using a protective shield to decrease splattering

17. The parents have chosen to have the child's wound closed with a tissue adhesive (TA). An advantage of using a TA is:
    - 0   A. TA administration causes significantly more pain than suturing
    - 0   B. The use of a TA costs more than suturing a facial wound
    - 0   C. The use of TA instead of suturing decreases the risk of wound infection
    - 0   D. The use of TA increases the risk of foreign body reactions

**18.** Tissue adhesives can be used for wound closure for all of the following *except:*

  0   A. Neck laceration

  0   B. Forehead lacerations

  0   C. Knee laceration

  0   D. Eyebrow laceration

**19.** Discharge instructions for the patient whose wound has been closed with a TA should include:

  0   A. The TA should be peeled off in 2 weeks

  0   B. The patient may shower, but should not soak the wound

  0   C. No explanation of signs and symptoms of infection

  0   D. Application of a moisturizing cream will enhance healing

**20.** Sutures placed in a patient's scalp should be removed:

  0   A. In 3 to 5 days

  0   B. In 4 to 6 days

  0   C. In 10 to 14 days

  0   D. In 7 to 10 days

## ANSWERS

1. **D. Assessment.** Crush injuries have the greatest potential to become infected because of the extent of injury and vascular compromise.[9]

2. **C. Assessment.** The foot is most likely to become infected because of differences in blood flow.[9]

3. **B. Assessment.** *Staphylococcus aureus* and streptococci are the most common pathogens on skin.[9]

4. **A. Intervention.** It has been over 10 years since the patient had a vaccination. The wound is clean and at a low risk for infection. A tetanus-diphtheria immunization is recommended.[8]

5. **C. Intervention.** Indications for antibiotic therapy for wound management include delay in wound closure of greater than 3 hours; pus in the wound; wounds contaminated with feces, saliva, or vaginal secretions; prevention of endocarditis; wounds over prosthetic joints; and bites to the hand.[9]

6. **B. Assessment.** Abrasions result from the skin being forced against a hard surface, such as a road. Injury can occur to both the epidermis and the dermis. The resultant injury is similar to a burn. Often, because of the mechanism of injury, these wounds are contaminated.[6]

7. **C. Assessment.** Asphalt is one of the most common contaminants found in an abrasion. If the abrasion is not properly cleansed and debrided, tattooing can occur because of the dark color of the asphalt. This can be especially disfiguring when the abrasion is on the patient's face.[5]

8. **A. Analysis.** Based on the initial assessment of this patient, the triage nurse's care would be based on the nursing diagnosis of fluid volume deficit related to blood loss from the wrist laceration.

9. **A. Assessment.** The extent and the potential complications that may result from a high-pressure injury (HPI) depend on the site of the injury (usually the nondominant hand), characteristics and amount of the substance injected (epinephrine, paint and paint solvents very toxic), and the underlying anatomy that will be affected.[10,11]

10. **D. Intervention.** The treatment of this type of injury requires immediate recognition of the type of injury it is (HPI) and preparation for further evaluation in the operating room. The wound should not be infiltrated or debrided in the emergency department. Occasionally, the patient may have a toxic reaction to the substance injected, requiring supportive care.[10]

11. **C. Assessment.** Risk factors that will contribute to delaying wound healing include inadequate blood supply; corticosteroid therapy; obesity; diabetes mellitus, poor general health, and anemia.[6]

12. **D. Avulsion.** Skin that has been peeled away from an extremity is a severe form of an avulsion also known as a degloving injury.[6]

13. **A. Analysis.** The initial care of this patient should be based on decreasing the risk for infection. The patient's skin is already impaired.[12]

14. **D. Assessment.** Examples of vegetative foreign bodies include thorns or wood. These foreign bodies are highly reactive and sometimes difficult to see.[12]

15. **C. Intervention.** Methods to decrease the pain of administering local anesthetic include: injecting the local anesthetic into the wound edges; warming the local anesthetic; buffering it with sodium bicarbonate at a 1:10 ratio; slowly injecting the medication; and pretreatment with a topical anesthetic.[8]

16. **D. Intervention.** Wound preparation includes removing hair follicles to decrease the risk of infection. However, eyebrows should not be shaved because they may not grow back and they may also be used for exact approximation of wound edges. Wounds should not be directly scrubbed with a hard brush or an undiluted solution because additional injury may be caused. Wounds should be

irrigated with normal saline. A splashguard should be applied to decrease splattering.[8]

17. **C. Analysis.** Tissue adhesives have been found to have a low rate of infection after their use. Other advantages include decreased pain with application compared with suturing; decreased foreign body reaction; and decreased cost with their use.[13]

18. **C. Assessment.** Tissue adhesives have problems with early bond weakness and are not recommended for use over joints or areas with increased mobility. Tissue adhesives are also susceptible to becoming ineffective in moist or wet environments.[13]

19. **B. Intervention.** Discharge instructions after application of tissue adhesives should include: avoid getting the area wet or applying creams or ointments that may loosen the adhesive, the patient may shower; signs and symptoms of wound infection; and the need to leave the tissue adhesive alone because it will fall off naturally within 2 weeks after application.[13]

20. **D. Intervention.** Sutures placed in the scalp should be removed 7 to 10 days after placement.[6]

### REFERENCES

1. Bates B: *A guide to physical examination and history taking,* ed 7, Philadelphia, 1999, Lippincott.
2. Engel J: *Pediatric assessment,* St Louis, 1993, Mosby.
3. Daly W, Munier-Sham J: Burns. In Kelley S, editor: *Pediatric emergency nursing,* Norwalk, 1994, Appleton & Lange.
4. Hackley L: Surface trauma. In Kitt S and others, editors: *Emergency nursing: a physiologic and clinical perspective,* Philadelphia, 1995, WB Saunders.
5. Trott A: *Wounds and lacerations: emergency care and closure,* ed 2, St Louis, 1997, Mosby.
6. Herman M, Newberry L: Wound management. In Newberry L, editor: *Sheehy's emergency nursing: principles and practice,* ed 4, St Louis, 1998, Mosby.
7. Harrahill M: Patterns of sharp force injury, *J Emerg Nurs* 18:355-356, 1992.
8. Hollander J, Singer A: Laceration management, *Ann Emerg Med* 34(3):356-365, 1999.
9. Eron L: Antimicrobial wound management in the emergency department: An educational supplement, *J Emerg Nurs* 17(1):189-195, 1999.
10. Stiles N: High-pressure injection injury of the hand: a surgical emergency, *J Emerg Nurs* 20:351-354, 1994.
11. Mol CJ, Gaver JC: A 39-year-old nurse with accidental discharge of an epinephrine autoinjection in the left index finger, *J Emerg Nurs* 18:306-307, 1992.
12. Mitchell B: Wound management emergencies. In Jordan KS, editor: *Emergency nursing core curriculum,* ed 5, Philadelphia, 2000, WB Saunders.
13. King M, Kinney A: Tissue adhesives: a new method of wound repair, *Nurs Pract* 24(10):66-74, 1999.

# Chapter 21

# Emergency Patient Transfer and Transport

## REVIEW OUTLINE

I. History of patient transport
   A. War transport
      1. European wars in the nineteenth century
      2. Civil War in the United States
      3. World War I
      4. World War II
      5. Korean War
      6. Vietnam War
   B. Civilian transport
      1. Hearse transport
      2. 1966 White paper, "Trauma, the Neglected Disease of Modern Society"
      3. Department of Transportation standards
      4. Emergency medical systems in the United States
   C. Air ambulance transport
      1. Balloons not used in the nineteenth century
      2. Air ambulance service in the early 1900s
      3. First military transport in 1945
      4. Korean War
      5. Vietnam War
      6. First hospital-based helicopter program in 1972

II. Components of an emergency medical service (EMS) transport system
   A. Human resources
      1. Levels of providers controlled by federal, state, local agencies
      2. Training: directed by level of provider
   B. Communications
   C. EMS response units
   D. Emergency facilities
   E. Critical care units
   F. Access to care
   G. Public information
   H. Disaster management and response
   I. Medical direction
   J. Prehospital triage

   K. Interhospital triage
   L. Policies and procedures for patient transport

III. Indications for transport
   A. Advanced level of care
      1. Level I or II trauma centers
      2. Pediatric care centers
      3. Cardiac care centers
      4. Neonatal care centers
      5. Transplant centers
      6. High-risk perinatal/neonatal centers
      7. Reimplantation centers
      8. Toxicological centers
   B. Indications for transport
      1. Patients who require a certain type of nursing and/or medical expertise not available at the initial care facility
      2. Patients who require diagnostic testing not available at the initial care facility
      3. Patients whose condition may deteriorate and who require care not available at the initial care facility
      4. Request by the patient's family that the patient be transferred to another facility
   C. Methods for making transport decisions
      1. Scoring systems
         a. Trauma score
         b. Pediatric trauma score
      2. Local protocols
      3. National standards
         a. Emergency Nurses Association (ENA)
         b. National Flight Nurses Association (NFNA) (now Air and Surface Transport Nurses Association)
         c. American College of Surgeons (ACS)
         d. American College of Emergency Physicians (ACEP)
         e. National Association of Emergency Medical Services Physicians (NAEMSP)
         f. Air Medical Physicians Association (AMPA)

IV. Consolidated Omnibus Budget Reconciliation Act (COBRA) (1986, 1989); Emergency Medical Treatment and Active Labor Act (EMTALA)

   A. All hospitals must examine all patients who come to the emergency department (ED) and provide necessary medical care

   B. Patients are not to be transferred until stabilized

   C. The referring center must be able to document that the medical benefits for the patient are greater at the receiving center

   D. The receiving facility must have available space and qualified personnel

   E. Ambulances, fixed-wing aircraft, and helicopters must have appropriate equipment and personnel to perform the transfer

V. Stabilization for transport

   A. Airway stabilization

   B. Ventilation

   C. Circulation (cardiac monitor, control of bleeding)

   D. Intravenous access

   E. Assessment of vital signs

   F. Neurological assessment

   G. Cervical spine and injured extremity immobilization

   H. History

   I. Temperature control

   J. Interhospital communication

   K. Family considerations

VI. Transport considerations

   A. Advantages of ground transport

      1. Availability

      2. Cost

      3. Space

   B. Disadvantages of ground transport

      1. Slower time

      2. Road conditions

   C. Advantages of air transport

      1. Decreased time

      2. Crew

      3. Advanced life support

   D. Disadvantages of air transport

      1. Availability

      2. Weather restrictions

      3. Cost

*I*n 1986, the Consolidated Omnibus Budget Reconciliation Act (COBRA) was passed, which, among other things, prohibits the "dumping" of patients by one hospital onto another. Several issues contributed to the development of this act, including an increase in the number of persons who do not have health insurance, the severity of the illnesses and injuries suffered by some people, and the cutting of health care budgets by both state and federal governments. The COBRA law contains major implications for the practice of emergency nursing and medicine, including the following[1]:

- All hospitals must examine all patients who come to the emergency department and provide necessary medical care.
- Patients should not be transferred until they are stabilized.
- It must be documented that the patient will receive better care at the receiving facility.
- The receiving facility must have available space and personnel to care for the patient.

Not all EDs, and the facilities that they are a part of, are able to take care of all the patients who are brought to them. The decision to transfer a patient should be based on many factors. Included in this decision-making process are the patient's need for additional expertise or diagnostic testing, possible deterioration in the patient's condition, and the family's request for transfer.

Specific physiological reasons have been identified to indicate a need for patient transfer.[2] These include:

- Serious injury to one or more organ systems
- Hypovolemic shock requiring more than one blood transfusion
- Spinal cord injuries
- Patients requiring advanced ventilatory support
- Head injuries with cerebrospinal fluid leakage, increased intracranial pressure (ICP), and a Glasgow Coma Scale (GCS) rating of less than 9

Before patients are transferred, they need to be stabilized. Stabilization is based on securing the patient's airway, providing ventilation, and maintaining adequate circulation. In addition to meeting the physical needs of the patient, the emergency department doing the transferring needs to arrange for a receiving facility. Having policies, agreements, transfer forms, and specific procedures already established makes transferring the patient much easier for those involved.[2,3]

The final step in the process of stabilization and transportation is deciding what mode of transportation should be used to get a patient to the receiving facility. There are both advantages and disadvantages to ground and air ambulances. Advantages of ground ambulances include space and the ability to move in most types of weather. Disadvantages of ground transport include the length of time it may require to transport the patient, poor road conditions, and the lack of availability of personnel trained in advanced life support (ALS).[3]

The advantages of air transport include saving of time, crews with advanced skills and experience, and generally a smoother ride for the patient. Disadvantages of air transport include a lack of available programs, weather restrictions, and limited space in which to provide patient care.[2,3]

## REVIEW QUESTIONS

*A 3-year-old child is brought to the emergency department after having been involved in a motor vehicle crash. Her injuries include a head injury with cerebrospinal fluid leakage, bruising in the left upper quadrant, and a fractured left femur. Her vital signs are B/P 80/50, P 140, and R 8. A decision is made to transfer the child to the pediatric trauma center about 100 miles away.*

1. In addition to documentation of the stabilization of the child's ABCs (airway, breathing, and circulation), what other component of the initial assessment should be documented?
   - 0   A. The weight of the child
   - 0   B. A neurological assessment
   - 0   C. Mechanism of injury
   - 0   D. Medical history

2. Based on the initial assessment of this child, the primary intervention the emergency nurse should prepare the patient for before transport is:
   - 0   A. Administering mannitol for ICP control
   - 0   B. Drawing blood for a type and crossmatch
   - 0   C. Intubation for airway management
   - 0   D. Applying MAST pants for hypotension

3. A tool that would be useful in the neurological evaluation of this patient is:
   - 0   A. Modified Glasgow Coma Scale
   - 0   B. A bedside EEG monitor
   - 0   C. Bedside cold water calorics
   - 0   D. Bedside oculocephalic reflexes

4. The most appropriate nursing diagnosis for the emergency nursing care of this patient is:
   - 0   A. Fluid volume deficit, high risk for, related to her multiple injuries
   - 0   B. Infection, high risk for, related to her multiple injuries
   - 0   C. Mobility, impaired physical, related to her head injury
   - 0   D. Thought processes, altered, related to her head injury

5. All of the following would indicate the need to transfer this patient *except:*
   - 0   A. Advanced diagnostic testing
   - 0   B. Nursing and medical expertise

   - 0   C. Lack of health insurance
   - 0   D. Serious injury to more than one organ system

*A 55-year-old man is brought to the ED complaining of severe left-sided chest pain. The patient is placed on a cardiac monitor, and the emergency nurse performs an ECG. There is significant ST elevation noted in leads II, III, and AvF. The patient is treated with rPA, but continues to have pain and ECG changes. He will require a cardiac catheterization and rescue angioplasty, which is not available at this facility.*

6. The COBRA law would not be breached by transferring this patient because:
   - 0   A. The patient has good health insurance and can afford to pay for the transfer
   - 0   B. Initial care has not been given to this patient at the referring facility
   - 0   C. The referring hospital cannot provide the care the patient needs and has stabilized the patient as much as their resources allow
   - 0   D. There are several critical care unit beds available at the receiving facility

7. An air medical transport program has been contacted to transport this patient to another ED. All of the following are advantages of helicopter transport for this patient *except:*
   - 0   A. A crew skilled in advanced life support care and the management of this type of patient
   - 0   B. Limited space in which to provide patient care in some helicopters
   - 0   C. Decreased transport time when flying by helicopter versus transferring the patient by ground
   - 0   D. Helicopter transport may provide a smoother trip for the patient

8. A disadvantage of using ground transport for this type of patient would be:
   - 0   A. Slower traveling time by ground transport than by air transport, especially in urban traffic
   - 0   B. The inside of the ground vehicle may provide total access to the patient
   - 0   C. A ground vehicle allows more crew mobility during transport if the patient would require additional procedures
   - 0   D. A ground vehicle is able to stop more quickly than an aircraft if the patient care requires it to

9. Of the following, the most important intervention in preparing this patient for transfer to another facility would be:
   0    A. Finding a facility willing to accept the patient
   0    B. Activating the transport system
   0    C. Initiating transport protocols
   0    D. Copying laboratory and radiography findings

10. The most appropriate nursing diagnosis for providing emergency nursing care when preparing this patient for transport would be:
   0    A. Injury, high risk for, related to the risks of transport
   0    B. Fluid volume excess, related to the physiologic impact of transport
   0    C. Activity intolerance, related to being secured for transport
   0    D. Cardiac output, decreased, related to the amount of injury to his heart

11. An advantage to allowing a family member to accompany a patient during transport is:
   0    A. The family member may distract the transport team during the transport
   0    B. The patient's family member takes up space and may get in the way of the patient's care
   0    C. If the patient dies, he or she will be with a family member, which is important to both the patient and the family
   0    D. The family member may become ill or have a fear of flying, which can be distracting to the transport team

*A 30-year-old man involved in a motor vehicle crash (MVC) is to be transferred from a hospital emergency department to a level I trauma center. Upon arrival of the transport team, the patient is found to have multiple rib fractures, subcutaneous emphysema, and moderate respiratory distress.*

12. Before taking this patient in the helicopter, the transport nurse should:
   0    A. Insert a central line for better intravenous access in case the patient requires blood during the transport
   0    B. Obtain a chest radiograph to be sure that the patient does not have a pneumothorax
   0    C. Perform a needle decompression of both sides of the patient's chest to manage his respiratory distress
   0    D. Place the patient on a pulse oximeter to monitor his oxygen saturation during flight

## ANSWERS

1. **B. Assessment.** Because of the child's severe head injury, the initial assessment should include an in-depth neurological assessment. The components of the neurological assessment should include the level of consciousness, pupillary response, motor response, sensory response, and vital signs.

2. **C. Intervention.** Because the child is hypoventilating—her respirations are 8—immediate control of the airway is indicated. Airway management may also help control any problems with ICP resulting from hyperventilation, as well as protect the child from aspiration.[2]

3. **A. Assessment.** A Modified GCS has been developed for the pediatric patient. The differences between the pediatric and adult GCS include "Best Verbal Response" and "Best Motor Response."[4]

4. **A. Analysis.** Because of the bruising on the child's upper left quadrant, the left fractured femur, and the initial vital signs, there is evidence that the child is at risk for the complications of hemorrhage shock. The emergency nursing care for this patient would be organized within the nursing diagnosis fluid volume deficit, high risk for.[2]

5. **C. Assessment.** One reason the COBRA law was drafted and passed in 1986 was to prevent hospitals from transferring or "dumping" patients for financial reasons. If a hospital is capable of providing needed patient services, it is obliged to do so. If this law is broken, the hospital may be fined $25,000 to $50,000 and lose its Medicare benefits. In addition, the injured party may be permitted to sue the hospital or anyone involved in his or her injury.[1]

6. **C. Intervention.** One of the major implications of the COBRA law is that patients should not be denied better medical care if it is available.[1]

7. **B. Intervention.** Using a helicopter to transfer this patient has the disadvantage of limited space in which to provide patient care.[2-4]

8. **A. Intervention.** The major advantage air transportation has over ground transportation is the saving of time. It takes approximately one-half to one-third the time to travel by air than it does by ground. When the patient requires a certain procedure or medication wherein time is important, the disadvantage of being slower could influence patient outcome.[2-4]

9. **A. Intervention.** The first step in preparing the patient for transport would be to identify and contact a facility willing to receive the patient. A great deal of time and trouble can be saved if protocols and transfer agreements have already been established before any problems arise.[2] The other issues

are important, but not initially important if there is no place to send the patient.

10. **D. Analysis.** Since this patient's potential complications would most likely stem from his cardiac problems, the most appropriate nursing diagnosis would be cardiac output, decreased. Some of the defining characteristics of this nursing diagnosis are dysrhythmia and ECG changes. ECG changes have already been documented.

11. **C. Assessment.** Advantages of allowing a family member to accompany a patient during transport include: emotionally beneficial to the patient and the family member; positive public relations; family presence if the patient dies; and family member available to give medical history or permission to treat.[5]

12. **B. Intervention.** Before taking a patient with significant chest trauma to altitude, the transport nurse should obtain a chest radiograph and evaluate whether there is a pneumothorax present and appropriately intervene if there is.[4]

## REFERENCES

1. Southard P: Legal and legislative considerations in emergency practice. In Kitt S et al, editors: *Emergency nursing: a physiologic and clinical approach,* Philadelphia, 1995, WB Saunders.
2. Haley K, Eckles N, Baker P: *Emergency nursing pediatric course,* Park Ridge, Ill, 1999, Emergency Nurses Association.
3. Harrahill M: Interfacility transfer. In Kitt S et al, editors: *Emergency nursing: a physiologic and clinical approach,* Philadelphia, 1995, WB Saunders.
4. Semonin Holleran R: *Prehospital nursing: a collaborative approach,* St Louis, 1994, Mosby.
5. Lewis M, Holditch-Davis D, Brunssen S: Parents as passengers during pediatric transport, *Air Med J* 16(2):38-43, 1997.

# Chapter 22

# Disaster Preparedness and Management

## REVIEW OUTLINE

I. General overview
  A. Disaster: any situation that overwhelms the existing resources of an institution, community, state, or nation.[1]
  B. Types of disaster
    1. Internal: i.e., institutional structure impaired, loss of electrical power as the result of a storm, terrorist activity, may require outside responders to assist
    2. External: takes place outside of the hospital, but has an impact on the hospital's operations, i.e., earthquake, flood, tornado, terrorist activity
  C. Emergency operations planning [1,2]
    1. Organized disaster committee
    2. Organized plan
      a. Authority: who or what activates the disaster plan
      b. Pre-established hospital operation centers
      c. Communication plan
      d. Coordination of patient care
      e. Security
      f. Deactivation
      g. Debriefing
  D. Effects of disaster(s)
    1. Loss of life
    2. Physical injuries
    3. Psychological trauma
    4. Property damage
    5. Environmental destruction
  E. National- and state-level interfaces
    1. Federal Emergency Management Agency (FEMA): the central point of contact in the federal government for a variety of emergency management activities with which hospitals may need to interface
    2. National Disaster Medical System (NDMS): federal-level system functioning to respond to major catastrophic disasters

    3. Joint Commission on the Accreditation of Healthcare Organizations' (JCAHO) requirements: hospitals must devise, implement, and practice a hospital-wide disaster plan
  F. Key components of emergency preparedness and emergency operations
    1. Disaster command center (DCC)
    2. Administrative operations center (AOC)
    3. Medical operations center
    4. Nursing operations center
    5. OR operations center
    6. Personnel operations center
    7. Security operations center
    8. ED operations center
    9. Public relations operations center
  G. Emergency disaster response
    1. Patient care
      a. Receiving, triaging, distributing
      b. Proper use of resources and facility
      c. Documenting care
      d. Evaluating care
    2. Communication
      a. Internal
      b. External
      c. News media
      d. Emergency operations center
    3. Resources
      a. Personnel
      b. Supplies
      c. Security
      d. Coordination
      e. Hospital resources
      f. Community resources
    4. Security, safety
      a. Traffic control
      b. Controlled access to department
    5. Coordination
      a. Local, state, federal
      b. Intradepartmental
      c. Interdepartmental

d. EMS community

e. Health care community

6. Documentation

a. Medical record

b. Disaster tags—(METTAG) the universal triage tag

c. Paper flow

H. Deactivation

1. Communication

2. Dispersal of additional resources

3. Community notification

I. Critical incident stress management (CISM)

1. Immediate reactions

2. Delayed reactions

3. Effect on care providers/community

II. Sources of disasters

A. Weapons of mass destruction and effect: nuclear, biological, chemical

1. Radiation

2. Routine industrial chemicals

3. Vesicants

4. Riot control agents

5. Nerve agents

6. Biological agents

7. Viral agents

8. Toxin agents

B. Terrorist activities

C. Nature: earthquakes, tornado, flood, and so on

III. Disaster preparedness

A. Philosophy related to disaster preparation and response

B. Disaster drills/exercises

C. Critique and education

A disaster has been defined as any situation, natural or manmade, that overwhelms an institution, community, state, or even a nation so that it is incapable of responding with existing resources.[1,2] Over the years, we have witnessed a variety of disasters, ranging from earthquakes and floods to terrorist attacks that include bombings and biological weapons. Generally, the emergency department is the initial place where victims will be transported. Emergency operations planning and disaster preparedness are integral pieces of emergency care.

The influx of casualties from a disaster can greatly tax or overwhelm the emergency department (ED). To prevent overwhelming the system, a plan is necessary to deal with the resultant increase in patient volume, increased workload, and the increased need for supplies and other resources. An Emergency Operations Plan is

an obligatory component of emergency department clinical operations and management.[2]

Hospitals are required by the Joint Commission on the Accreditation of Healthcare Organizations (JCAHO) to prepare for disaster situations. The JCAHO requires hospitals to have a documented plan for the environment of care that (1) addresses emergency preparedness, (2) has an orientation and education component, (3) establishes performance standards to measure its effectiveness on the environment of care, and (4) ensures the organization conducts emergency drills to test the responsiveness to emergency situations[3] (see Environment of Care and Human Resource Standards in JCAHO Manual).

The emergency department disaster preparedness plan must include detailed guidelines that collaboratively interface with both the hospital and the community plans. Key components of the disaster plan include patient care, communication, resources, safety or security, coordination, and documentation. Recent attention has also been focused on both national and international response to disasters, particularly those caused by chemical or biological weapons.[3]

Greater risks for disaster situations exist in the world today. ED personnel must be familiar with their disaster plan and know their role in executing the plan when needed. They also need to understand the stages of a disaster so they can better understand what has happened to patients before their arrival to the ED and what they will likely experience after treatment and admission to the hospital or discharge from the hospital. They need to be able to assess the impact of a disaster upon themselves, their co-workers, and the rescue personnel and assist them in coping with the effects of the disaster experience.

The role of the emergency department nurse in disaster preparedness and management involves many areas: (1) development and practice of the plan, (2) implementation of the plan, (3) development of an emergency operations center to serve as a communications link with the hospital and external environment, (4) triage activities, (5) secondary triage, (6) stabilization, and (7) critical incident stress management (CISM). Emergency nurses are well equipped for disaster preparedness and management because of their rapid assessment and triage skills, crisis management abilities, and linkages with community resource persons.

Of specific concern is knowing how to handle weapons of mass destruction that include chemical, biological, and radiation disaster situations. Donning the personal protective gear, using the proper procedures, and evaluating the disaster drills in which one participates are all important to the efficient functioning of the staff during a real situation. Practice helps keep the staff and patients safe and makes for a smoother operation when a real disaster occurs.

The ED plan must provide for the efficient management of incoming casualties and must include charge nurse responsibilities, disposition of patients currently in the department, preparation of triage site, patient flow, extent of initial and ongoing treatment, alternate patient care areas, and staffing and supply needs.

Sanford describes the eight principles of disaster management: preventing the occurrences of a disaster, minimizing the number of casualties, rescuing, providing first aid, evacuating the injured, providing definitive care, facilitating reconstruction, and recovery.[4] Whether in the prehospital care arena or in the ED, the emergency nurse is best prepared to handle disaster situations. It is important, however, for the nurse to be aware of the differences in triage priorities "in the field" versus in the ED.

Comprehensive disaster preparedness incorporates the community, the hospital, the ED, and the local, state, and federal domain. Disaster preparedness and management requires careful planning, frequent practice, critiques, and ongoing improvement/revisions. The ED nurse must be knowledgeable about these disaster systems and be in a constant state of readiness to quickly implement and execute the plan.

## REVIEW QUESTIONS

*There has been an explosion at a chemical plant in an inner-city area. Employees, persons passing by in cars, and people in nearby houses and buildings have been injured. The number of injuries is unknown. The emergency nurse has been called to assist with field triage and, on arrival, finds the following victims:*

- *No. 1: 28-year-old man in acute respiratory distress who is cyanotic and diaphoretic. Vital signs are B/P 70/40, P 140, and R 40, with labored respirations. There is bruising on the left side of his chest.*
- *No. 2: 64-year-old man in cardiac arrest with dilated and fixed pupils. There is no pulse or respiration. There are no physical signs of injury.*
- *No. 3: 30-year-old pregnant woman who is full term and in active labor with contractions every 5 minutes. This is her fourth child. She is upset and crying. There are no physical signs of injury.*
- *No. 4: 35-year-old woman with head, face, and leg lacerations with bleeding. She is incoherent. Her vital signs are B/P 96/60, P 110, and R 30.*

- *No. 5: 60-year-old man with a head laceration who is unresponsive to verbal or painful stimuli. Vital signs are B/P 100/70, P 96, R 24.*

1. Which patient should be cared for first?
   - 0   A. Patient no. 1
   - 0   B. Patient no. 2
   - 0   C. Patient no. 3
   - 0   D. Patient no. 4

2. The most obvious nursing diagnosis for patient no. 1 in this scenario is:
   - 0   A. Airway clearance, ineffective
   - 0   B. Tissue perfusion, altered
   - 0   C. Gas exchange, impaired
   - 0   D. Cardiac output, decreased

3. Which patient in this scenario should receive last priority for treatment?
   - 0   A. Patient no. 2
   - 0   B. Patient no. 3
   - 0   C. Patient no. 4
   - 0   D. Patient no. 5

4. Disaster management principles include:
   - 0   A. Maximize the number of casualties
   - 0   B. Prevent occurrence of a disaster
   - 0   C. Treating all injured at the scene
   - 0   D. Only one form of communication

5. The nurse who enters an internal disaster scene begins an evaluation to control the disaster. The first and foremost step for the emergency nurse to take is to:
   - 0   A. Take photographs of the situation so that mechanism of injury can be identified
   - 0   B. Tell everyone else to stand back while the nurse cares for the victims
   - 0   C. Assure that the area where the disaster occurred is safe before entering
   - 0   D. Notify the National Disaster Management Services (NDMS) before entering

6. The emergency nurse receives a patient who has been exposed to radiation into the decontamination room. The largest part of the decontamination procedure is accomplished by:
   - 0   A. Removing the patient's clothing and placing in a sealed container
   - 0   B. Washing the patient with soap and water before removing their clothes

O  C. Washing the patient with water only after removing their clothes

O  D. Using a specific antidote for decontaminating radiation materials

7. The initial care of the patient who has suffered a radiation exposure includes:

O  A. Preventing further exposure to the radiation

O  B. Treatment of life-threatening emergencies

O  C. Notifying the patient's family about the exposure

O  D. Calling the state health and safety regulatory agency immediately

8. Personal protective equipment (PPE) for caregivers involved in radiation decontamination consists of:

O  A. Surgical hood over a cotton uniform, waterproof shoes

O  B. Cotton uniform, face mask, waterproof shoes

O  C. Surgical trousers and top covered by a surgical gown

O  D. Two pairs of gloves taped to sleeves and cuffs

9. The primary method of decontamination for most chemical exposures is:

O  A. Application of a specific antidote to the affected area

O  B. Placement in a hyperbaric chamber for oxygenation

O  C. Administration of a aerosolized specific antidote

O  D. Showering with large quantities of water to dilute the agent

10. A 23-year-old patient arrives from a construction site cave-in in critical condition. Which triage tag would indicate his condition to the triage nurse?

O  A. Yellow tag

O  B. Red tag

O  C. Black tag

O  D. Green tag

11. Which of the following bacterial agents has been used in military and civilian populations?

O  A. Smallpox

O  B. Sarin

O  C. Cyanide

O  D. Anthrax

12. The critique following a disaster exercise should include:

O  A. Patient triage and tracking

O  B. Security operations

O  C. Deactivation of the disaster

O  D. All of the above

13. Following a disaster, the staff may need to deal with their feelings about the situation and the patients they cared for. This could best be accomplished by:

O  A. Calling the chaplain to come to the emergency department and conduct a debriefing

O  B. Asking the staff to talk openly in a group session with the nurse manager

O  C. Calling the CISM team to conduct a defusing

O  D. Asking a physician to prescribe sleeping medication for all personnel who request it

14. The most important tool to have in the ED to serve as a first line of defense for disasters is:

O  A. A well-organized disaster plan, which has been rehearsed

O  B. A medical director who has disaster medicine experience

O  C. Red Cross nurse on staff who works with the MAT

O  D. Alarm system that connects to the local fire department

15. JCAHO requires:

O  A. All hospitals experience one real disaster a year in order to be accredited

O  B. All hospitals schedule a disaster drill each year in order to remain current

O  C. All hospitals experience two drills (one with patients) or actual events each year

O  D. That hospitals do not have to have any drills if they feel qualified

## ANSWERS

1. **A. Assessment.** Always remember the airway, breathing, circulation rule and that field triage is geared toward saving the greatest number of lives using the simplest measures possible. Triage in the ED is focused on doing the greatest good for the greatest number. For patient no. 1, an airway needs to be established or cleared; the patient then needs to be transported to the emergency department.[1,2]

2. **A. Analysis.** The patient's airway is not patent. The airway must be opened so that breathing and circulation issues can be further assessed.[1]

3. **A. Assessment.** The life of this patient could not be saved "simply" or in a short period of time. Other patients whose lives might be saved would have to wait if this patient were dealt with first.[2,4-6]

4. **B. Assessment.** The principles of disaster management include prevent the occurrence of a disaster; minimize casualties; prevent further casualties; rescue the injured; provide first aid; evacuate the injured; provide definitive care; and facilitate recovery.[2]

5. **C. Intervention.** The nurse who goes to a disaster situation should do a three-step evaluation of (1) the safety of the area, (2) the organization of the disaster system, and (3) the provision of the most appropriate patient care.[1]

6. **A. Intervention.** Ninety to ninety-five percent of the decontamination procedure is accomplished by removing the patient's clothing. The clothing is placed in bags, tagged, and removed to a remote section of the contaminated area to be disposed of later by qualified personnel. The remaining decontamination is accomplished by washing the patient with soap and water.[1]

7. **B. Intervention.** The initial management of the patient who has been exposed to radiation is the treatment of any life-threatening emergencies, management of the patient's ABCs, and decontamination.[1]

8. **C. Intervention.** Personal protective equipment for caregivers caring for a radiation exposure includes surgical trousers and top covered by a surgical gown, two pairs of gloves with one pair secured with tape to sleeves and cuffs, so that one pair can be removed when contaminated, surgical mask, and eye protection.[1]

9. **D. Intervention.** An effective method of decontamination for most chemical exposures consists of showering with large quantities of water.[1]

10. **B. Assessment.** A colored tag system should be utilized to identify patient priority. One of the most common is based on red–critical; yellow–serious condition; green–stable condition; and black–dead.[5]

11. **D. Assessment.** Anthrax, or *bacillus anthracis,* is a bacterial agent that has been used in both military and civilian populations.[6]

12. **D. Evaluation.** Critique of a disaster exercise should include ED operations; ED staff; communications; security operations; patient management and tracking; and deactivation.[1]

13. **C. Intervention.** The debriefing team is best prepared to handle this situation. Team members remain objective and are most helpful to the staff, enabling them to discuss their feelings and providing a tool to prevent and alleviate symptoms created by the event. This offers immediate crisis intervention, helping the staff to return to their precrisis level of functioning.[1,2,6]

14. **A. Evaluation.** A well-defined disaster plan that has been practiced and critiqued will provide emergency nurses with guidelines for dealing with real disaster situations.[6]

15. **C. Intervention.** The JCAHO requires that hospitals have two drills (one with patients) or actual events each year.[1]

## REFERENCES

1. Klein J: Disaster preparedness/disaster management. In Jorgan K, editor: *Emergency nursing core curriculum,* ed 5, Philadelphia, 2000, WB Saunders.

2. Wilson, EM: Emergency operations preparedness. In Newberry L, editor: *Emergency nursing principles and practice,* ed 4, St Louis, 1998, Mosby.

3. Institute of Medicine and Board on Environmental Studies and Toxicology: National Research Council: *Chemical and biological terrorism. Research and development to improve civilian medical response,* Washington, DC, 1999, National Academy Press.

4. Elliot D, Cushing B: Mass casualty incidents. In Maull K, Rodriguez A, Wiles C, editors: *Complications in trauma and critical care,* Philadelphia, 1996, WB Saunders.

5. Moatman D, Alson R, Baldwin J, Stevens J: Multi-casualty incidents and triage. In Campbell J, editor: *Basic trauma life support,* ed 4, Upper Saddle River, NJ, 2000, Brady/Prentice Hall Health.

6. Proper C and Solotkin K: One urban hospital's experience with false anthrax exposure disaster response. *J Emerg Nurs* 25(6): 501-504, 1999.

## ADDITIONAL READINGS

Lanros N: *Assessment and intervention in emergency nursing,* ed 2, Bowie, Md, 1983, Robert J. Brady.

National Council on Radiation Protection and Measurements: Management of persons accidentally contaminated with radionuclides, Report No 65, Bethesda, Md, 1985, US Government Printing Office.

Wash M: *Accident and emergency nursing: a new approach,* ed 2, Oxford, 1990, Honeymoon Medical.

# Chapter 23

# Legal and Ethical Issues in Emergency and Transport Nursing

## REVIEW OUTLINE

I. Legal issues in emergency and transport nursing
  A. General overview
    1. Hospital's duty to provide care[1]
      a. *Wilmington General Hospital vs. Manlove* (1961): the hospital's duty to provide care outweighs the hospital's internal policies
      b. Hill-Burton Act (1946): if the hospital receives federal funds under this act, it must provide care regardless of the patient's ability to pay or the nature of the presenting complaint
    2. Nurse's duty to provide care
      a. State nurse practice act: duty, responsibility, and scope of practice defined
      b. Hospital employment policies: obligation to follow directions and fulfill duties
    3. Sources of law[2]
      a. Constitutional: determines the validity of both the statutory decision and the case law within the provisions of the fourth, fifth, and fourteenth constitutional amendments
      b. Statutory: law enacted by a legislative body
      c. Regulatory: regulations developed by an official under empowerment by statutory law
      d. Case (common): interpretation by the courts on statutes, administrative rules, and common law
      e. Contract: written, oral, or implied agreement between parties
      f. Administrative: laws created by administrative agencies through power delegated to them by state or federal legislature

    4. Types of law
      a. Civil law: addresses injury to individual and/or their property
      b. Criminal law: addresses injury to society
    5. General legal terms, concepts
      a. Standards of care
        (1) Provides guidelines
        (2) Ordinary, reasonable, prudent person (ORPP) with like or similar training in like or similar circumstances
      b. Negligence: omission or commission of an act that should or should not have been performed coupled with unreasonableness and/or imprudence on the part of the doer
        (1) Standard
        (2) Deviation from standard
        (3) Elements of negligence (nonintentional tort)
      c. Malpractice: negligence on the part of a professional when his or her misconduct, lack of skill, omission, or misjudgment in the commission of duty causes harm to the person or property of the recipient of services
      d. Tort: unintentional negligent act on the person of another that results in injury to that person
    6. Assault: threat to do harm to another without the actual performance of that threatened harm
    7. Battery: actual touching of another person without the person's consent
    8. False imprisonment: restrictions of a person's right to freedom of movement
    9. Good Samaritan law: law passed to encourage assistance to be rendered in emergency

conditions without fear of liability for the assistance provided

10. Respondent superior: liability that employers have for the negligent acts of their employees who act within the scope of their employment

B. Consent issues

1. Types of consent

a. Express consent: voluntary consent of an individual seeking medical treatment—patient must be competent to provide consent

b. Implied consent: individual is in life- or limb-threatening situation and is unable, because of unconsciousness or incompetence, to provide express consent

c. Involuntary consent: individual refuses to consent to needed medical treatment and yet another individual (physician or police) can ensure that the individual receives treatment

d. Informed consent: has three components that must be presented to the patient by the physician prior to the procedure. For the patient to make an informed decision, the physician must describe the procedure to be performed, explain the alternative available, and detail the risks of the procedure

2. Consent-related issues

a. Minors

b. Religious implications

c. Against medical advice (AMA)

d. Withholding or withdrawing life support

e. Living wills

f. Patient Self-Determination Act: A December 1991 federal law that provides hospitalized patients with the ability to make decisions regarding termination or continuation of life support

g. Durable power of attorney for health care decision/living wills: allows individuals to select someone to act for them in the area of health care decisions should they become unable to make their own decisions

C. Reporting requirements

1. Medical record documentation

2. Discharge instructions

3. Handling information/confidentiality

4. Reportable events/situations

a. Local, state, and federal regulations

b. Hospital policies and procedures

D. ED record

1. JCAHO requirements

2. Hospital documentation requirements

3. Confidentiality

4. Release of information

a. Privacy act

b. Rights of press

c. Hospital policy

5. Patient transfers: Consolidated Omnibus Budget Reconciliation Act (COBRA)/ Omnibus Budget Reconciliation Act (OBRA)[3]

a. OBRA: Part of the Medicare law preventing inappropriate transfers of individuals who seek emergency department care (anti-dumping law)[4]

(1) ED requirements

(2) Transfer requirements

(3) Penalties

(4) Special requirements

6. Patient discharge and instructions: oral and written

7. Chain of evidence collection

E. Specific emergency situations

1. Triage guidelines

a. Hospital policy—triage guidelines

b. State law

c. Nurse practice act

2. Telephone advice

a. Hospital policy/procedure

b. Documentation

3. Restraining of patients

a. Out-of-control behavior

b. Danger to self or others

c. Nursing considerations

d. Documentation

4. Psychiatric patients

a. Assess danger to self or others

b. Knowledgeable of policies/procedures/ laws regarding "holds"

5. Blood alcohol/drug screening

a. Hospital policy

b. State law

c. Medical purposes vs. police request

6. Assault/abuse situations

a. Sexual assault

(1) Policies/procedures

(2) Documentation

(3) Collaboration with team members

(4) Preserving evidence/chain of evidence collection

(5) Referring of evidence collection for appropriate follow-up

      b. Abuse and neglect
        (1) Child
        (2) Elderly
II. Going to court[5]
  A. Expert witness
    1. Practicing clinician
    2. Experience relevant to the case
    3. Communication skills
    4. Experience with testifying in court
    5. Certification in specialty
  B. Patient-related issues
    1. SANE testimony
    2. Evidence
  C. Components of a lawsuit
    1. Complaint
    2. Discovery
    3. Trial
III. Transport law[6]
  A. Emergency Medical Treatment and Active Labor Act (EMTALA)
    1. Appropriate medical screening must occur before transport
    2. Written consent should be obtained from patient or person acting for the patient for the transfer
    3. Agreement for the receiving facility to accept the patient
    4. Transfer in the most appropriate transport vehicle
    5. Qualified transport crews
    6. Copies of documentation
  B. Responsibility for medical direction during transport
  C. Whose patient is it during transport?
IV. Ethical issues
  A. Sources of issues
    1. Patients
    2. Families
    3. Institutions
    4. Communities
    5. Co-workers
  B. Ethical decision-making model
    1. Problem identification
    2. List alternatives
    3. List ethical values related to the problem
        a. Beneficence
        b. Fairness
        c. Patient self-determination
        d. Reparation
        e. Alternative
    4. Frame an ethical statement
    5. List consequences of actions
    6. Examine personal values
    7. Compare consequences to values

    8. Are the consequences consistent or inconsistent with values
    9. Make a decision
    10. Act on the decision
  C. Resuscitation
    1. Advanced directives
    2. Do not resuscitate (DNR) orders
    3. Transporting under full cardiopulmonary arrest
    4. Pronouncing patients dead in the field
    5. Pronouncing patients dead in other institutions
  D. Resources
    1. Hospital ethics committee
    2. Case presentations
    3. National associations
    4. American Nurses Association (ANA) Code of Ethics
    5. Personal philosophy, spirituality, religion

The legal and ethical issues encountered by emergency and transport nurses are many and varied. Nursing practice is governed by state nursing practice acts and guided by standards of care from professional nursing associations, previous court opinions, administration regulations, authoritative nursing texts and journals, and other associations such as JCAHO.[7] Nurses need to be aware of the legal issues that influence their practice and be prepared to be held accountable for their practice.

Legal issues faced by both emergency and transport nurses include consent, confidentiality, and evidence collection. Consent can be particularly challenging, since in emergency situations, the patient may be unable to give consent, and family or legal guardians may not be available. There are three types of consent: expressed consent; implied consent; and informed consent. Many emergency and transport care circumstances involve implied consent, or, if the patient was able, he would consent to the care that is being rendered to him.

The prehospital care environment and the ED frequently are in the public spotlight because of both the nature of the incidents that occur and simple human curiosity. Nurses need to ensure that the patient's illness or injury is afforded as much privacy as possible. Federal, state, and local laws require that certain situations have to be reported. Suspicion of child maltreatment, attempted suicide or homicide, and sexual assault are some examples of incidents that must be reported.

Nurses who practice in the ED and prehospital care environment will become involved in the collection of evidence. Evidence that may be collected by nurses includes clothing, weapons, and body fluids. Photographs of injuries are also examples of evidence.

Evidence such as clothing and some body fluids should be air-dried, labeled, and stored in paper bags. All evidence needs to be labeled with its source, date and time of collection, name of the patient, and place of storage in order to maintain a chain of custody.

Emergency and transport nurses' practice are based on and evaluated by standards set by their professional associations. Emergency Nurses Standards of Care and the National Flight Nurses Standards of Care are based upon the nursing process. Both are revised and reflect the current practice environments.

In 1950, the ANA adopted a code of ethical nursing practice that offered a description and guidelines for the ethical practice of nursing.[8] Ethical decision making in nursing practice is influenced by several entities, including the nurse's obligation to care, standards of care, legal direction, and the nurse's life experiences.[8]

Ethical decisions may be based on four principles. These are beneficence (i.e., does the care or procedure benefit the patient), nonmaleficence (i.e., will the care or procedure harm the patient), autonomy (i.e., the patient's ability to participate in the decision making), and fidelity.[8]

Common ethical dilemmas encountered by emergency and transport nurses include refusal of treatment or transport, resuscitation issues, and transport of patients undergoing CPR.

One of the primary roles of nursing practice today is to act as patient advocates.[10] Many patients present to the health care system with limited knowledge about their rights and the type of care they are about to receive. Emergency and transport nurses meet patients in crisis situations. The volatility of these situations require that both emergency and transport nurses be prepared to assist families as well as become a part of ethical decision making.

The practice of emergency and transport nursing continues to provide both legal and ethical challenges that we must be prepared to effectively deal with. Our patients and their families depend on us to be their voices and guides through very difficult and challenging life predicaments.

## REVIEW QUESTIONS

*A 75-year-old man with a history of intermittent confusion and disorientation is brought to the ED. The nursing home record confirms the report given by EMS personnel that the patient has wandered about the nursing home during periods of confusion and disorientation and fallen without injury on more than one occasion. On admission, the*

*patient is alert, oriented, and joking with the nurse about how young he feels. Fifteen minutes later, he becomes confused and disoriented, trying to get out of bed to turn on the radio.*

1. The nursing diagnosis for this patient that calls for immediate nursing intervention is:
   0    A. Thought processes, altered related to his confusion
   0    B. Injury, high risk for, physical related to his confusion
   0    C. Mobility, impaired physical related to his confusion
   0    D. Infection, high risk for related to his confusion

2. Nursing interventions for this patient should include:
   0    A. Side rails and soft restraints
   0    B. Side rails, restraints, and sedation
   0    C. Four-point leather restraints and sedation
   0    D. Watching the patient closely without restraint

3. The nurse caring for this patient fails to put up one of the side rails and appropriately restrain the patient. The patient falls out of bed. Radiographs reveal a fractured hip and wrist. The patient's family files a lawsuit. The lawsuit would most likely accuse the emergency nurse of:
   0    A. Negligence
   0    B. Malpractice
   0    C. Battery
   0    D. Felony

4. In order to claim negligence, which of the following must be proven?
   0    A. The emergency nurse did not have a duty to care for this patient
   0    B. The emergency nurse did follow current standards related to patient restraint
   0    C. The emergency nurse's action did cause the patient's injuries
   0    D. The damage the patient suffered was not related to his fall in the ED

5. When an emergency or transport nurse is notified by a lawyer that she is going to be sued, she should first:
   0    A. Contact her own legal counsel
   0    B. Obtain malpractice insurance
   0    C. Talk with her co-workers about the case
   0    D. Contact her employer's risk manager

6. One of the best ways to prevent misinterpretation of patient care situations is:
   O  A. Clearly and concisely document what happened
   O  B. Call the supervisor to witness any unusual events
   O  C. Ask the physician to add information to her dictation
   O  D. Complete an exception report as a routine part of the chart

7. On entering the trauma room, the emergency nurse finds the surgical resident beginning to start a research protocol drug on the patient who has just arrived. The patient is alert and oriented. What should the emergency nurse's first reaction be?
   O  A. To ask the resident if the patient has been informed about the study and has signed a consent form
   O  B. To not worry about bothering the patient with paperwork, since the patient is a trauma patient
   O  C. To ask the patient if he knows whether the resident is allowed to perform the research study the patient is about to be involved in
   O  D. To notify the resident's superior as soon as the research protocol has been initiated in the emergency

8. A 15-year-old boy is brought to the ED by his 18-year-old sister. He is complaining of flulike symptoms. Permission to treat should be received from the:
   O  A. Patient's parents
   O  B. Patient's sister
   O  C. Hospital administrator
   O  D. Local court system

9. A 46-year-old woman is brought into the ED. She has the smell of alcohol on her breath. On transfer to the treatment stretcher, she becomes violent, cursing at the staff and attempting to hit anyone nearby. The first priority of the ED nurse would be to:
   O  A. Call security and have the patient taken to jail
   O  B. Try to calm the patient by establishing rapport
   O  C. Protect the patient, family, and staff from physical harm
   O  D. Prepare the patient for transfer to a psychiatric facility

10. A 24-year-old woman known to have diabetes passes out at work and hits her head. She is incoherent for a few seconds after she is awakened from the incident and is brought to the ED. After the nurse and physician see the patient, blood is drawn for laboratory studies and x-ray films are ordered. In a short while the patient tells the nurse she is tired of waiting and is going home. What is the first and most important step for the nurse to take in this AMA situation?
    O  A. Determine the patient's competency to decide refusal
    O  B. Assist the patient in understanding the risks involved in leaving
    O  C. Have the patient sign the AMA form on her way out
    O  D. Try to convince the patient to stay

11. A 21-year-old uninsured paranoid schizophrenic patient who has been deeply depressed has attempted suicide. She is brought to the community hospital emergency department with a large laceration on the right side of her neck and one on her left upper arm. She has some active bleeding from the arm, which is controlled with a pressure bandage. The emergency department physician asks the nurse to arrange a transfer to the county hospital because they have emergency psychiatric services available. Before transport, the most important thing the nurse should ensure is that the:
    O  A. Patient consents to the transfer to another facility and is not concerned that she is being transferred to a psychiatric facility
    O  B. Receiving hospital agrees to the transfer of this patient and has a bed available for the patient
    O  C. Reason for the transfer is clear and justifiable on the transport document
    O  D. Patient is stabilized prior to the transfer and deemed safe for transport to another facility willing to accept her

12. A 28-day-old infant is brought to the ED by his parents. They are concerned because he has been lethargic and feeding poorly for the last 24 hours. The infant is lethargic and pale. He has weak peripheral pulses. Oxygen by mask is applied, an intraosseous needle is inserted, and the patient is given a 20 ml/kg fluid bolus. His condition shows little improvement, and the

emergency physician contacts the pediatric center 50 miles away. The receiving physician recommends that the referring ED wait for the pediatric transport team to transfer the patient. The referring physician sends the infant with a basic life support squad instead. Which component of EMTALA has this physician violated?

- ○   A. The hospital must examine all patients who present to the emergency department no matter what their insurance status
- ○   B. The transport vehicle should be equipped with appropriate personnel and equipment to safely transfer the patient
- ○   C. All patients who present to the emergency department must be stabilized before transfer to another facility
- ○   D. The receiving facility should agree to accept and have a bed available for the patient

13. During the transport, the infant suffers a respiratory arrest. The EMT initiates bag-valve-mask ventilation, but the child arrives in full arrest at the receiving facility. Who is responsible for any further injury that may have occurred to the infant during transport?
- ○   A. The EMT who initiated resuscitation
- ○   B. The receiving emergency department
- ○   C. The referring emergency physician
- ○   D. The infant's parents or caregivers

14. When does the receiving facility's liability begin related to patient transport?
- ○   A. When the referring institution initiates resuscitation measures before calling the receiving facility
- ○   B. When the referring facility's physician refuses to carry out the receiving physician's recommendation
- ○   C. When the referring facility transports the patient before notifying the receiving facility about the patient transfer
- ○   D. When the receiving facility's transport team prepares the patient for transport to the receiving hospital

15. A 32-year-old man is transferred from the ED to the PACU to await an emergent appendectomy. The surgeon explains the procedure to the

patient, as well as the risks. Which type of consent is the patient giving for this procedure?
- ○   A. Informed authorization
- ○   B. Implied consent
- ○   C. Expressed consent
- ○   D. Informed consent

16. When cutting clothes off a victim who has sustained a gunshot wound to the chest, the nurse should:
- ○   A. Cut through the area of the gunshot wound and place the clothes in an unlabeled plastic bag
- ○   B. Leave the patient's clothes on the patient until the police arrive to remove them and label them as evidence
- ○   C. Cut around the gunshot wound and place the clothes in a labeled plastic bag until the police arrive
- ○   D. Cut around the area of the wound and place the patient's clothes in a labeled paper bag

17. When testifying in court related to a patient care case in which the flight nurse provided care, the flight nurse should:
- ○   A. Not read the patient care record or any related documents before appearing in court
- ○   B. Provide an elaborate description of the incident, including current medical definitions
- ○   C. Answer only the questions that have been asked and not offer any additional information
- ○   D. Answer only the questions that the flight nurse believes that the hospital would like him to answer

18. Cardiopulmonary resuscitation should not be performed:
- ○   A. If the patient is incompetent
- ○   B. If the patient has written DNR orders
- ○   C. If the patient has verbal DNR orders
- ○   D. If the patient has not suffered a decapitation

19. The principle that respects the patient's ability to make his own decisions is:
- ○   A. The ethical principle of beneficence
- ○   B. The ethical principle of fidelity
- ○   C. The ethical principle of autonomy
- ○   D. The ethical principle of nonmaleficence

20. The flight team has been called to a referring facility to transport a 73-year-old female in congestive heart failure and chronic renal failure. Upon arrival at the referring facility, the flight teams find a patient in severe respiratory distress with no palpable blood pressure. The flight team elects to intubate the patient before placing her in the aircraft. The referring emergency department physician states that the patient has a written DNR order. What should the flight team do?

  O  A. Ask the patient if she understands that in order to be safely transported, she must be intubated

  O  B. Attempt to contact the patient's family to determine what their wishes are related to the care of this patient

  O  C. Explain to the referring physician that the patient must be intubated in order to safely transport her no matter what her wishes are

  O  D. Intubate the patient because flight team members do not have to honor do-not-resuscitate orders outside of their hospital

## ANSWERS

1. **B. Analysis.** Based on the patient's history and assessment, he is at great risk for falling and causing physical injury to himself.[7,8]

2. **A. Intervention.** Side rails up and locked in place, along with a jacket restraint device, are needed to prevent possible falls.[7,8]

3. **A. Analysis.** Negligence, to be alleged and proved in court, must consist of four elements: (1) duty (accepting responsibility for care and then being obligated to provide acceptable care); (2) breach of duty (not providing care according to accepted standards); (3) damage or injury (damage must have occurred); and (4) proximate cause (a cause-and-effect relationship between damage and breach of duty must exist). In this case the nurse had a duty to protect this patient with an altered mental status from harm and injury. She neither put up the side rail nor restrained the patient. The damage (fractured hip and wrist) resulted because of this negligence, although it was unintentional on the part of the nurse.[5,7]

4. **C. Intervention.** See discussion in question 3.

5. **D. Intervention.** When a nurse is informed that she is to be involved in any legal matter related to her work, she should immediately contact her institution's risk manager. It is a good idea to have malpractice insurance before an incident occurs.[5,7]

6. **A. Intervention.** Documentation of what happened, clearly and concisely, is the best way to prevent misinterpretation of what happened.[7,9]

7. **A. Intervention.** The rights of human subjects must be a priority in research endeavors. If the research protocol has outlined that consent is to be signed, that policy must be adhered to. The role of the emergency department nurse in conjunction with research endeavors is often one of ensuring patient safety.[11]

8. **A. Intervention.** If a minor is brought to the emergency department by anyone other than the parents, all attempts must be made to contact the parents before treatment is rendered unless a life-threatening situation exists.[12]

9. **C. Intervention.** The first priority should be safety for all parties involved in providing emergency care.[7-10]

10. **A. Intervention.** The patient's competency to leave against medical advice must be determined. A competent, conscious patient has the right to refuse treatment if he or she understands the consequences of refusal. This should be confirmed by a signature on the AMA form. The patient's chart should include documentation that the risks and/or consequences of leaving against medical advice were explained.[8,12]

11. **D. Intervention.** While all of these steps must be taken, the most important is the safety of the patient. The COBRA law requires that any hospital receiving Medicare funds must evaluate all emergency patients to determine whether an emergency condition exists. If it does, the hospital must provide immediate and stabilizing care before a transfer is considered.[12]

12. **B. Intervention.** When a patient is to be transferred to another facility, the level of care and equipment needed for safe transport should be available and provided. A pediatric patient, particularly an infant, requires educated and trained individuals who can ensure safe care for this child.[6,13]

13. **C. Intervention.** The referring emergency physician would be responsible for any injury that occurred to the infant during the transport. However, the emergency nurse at the referring facility should have documented any objections to this patient's care and attempted to stop it by notification of the appropriate authorities.[6,13,14]

14. **D. Assessment.** The liability of the receiving facility begins when the receiving hospital accepts the patient. The transport team is responsible for the

patient once the team arrives at the receiving facility and begins providing care for the patient. It can be assumed that the patient has been admitted to the receiving facility.[13,14]

15. **D. Intervention.** The patient is giving informed consent. Informed consent consists of providing a description of the procedure, a discussion of any alternative treatments, and a discussion of the risks of the procedure.[2]

16. **D.** The nurse should cut around any bullet or knife wound holes in clothing. All clothing should be labeled as to their source, the patient's name, age, date, and time collected and placed in a paper bag to preserve evidence.[15]

17. **C.** When testifying, the flight nurse should review the chart and any related materials before appearing in court, answer the questions (keeping the terminology simple and direct), answer only the questions, and always tell the truth.[16]

18. **B. Intervention.** Cardiopulmonary resuscitation should not be performed if the patient is competent and refuses it, has written DNR orders, is decapitated, or has rigor mortis or tissue decomposition.[17,18]

19. **C. Autonomy.**[8]

20. **A.** Speak with the patient to be sure that she understands that she must be intubated to safely transport her. If the patient were unconscious or unable to understand, even though her wishes would be legally honored in most states, it would be wise to contact the patient's family and explain the situation. Discussing the case with medical direction would also be of assistance in this difficult situation.[18]

## REFERENCES

1. *Wilmington General Hospital v. Manlove,* 194A. 2d 135, State Court, Delaware, 1961.

2. Lee G: Legal issues. In Jordan K, editor: *Emergency nursing core curriculum,* ed 4, Philadelphia, 2000, WB Saunders.

3. Consolidated Omnibus Budget Reconciliation Act (COBRA) of 1985 (42 U.S.C.A. Section 1395 dd) as amended by the Omnibus Budget Reconciliation Act (OBRA) of 1987, 1989, and 1990.

4. Omnibus Budget Reconciliation Act of 1989, Pub. L. No. 101-239, Washington, DC, Government Printing Office.

5. Sheehy S: Understanding the legal process: your best defense. *J Emerg Nurs* 25(6):492-495, 1999.

6. Niersbach C: EMTALA, *J Emerg Nurs* 25(6):541-543, 1999.

7. Showers JL: What you need to know about negligence lawsuits, *Nursing 2000* 30(2):45-48, 2000.

8. Pryor-McCann JM: Ethics in trauma nursing. In Cardona V and others, editors: *Trauma nursing: from resuscitation to rehabilitation,* ed 2, Philadelphia, 1994, WB Saunders.

9. Sheehy S: A duty to follow-up on laboratory reports, *J Emerg Nurs* 26(1):56-57, 2000.

10. George J, Quattrone M, Goldstone M: Nursing judgment—Is it alive? *J Emerg Nurs* 25(1):43-44, 1999.

11. Cole F: Research. In Jordan K, editor: *Emergency nursing core curriculum,* ed 5, Philadelphia, 2000, WB Saunders.

12. Southard P: Legal and legislative considerations in emergency practice. In Kitt S and others, editors: *Emergency nursing: A physiologic and clinical approach,* ed 2, Philadelphia, 1995, WB Saunders.

13. McCloskey K: *Guidelines for air and ground transport of neonatal and pediatric patients,* Elk Grove Village, IL, 1999, American Academy of Pediatrics.

14. Akoi B, McCloskey K: *Evaluation, stabilization, and transport of the critically ill child,* St Louis, 1992, Mosby.

15. DeJarnette R, editor: *Flight nursing advanced trauma manual,* Thorofare, NJ, 1994, National Flight Nurses.

16. Krupa D, editor: *Flight nursing core curriculum,* Park Ridge, MD, 1997, Road Runner Press.

17. Jecker N: Ceasing futile resuscitation in the field. Ethical considerations, *Arch Intern Med* 11:139-142, 1992.

18. Haynor P: Meeting the challenge of advanced directives, *AJN* 98(3):26-32, 1998.

# Chapter 24
# Research

**REVIEW OUTLINE**

I. Purpose of research
   A. Describes the characteristics of a particular problem
   B. Explains phenomena
   C. Predicts outcome
   D. Controls occurrences of undesired outcomes
II. Purpose of emergency nursing research
   A. Identifies and describes nursing knowledge
   B. Discovers whether nursing care does make a difference
   C. Provides scientific explanations for emergency nursing actions
   D. Discovers emergency nursing's professional identity
III. Two approaches to research in emergency nursing
   A. Quantitative
      1. Explores causes and makes predictions
      2. Objective perspective
      3. Requires large sample sizes
      4. Data collection based on some objective instrument
      5. Data analysis is statistical
   B. Qualitative
      1. Phenomenology
      2. Grounded theory
      3. Ethnography
      4. Historical
IV. Research process
   A. Identification of the research question or problem
      1. From practice
      2. Duplication of previous study
      3. Literature
      4. Case study
      5. Continuous quality improvement
   B. Review of the literature
   C. Implementation of a new procedure
   D. Need for change
   E. Theories
      1. Theory-practice-theory
      2. Practice-theory

3. Research-theory
4. Theory-research-theory
5. Modified-practice-theory
   F. Conceptual models
      1. Johnson's behavioral systems model
      2. Leninger's sunrise model
      3. Watson's caring constructs
      4. King's open systems model
      5. Levine's conservation model
      6. Orem's model of self-care
   G. Review of the current literature
   H. Defining research variables or definition of terms
      1. Dependent variables
      2. Independent variables
      3. Extraneous variables
   I. Hypothesis or research questions
   J. Research design
      1. Experimental
      2. Quasi-experimental
      3. Descriptive
      4. Exploratory
      5. Methodological
      6. Historical
   K. Methods of data collection
      1. Identification of the research population
         a. Consent issues
      2. Methods
         a. Observation
         b. Self-report methods
         c. Physiologic measurements
         d. Scales
         e. Sorts
         f. Chart reviews
      3. Reliability and validity issues
      4. Data entry
   L. Analysis of the data
      1. Descriptive statistics
      2. Inferential statistics
      3. Multivariate statistical analysis
   M. Interpretation of the results

N. Communication of the results
   1. Introduction
   2. Methods
   3. Results
   4. Discussion
   5. Implications to nursing practice
O. Critiquing research
   1. Research question/hypothesis/problem
   2. Methods used to collect data
   3. Ethical issues
   4. Interpretation of the results
   5. Presentation of the results
   6. Conclusions drawn from the study
P. Applying research to practice
   1. Identification of sources of research
   2. Evaluating research findings in practice
   3. Ethical issues

Research always begins with a question or a problem to be solved, and research in nursing practice begins with questions or problems in nursing practice.[1,2] Research provides a means of discovering and evaluating old and new ideas (knowledge) in the practice of emergency nursing. The practice of emergency nursing offers multiple sources for research opportunities. Evidence-based research has emerged as an important method of validating what the practice of emergency nursing is and does.[3] Research studies also provide a framework to discover new methods of providing patient care and enhancing clinical practice. Research helps us discover who we are and what difference we make in patient care.

There are two general approaches to research: quantitative and qualitative. Quantitative research explores causes in order to make predictions. It depends on control, reproducibility, and generalizability. The qualitative approach to research is perceptual and exploratory and produces themes that may or may not be generalizable. It is fluid and many times is better at describing what nursing is all about.[4,5]

There are myriad ways to discover knowledge in clinical practice, including observing, measuring, or describing phenomena. The equipment that emergency nurses use on a daily basis, such as monitors, or the procedures that are employed to care for patients, offer rich sources of data. However, the emergency nurse must always put the rights of the patient or patients before the need of the study. Patients and staff may always refuse to participate.

The research process is composed of multiple steps, including identification of the problem, review of the literature, development of a theoretical framework, defi-nition of research variables, hypothesis formation or formation of research questions, selection of a research design, sample selection, measurement of variables, collection of the data, data analysis, interpretation of the results, and communication of the research findings.[1-4]

It is important for emergency nurses to read and evaluate research. Because of the multiple sources of knowledge needed to practice emergency nursing, research studies in medicine, psychology, and sociology, for example, should be reviewed. Learning to apply research findings to emergency nursing practice will serve to expand not only nursing's knowledge but the other disciplines that collaborate with us as well.[6,7]

## REVIEW QUESTIONS

1. The primary purpose of nursing research is:
   - O  A. To discover what care activities patients do not require while in the ED
   - O  B. To understand which care providers make the most difference in the ED
   - O  C. To develop a collaborative framework to describe patient care in the ED
   - O  D. To describe and validate nursing knowledge and nursing practice

2. The advocacy role the emergency nurse plays in any research study is:
   - O  A. Collection of data according to protocol
   - O  B. Interpretation of data after data collection is complete
   - O  C. Protection of patients' rights before and during the research process
   - O  D. Deciding the study design in collaboration with the primary investigator

3. The first step in the research process is:
   - O  A. Obtaining patient consent for data collection
   - O  B. Identifying the research problem or question
   - O  C. Reviewing the current literature related to the research problem
   - O  D. Selecting a research design before identifying the research question

4. All the following are examples of an instrument that may be used to collect data *except:*
   - O  A. Literature review
   - O  B. Pulse oximeter
   - O  C. Focused interviews
   - O  D. Questionnaires

5. When using biophysiological instruments to collect data, the emergency nurse must first evaluate the instruments':
   - 0    A. Battery life
   - 0    B. Reliability
   - 0    C. Cost
   - 0    D. Validity

6. In the discussion section of a research report, the researcher:
   - 0    A. Tells the reader the significance of the work to nursing practice and links the results with previous studies
   - 0    B. Presents the results of the data collection in tables, graphs, or selected reproduction of data that were collected
   - 0    C. Tells the reader about the reliability and validity of the instruments used to collect data
   - 0    D. Discusses the definition of the variables that are to be studied during the research process

7. In the study, "Does heparin flush or normal saline flush keep an intravenous line patent longer?" what is the dependent variable?
   - 0    A. Heparin flush
   - 0    B. Normal saline flush
   - 0    C. Intravenous line
   - 0    D. There is no dependent variable

8. A sample of 513 patients was chosen to evaluate pain medication used to manage fractured arms. Using an exploratory design, the researchers found that only 30% of the patients received any pain medication. What type of statistics did the researchers use to present their results?
   - 0    A. Inferential statistics
   - 0    B. Descriptive statistics
   - 0    C. Correlational statistics
   - 0    D. Multiple regression statistics

9. Questions that may be used to validate nursing practice by using the results of previous research include:
   - 0    A. What do you want to change about your emergency nursing practice?
   - 0    B. How similar is the study sample to your own work environment?
   - 0    C. Is there a risk to patients with any change in emergency nursing practice?
   - 0    D. All of the above questions would be pertinent to the validation process

10. Characteristics of an experimental research design include:
    - 0    A. Equal group participation
    - 0    B. There is no comparison group
    - 0    C. Subjects are randomly assigned
    - 0    D. Variables are not controlled

11. A common "pitfall" encountered by researchers is:
    - 0    A. Building co-worker support for the research project within the ED
    - 0    B. Providing adequate time to plan and educate all of the affected personnel in the ED
    - 0    C. Making the entire research process as user friendly as possibly
    - 0    D. Choosing an inappropriate research focus for evaluation in the ED

12. A difference between clinical problem solving and a research study is:
    - 0    A. Clinical problem solving involves a formal plan to solve problems
    - 0    B. Clinical problem solving is based upon a specific nursing theory
    - 0    C. A research study is concerned with issues of validity and reliability
    - 0    D. Clinical problem solving looks for several solutions simultaneously

13. A pharmaceutical company has contracted with the ED to evaluate the effectiveness of their new drug. The ED researchers are ethically accountable for:
    - 0    A. Hiding the disadvantages of the pharmaceutical company's medication
    - 0    B. Acknowledging the source of their funding for the research project
    - 0    C. Allowing the pharmaceutical company to make all the decisions about the design
    - 0    D. Using the funding only if the results please the pharmaceutical company

14. An emergency nurse wants to study the patient's experience related to pain in the emergency department. Which methodology would be most appropriate?
    - 0    A. Grounded theory
    - 0    B. Ethnography
    - 0    C. Phenomenology
    - 0    D. Historical

**15.** A statistical test that determines whether there is a difference between the means between two groups is:

0   A. t-test
0   B. ANOVA
0   C. Chi-square test
0   D. Correlation coefficient

## ANSWERS

1. **D.** The major purpose of nursing research is to identify and discover what is nursing knowledge. Other purposes of nursing research include discovering whether nursing care makes a difference, providing scientific explanations of nursing procedures, and helping establish a professional identity for nursing.[1]

2. **C.** One of the most important roles that the emergency nurse plays in the research process—whether or not he or she is conducting the study—is the assurance of the protection of human subjects. ED patients are a very vulnerable group of people. The emergency nurse may need to act as an advocate not only to be sure that the patient understands the study but also to support a patient if he or she chooses not to participate.[1,4]

3. **B.** The first step in the research process is identifying the problem or formulating the question. Before one can begin the process, one needs to first identify what one is going to study. Important delineations to make when identifying a nursing research problem or question include whether the problem or question will add to the body of nursing knowledge, will improve nursing practice, or will provide solutions to explain, describe, identify, or predict behavior.[4]

4. **A.** Review of the literature is a step in the research process. The other answers provide examples of instruments the emergency nurse may use to gather data about a research problem in the ED.

5. **B.** The reliability of biophysiological instruments is very important in the collection of data. The instrument must be able to accurately measure what it has been designated to measure. This would be very important in the ED where multiple individuals may be involved in the use of a particular instrument.[1]

6. **A.** The discussion section of a research report should tell the reader about the significance of the research. In addition, particularly in nursing research, there should be a discussion of how the research can be applied to nursing practice.[1,4]

7. **C.** The intravenous line is the dependent variable. The dependent variable is the outcome variable of interest; in other words, the emergency nurse is interested in what will keep the intravenous line patent. The independent variables are the procedures (heparin vs. saline flush) that will be used to keep it patent.[1]

8. **B.** Descriptive statistics such as the median, mean, or mode are used to describe what has been found in the research population. In this case, the researchers found that only 30% of the patients with fractured arms received some type of pain medication.[1,4]

9. **D.** Developing a model on which to validate emergency nursing practice should be based on multiple questions. One model that has been presented and evaluated by practicing nurses is the Stetler/Marram Model, discussed in the Carlson and Rouse article.[7]

10. **C.** The characteristics of an experimental design include random assignment of subjects and control of the independent variable.[1]

11. **D.** Pearls related to research include A,B,C. A common pitfall encountered by researchers is choosing an inappropriate or ill-defined research question.[8]

12. **C.** A research study is concerned with issues of reliability and validity, looks for several solutions simultaneously, and uses a formal plan of study.[4]

13. **B.** When conducting research with a pharmaceutical company, the researcher is ethically accountable for acknowledging where the funding came from; actively participating in the design of the research; reporting the results accurately; and reporting both the positive and negative results of the study.[9]

14. **C.** Phenomenology provides a framework to study and describe patient experiences.[4,5]

15. **A.** A t-test determines the difference between the means of two groups. ANOVA determines the difference among the means of two or more groups. A chi-square test is a nonparametric test used when two sets of data fall into various categories. A correlation coefficient is used to describe the relationship between two measures.[10]

## REFERENCES

1. Polit D, Hungler B: *Essentials of nursing research,* Philadelphia, 1995, Lippincott.
2. Mateo MA, Kirchoff KT: *Conducting and using nursing research in the clinical setting,* Baltimore, 1991, Williams & Wilkins.
3. Manton A: Validation of what we do: a word about evidence-based practice, *J Emerg Nurs* 24(1):1-2, 1998.

4. Cole F: Research. In Jordan K, editor: *Emergency nursing core curriculum,* ed 5, Philadelphia, 2000, WB Saunders.

5. Thompson C, Walker L: Basics of research (Part 12): qualitative research. *Air Med J* 17(2):65-70, 1998.

6. Rea R, Vancini M, Perdue S: Research in emergency nursing. In Kitt S et al, editors: *Emergency nursing: a physiologic and clinical perspective,* Philadelphia, 1995, WB Saunders.

7. Carlson D, Rouse C: Staff nurses: Using research in everyday practice, *J Emerg Nurs* 25(6):564-568, 1999.

8. Panacek E: Basics of research (Part 9): practical aspects of performing clinical research, *Air Med J* 16(1):19-23, 1997.

9. Malone R: Ethical issues in industry-sponsored research, *J Emerg Nurs* 24(2):193-196, 1998.

10. Lenaghan P: Research. In Newberry L, editor: *Sheehy's emergency nursing principles and practice,* St Louis, 1998, Mosby.

# Chapter 25

# Education: Patient, Family, Community

## REVIEW OUTLINE

I. Teaching/learning process
  A. Identification of learning needs
  B. Assessment of the learner
    1. Readiness to learn
    2. Present anxiety level
    3. Capability to learn
    4. Motivation
  C. Establishment of goals
  D. Selection of teaching methods
    1. Verbal
    2. Written
      a. Home care instruction sheets
      b. Patient-specific instructions
    3. Visual aids
    4. Question-and-answer session
    5. Return demonstration
  E. Provision of adequate time
  F. Barriers to teaching/learning in the emergency and transport environments
    1. Pain
    2. Age of the patient
    3. Gravity of the current situation
    4. Language and communication
    5. Visual and auditory
    6. Illiteracy
    7. Fear of personal safety, death, long-term consequences of illness or injury
    8. Noise level
    9. Personality factors
    10. Nurses' knowledge deficit
II. Content
  A. Disease, disorder, or injury
    1. Causes
    2. Predisposing and precipitating factors
    3. Expected course
    4. Plan of care
  B. Diagnostic test or procedure
    1. Equipment
    2. Activity
    3. Outcome
  C. Discharge, home care
    1. Equipment and supplies needed
    2. Step-by-step procedure
    3. Specifics regarding medications
    4. Pertinent observations
    5. Appropriate follow-up
    6. Changes requiring immediate intervention
    7. Community resource referral, if indicated
  D. Prevention
    1. Prevention of recurrence
    2. Prevention of infection
    3. General hygiene
  E. Pretransportation orientation
    1. Rotary wing
    2. Fixed wing
    3. Ground transport
    4. Other methods of transport
  F. Orientation of patient and family accompanying the patient during transport
    1. Orientation to transport vehicle
    2. Safety briefing
    3. Follow-up visits after the transport
III. Community education
  A. Educational pamphlets
  B. Educational videos
  C. Educational spots on television and radio
  D. Injury prevention
    1. Motor vehicle injuries
    2. Falls
    3. Poisonings
    4. Burns
    5. Recreational injuries
    6. Abuse and assault
    7. Suicide
    8. Violence
    9. Firearm injuries
    10. Occupational injuries
  E. Health and wellness education
  F. Public relations visits

G. Safety presentations
1. Operations around transport vehicles
2. Landing zones
3. Patient preparation

An important component of emergency and transport nursing is education. The nurse assumes the role of health teacher in preparing each patient and/or significant other to assume patient care on leaving the ED. This is a vital nursing task, essential to the practice of emergency nursing. The transport nurse educates patients, families, and communities about the transport process. They also play an active role in community intervention programs.

One must be familiar with the process of teaching and use the time available to prepare the patient for discharge. Ideally, patient teaching begins at the first nurse-patient encounter and continues throughout the patient's stay. Saving all the information until actual discharge can be overwhelming to both patient and nurse. It is much more effective to do nursing care teaching in parts during the patient's stay so that the patient has time to digest information and ask questions. Discharge is best used as a time of summary and return verbalization of instructions by the patient to ensure understanding. There are a number of obstacles to overcome in preparing patients to successfully care for themselves. The stress of a busy, noisy department can increase the anxiety already felt by the patient, and a high anxiety level clouds the learning process. The nurse helps to decrease this stress through both verbal and nonverbal means. Simple acts such as explaining tests and procedures in understandable terms and listening carefully to what the patient has to say can allay anxiety. Likewise, nonverbal communication in facial expression, touch, and body language is effective.[1]

The vast array of health problems encountered in the emergency and transport settings makes it imperative for the nurse to have a broad range of teaching skills. Whereas the obstetrical nurse or orthopedic nurse is usually dealing with a single issue, the emergency nurse must be able to prepare patients with a variety of health problems for home care.[1]

Issues of importance to be taught during the patient's emergency visit include cause and prevention of the injury or illness and possible complications. Lengthy explanations are not necessary; simple descriptions usually suffice. The patient who understands something about what has happened is more likely to be compliant with treatment and more likely to know how to work toward prevention of a similar episode in the future. This information also assists the patient in recognizing any complications that may arise and in seeking further intervention as necessary.

Obviously, the patient must learn about nursing care measures specific to his or her problem. Discharge instructions given by the physician are not sufficient. Nursing care is best taught by nurses. Items such as wound care, fever control, and walking with crutches are examples of the many things patients must understand in order to get well at home. Also, the nurse must have learned enough about the patient's home situation to help the patient adapt care routines to his or her needs. For example, does the patient with a leg cast have stairs that must be traveled at home? Does the mother of a febrile child have a thermometer, and does she know how to use it? These are nursing problems that need to be solved before the patient leaves the ED.

Another educational need the nurse meets in preparing the patient for discharge concerns prescribed medications. It is important that the patient understand the expected actions and possible side effects, as well as specifics for taking or using the medication. Reviewing with the patient how to use a suppository, or the importance of taking a particular drug with food, can ensure compliance.

Finally, documentation of patient education must be recorded. Many institutions have standardized care instructions available for specific uses, such as wound care and head injury observation. Notation is made that these are given to the patient. Instructions specific to the individual are written, ideally with a duplicate for the patient to take home. Again, it is important that these instructions be in terms the patient can understand, and, of course, they must be legible. The nurse notes on the patient's records who received the instructions and that the receiver verbalized understanding. The chart should be signed by the patient or significant other, verifying this.

One of the primary roles of providing education in transport nursing is teaching those who use a particular mode of transport how to safely work around it. For example, how to set up a well marked, clear landing area. Community outreach programs also afford transport nurses an opportunity to teach about prevention.

Patient teaching in the emergency and transport settings is essential to good care. Patients who leave the emergency department with an adequate understanding of how to care for their problem at home are more likely to recover without complications. Good discharge information often prevents unnecessary return visits and time-consuming phone calls back to the facility.

Community and outreach education help to ensure safe transport operations as well as assist in the appropriate utilization of resources. Education is a fluid, on-going process in which all emergency and transport nurses must take an active role. Patient and community satisfaction are enhanced when educational needs are met.

## REVIEW QUESTIONS

1. An 8-month-old girl is being discharged from the ED with bilateral otitis media. In addition to instructions for fever management and medication administration, the nurse tells the mother to:
    0   A. Weigh the baby daily in the morning before her breakfast
    0   B. Isolate the baby from other children until the fever is gone
    0   C. Discontinue formula, substituting clear liquids
    0   D. Avoid putting the baby to bed with a bottle

2. When providing the baby's mother with information about the antibiotic that has been prescribed for the child, the emergency nurse should:
    0   A. Use both the generic and commercial name of the antibiotic so the mother will not become confused
    0   B. Use an instruction sheet that assumes that the mother has graduated from a four-year college
    0   C. Use examples to clarify how to administer the antibiotic to the baby, i.e., syringe administration to a doll
    0   D. Tell the mother to never return to the ED if she has any problems because the baby's illness has already been treated

3. In reviewing fever control measures with the parent, the nurse learns that the parent has no acetaminophen but does have baby aspirin. Based on the baby's age and weight of 19 pounds, the appropriate dose of aspirin is:
    0   A. Half a baby aspirin every 4 hours
    0   B. Half a baby aspirin every 6 hours
    0   C. One baby aspirin every 6 hours
    0   D. Infants should not receive aspirin

4. A 32-year-old man is being discharged from the ED with a diagnosis of left corneal abrasion sustained at work. He has a patch in place and has been given antibiotic ointment to use. The most important teaching to be done for this patient would be:
    0   A. Stressing the importance of not driving or operating other machinery while wearing the patch
    0   B. Teaching him how to apply the ointment to his eyes so that his family will not have to do it for him
    0   C. Reminding him how long the patch is to be worn and when to follow-up with his family doctor
    0   D. Stressing the importance of wearing goggles at work to prevent recurrence of this injury

5. A 10-year-old boy is being discharged from the ED with a right forearm fracture sustained in a fall. He has a splint applied to his arm, and his mother is taught how to do circulation checks every 4 hours until he is seen by the orthopedic surgeon in the morning. The emergency nurse may evaluate the effectiveness of her instruction by:
    0   A. Asking the mother to read the written instructions back to you or the doctor
    0   B. Giving the mother a video about orthopedic injuries to take home with her
    0   C. Asking the mother to demonstrate how to do a circulation check on her son's arm
    0   D. Discharging the mother before evaluating her skills and calling her on the phone later

6. Another bit of advice pertinent for this patient would be:
    0   A. How to trim excess padding from around the cast
    0   B. To avoid striking the cast against anything
    0   C. How to dry the cast if it gets wet
    0   D. That writing on the cast can begin on arrival home

7. A 42-year-old man is being discharged from the ED with a diagnosis of low back strain after lifting a refrigerator. His discharge instructions are based on which of the following nursing diagnoses?
    0   A. Pain related to his back injury
    0   B. Activity intolerance related to his back injury

    0  C. Mobility, impaired physical related to his back injury

    0  D. All of the above would be applicable

8. Methods that the emergency nurse may use to reinforce discharge instructions include:

    0  A. Give only oral instructions when discharging a patient from the emergency department

    0  B. Tell the patient to call his physician or nurse practitioner if there is anything he does not understand about his care in the emergency department

    0  C. Involve the patient's family or significant others in the discharge instructions that are being given to the patient

    0  D. If the patient does not speak English, encourage him to contact a translator when he returns home to explain the instructions to him

9. A 52-year-old woman has been treated in the ED for stable angina and is ready for discharge with sublingual nitroglycerin. The most important instruction she receives is:

    0  A. How to take nitroglycerin when she is on vacation in another state or country

    0  B. How to restrict activity when she is having any type of chest pain

    0  C. When to follow up with her private physician after this emergency visit

    0  D. To seek medical attention immediately if pain persists after taking three nitroglycerins

10. Side effects of nitroglycerin to be reviewed with this patient include:

    0  A. Dizziness, transient headache, blurred vision, flushing

    0  B. Dizziness, lightheadedness, transient headache, flushing

    0  C. Lightheadedness, persistent headache, blurred vision, rash

    0  D. Dizziness, fainting, transient headache, rash

11. Assumptions about adult learners include:

    0  A. The adult learner has no previous experience on which to base her learning

    0  B. Adult learning can only be accomplished through the use of lecture and discussion

    0  C. Adults learn best from problem-centered educational experiences

    0  D. Adults can only learn when they are motivated by a potential salary increase

12. Methods that may be used to enhance teaching/learning in the prehospital and emergency department environments include:

    0  A. Lack of privacy

    0  B. Adequate time

    0  C. Well-lit environment

    0  D. Involving the family

## ANSWERS

1. **D. Intervention.** Babies who are routinely put to bed with a bottle are more prone to recurrent bouts of otitis media. They often fall asleep in the act of sucking, which increases pressure in the eustachian tubes, inhibiting free drainage and providing a source of infection. Parents should be encouraged to hold the baby until the bottle is finished. This will prevent prolonged negative pressure in the eustachian tubes, as well as promote bonding between parent and infant.

2. **C. Intervention.** When providing patients and families with discharge instructions, the emergency nurse should use simple, nontechnical terms to describe medications; assure that the discharge instructions are at an educational level so that the patient and family understands (usually between fourth to sixth grade); and offer examples to clarify the instructions.[1,2]

3. **D. Intervention.** The use of aspirin for fever control in infants and children has been linked to the development of Reye's syndrome and is therefore contraindicated. Acetaminophen will reduce fever without harmful side effects in appropriate dosage. Methods for obtaining this drug, preferably in elixir form, should be explored with the mother before she goes home.

4. **A. Intervention.** When one eye is patched, depth perception is severely altered. To prevent injury to himself and others, the patient should avoid activity in which intact vision is crucial to safety.

5. **C. Intervention.** There are several ways that the emergency nurse could evaluate the effectiveness of her teaching. These include asking the mother questions about the procedure, providing a follow-up call and having the parent perform a return demonstration of the procedure.

6. **B. Intervention.** A plaster cast is to be kept dry and all padding left as is. A 24-hour drying time is

needed, and during that time handling of the cast should be careful and minimal; therefore, writing on it should be deferred until after that time. This patient's age, sex, and mechanism of injury should alert the nurse to the need to stress that the cast is not to be used as a weapon to strike objects or other people. Active children and young men seem prone to this activity and need to be discouraged from it. On impact, the cast may be damaged, causing further damage to the already injured area. Of course, the possibility of harm to other people or objects is obvious.

7. **D. Analysis.** This patient's instructions will include use of prescribed medications and nursing comfort measures to be followed at home, as well as prevention of future similar injury. In discussing each of these points with the patient, the nurse is imparting knowledge specific to him and his current problem.

8. **C. Intervention.** Methods that the emergency nurse can use to reinforce discharge instructions include: providing written as well as oral instructions; answering and clarifying all questions the patient may have before leaving the emergency department; and providing the instructions in a way the patient may understand, i.e., language, visual, etc.[3]

9. **D. Intervention.** Pain not relieved with rest and three successive nitroglycerin tablets may forecast a serious myocardial event. A patient with angina should be reminded of when and how to seek help.

10. **B. Evaluation.** The vasodilating effects of this drug are responsible for the transient dizziness, lightheadedness, headache, and flushing of the face and neck that some people experience. The duration of action with sublingual nitroglycerin is very short; therefore any persistent events such as blurred vision, fainting, rash, or prolonged headache should be reported to the physician.

11. **C. Intervention.** Adult learners have multiple life experiences, prefer to learn through a number of different types of activities (group and individual); enjoy problem centered teaching, and are motivated to learn by both intrinsic and extrinsic motivators.[3,4]

12. **A. Assessment.** Lack of privacy is a detractor to the teaching/learning process.

**REFERENCES**

1. Rush C: Patient education. In Newberry L, editor, *Sheehy's emergency nursing principles and practice,* ed 4, St Louis, 1998, Mosby.
2. Duffy M, Snyder K: Can ED patients read your patient education materials? *J Emerg Nurs* 25(4):294-297, 1999.
3. Bracken L, Martinez R: Education. In Jordan K, editor: *Emergency nursing core curriculum,* ed 5, Philadelphia, 2000, WB Saunders.
4. Krupa D, editor: *Flight nursing core curriculum,* Park Ridge, Md, 1997, Road Runner Press.

# Part Two

# TRANSPORT NURSING

# Chapter 26

# Flight Physiology

## REVIEW OUTLINE

I. Gas laws
   A. Boyle's law (law of gaseous expansion)—defines the relationship between gas volume and barometric pressure
   B. Charles' law—defines the relationship between gas volume and temperature
   C. Universal gas law—combines Boyle's and Charles' laws
   D. Henry's law (law of gases in solution)—defines the effect of barometric pressure on volume of gas dissolved in fluids
   E. Dalton's law—law of partial pressures
   F. Law of gaseous diffusion-gasses diffuse from area of higher concentration to an area of lower concentration

II. The earth's atmosphere
   A. Atmospheric gas composition
      1. Oxygen–21%
      2. Nitrogen–78%
      3. Other gases–1%
   B. Atmospheric gas distribution
      1. Altitude
      2. Latitude
      3. Temperature
      4. Humidity

III. Stresses of flight
   A. Barometric pressure change
      1. Temperature effect
      2. Latitude effect
      3. Moisture effect
      4. Rotary vs. fixed wing
      5. Rapid decompression
   B. Physiological effects of barometric pressure change
      1. Middle ear
      2. Facial sinuses
      3. Teeth
      4. GI tract
      5. Respiratory system
      6. Circulatory system
      7. Extremities
      8. Decompression sickness
      9. Medical equipment considerations
   C. Hypoxia
      1. Hypoxic
      2. Hypemic
      3. Histotoxic
      4. Stagnant
      5. Altitude-related hypoxia
      6. Time of useful consciousness (TUC)
      7. Oxygen requirements at altitude
   D. Thermal stress
      1. Heat loss
      2. Heat production
      3. Heat conservation
      4. Minimizing heat loss in flight
   E. Gravitational forces
      1. Classification of G-forces
      2. Physiological effects
   F. Humidity
      1. The flight environment
      2. Physiological effects
   G. Noise
      1. Effects of noise exposure
      2. Hearing loss
      3. Noise attenuation
   H. Vibration
      1. Exposure
      2. Physiological effects
   I. Fatigue
      1. Cumulative effects
      2. Self-imposed

In order to provide an efficient, therapeutic patient care environment at altitude, one must understand characteristics of atmospheric variation associated with flight. The transport team who flies should develop a practical understanding of physical changes that occur during flight that can create and contribute to physiological stress. Medical flight crew members must understand how and to what extent these stressors can affect the already physiologically compromised patient being transported by fixed- or rotary-wing aircraft. In addition, the effect of flight on crew members must be considered in order to provide a medical crew that can deliver high-quality patient care while anticipating and effectively dealing with those physiological stressors that impact patients, other crew members, and themselves.[1]

## REVIEW QUESTIONS

*You are transporting a patient with an acute anterior myocardial infarction in a fixed-wing aircraft. At 28,000 feet the aircraft experiences a rapid decompression emergency.*

1. An oxygen mask should be placed first on:
   - 0  A. The pilot
   - 0  B. The patient
   - 0  C. Yourself
   - 0  D. Your partner

2. Areas of the body affected by changes in barometric pressure include all of the following *except:*
   - 0  A. Middle ear
   - 0  B. Teeth
   - 0  C. Sinuses
   - 0  D. Liver

3. When rapid decompression occurs at 25,000 feet, the transport team members have how much TUC?
   - 0  A. <15 seconds
   - 0  B. 20 to 30 minutes
   - 0  C. 30 to 60 seconds
   - 0  D. 3 to 5 minutes

4. Factors that affect the development of hypoxia in crew members include all of the following *except*:
   - 0  A. Altitude of 2000 feet or less
   - 0  B. Individual tolerance to altitude changes
   - 0  C. Physical fitness of the crew member
   - 0  D. Changes in environmental temperature

5. Two hours after the aircraft lands, the pilot complains of pain in his left knee. Appropriate actions would include:
   - 0  A. Range of motion to decrease stiffness
   - 0  B. Splinting the affected limb
   - 0  C. Applying nasal cannula oxygen
   - 0  D. Treating the pain with aspirin

6. The evolution of gas bubbles within the body at high altitudes is best explained by:
   - 0  A. Boyle's law
   - 0  B. Charles' law
   - 0  C. Henry's law
   - 0  D. Dalton's law

7. The sharp temperature drop associated with a rapid decompression is best explained by:
   - 0  A. Boyle's law
   - 0  B. Charles' law
   - 0  C. Henry's law
   - 0  D. Dalton's law

*A 62-year-old man was found unresponsive in his car in an enclosed garage. He is intubated and transported by helicopter to the closest trauma center.*

8. This patient would most likely be suffering from which type of hypoxia?
   - 0  A. Hypoxic hypoxia
   - 0  B. Hypemic hypoxia
   - 0  C. Stagnant hypoxia
   - 0  D. Histotoxic hypoxia

9. The most common form of hypoxia associated with flight is:
   - 0  A. Hypoxic hypoxia
   - 0  B. Hypemic hypoxia
   - 0  C. Histotoxic hypoxia
   - 0  D. Stagnant hypoxia

10. A patient is suspected of having a large right pneumothorax. In order to be transported to a trauma center, the patient must be flown from sea level to 4000 ft in an unpressurized aircraft. The driving force behind volume expansion of the pneumothorax is estimated to be about:
    - 0  A. 100 mm Hg
    - 0  B. 10 mm Hg
    - 0  C. 400 mm Hg
    - 0  D. 25 mm Hg

11. The limitations of using a pulse oximeter to measure a patient's oxygen saturation during transport include:
    - 0  A. Hypothermia increases the instrument's ability to measure oxygen saturation
    - 0  B. Digits are always the best place to put the pulse oximeter probe during transport
    - 0  C. Pulse oximetry accuracy will decline in patient's with high perfusion states
    - 0  D. Motion does not affect the accuracy of the pulse oximeter during transport

12. After extrication, a MAST suit is placed to stabilize suspected pelvic and lower extremity fractures. On ascent, the patient complains of increased pressure and pain under the MAST suit. This is best explained by:
    - 0  A. Boyle's law
    - 0  B. Charles' law
    - 0  C. Henry's law
    - 0  D. Dalton's law

13. In reviewing the incidence of ear problems among flight crew members, it is noted that there is a much higher incidence of barotitis media during the cold winter months when compared with the warmer summer months. This is best explained by:
    - 0  A. Boyle's law
    - 0  B. Charles' law
    - 0  C. Henry's law
    - 0  D. Dalton's law

14. Barotitis media would most likely occur in which one of the following situations:
    - 0  A. A rapid ascent from 5000 to 10,000 ft
    - 0  B. A rapid descent from 25,000 to 20,000 ft
    - 0  C. A slow descent from 10,000 to 5000 ft
    - 0  D. A rapid descent from 5000 ft to sea level

15. The noise level within the cabin of a fixed-wing aircraft is measured at 92 dB. The flight crew member without hearing protection would exceed maximum recommended daily exposure in about:
    - 0  A. 16 hours
    - 0  B. 30 minutes
    - 0  C. 4 hours
    - 0  D. 2 hours

16. A crew member wears both a pair of earplugs with a noise attenuation of 15 dB and a helmet with an attenuation level of 25 dB. The level of noise attenuation achieved by this combination would be:
    - 0  A. 25 dB
    - 0  B. 15 dB
    - 0  C. 10 dB
    - 0  D. 40 dB

*Your flight team responds to a small rural clinic where they find a 5-year-old boy who was injured in an explosion and subsequent fire. He has sustained second- and third-degree burns to approximately 75% of his body surface area. The patient's nasal hairs are singed and he complains of mild shortness of breath.*

17. Which of the following factors would not be a mechanism of heat loss for this patient?
    - 0  A. Radiation
    - 0  B. Conduction
    - 0  C. Vasoconstriction
    - 0  D. Evaporation

18. Under which conditions would this patient most likely be exposed to physiological stress associated with decreased humidity?
    - 0  A. 1 hour flight at 1000 ft in a rotary-wing aircraft
    - 0  B. 3 hour flight in an unpressurized plane at 5000 ft
    - 0  C. 1 hour flight in a pressurized plane at 15,000 ft
    - 0  D. 6 hour flight in a pressurized plane at 25,000 ft

19. The patient must be flown at an altitude of 11,150 ft in an unpressurized aircraft in order to reach a burn unit. The $pO_2$ at 11,150 ft would be approximately:
    - 0  A. 18.5%
    - 0  B. 21%
    - 0  C. 24%
    - 0  D. 15.5%

20. Most healthy adults begin to develop signs and symptoms of hypoxia at which altitude:
    - 0  A. 8000 ft
    - 0  B. 10,000 ft
    - 0  C. 16,000 ft
    - 0  D. 18,000 ft

21. Factors that contribute to a decrease in patient temperature during transport include:
    - 0  A. Wrapping the patient in a down-filled transport blanket before lift-off
    - 0  B. Removing all wet clothing before transport in a rotary-wing aircraft
    - 0  C. Patients who are normothermic before short rotary-wing transport occurs
    - 0  D. Patients who have received neuromuscular blocking agents before transport

22. Methods to manage motion sickness include:
    - 0  A. Not eating before taking a rotary-wing flight
    - 0  B. Taking slow, deep breaths to decrease nausea
    - 0  C. Making sudden and rapid head movements
    - 0  D. Blowing warm air on the person's face

**23.** Positive G (gravitational) forces cause:

   **0**  A. Blood pooling in the lower extremities

   **0**  B. Blood pooling in the upper extremities

   **0**  C. Decreased intravascular pressures

   **0**  D. Histotoxic hypoxia

**24.** A medical crew member is treated with hyperbaric oxygen for decompression sickness. A serious complication of hyperbaric therapy is:

   **0**  A. Occasional dry cough

   **0**  B. Confinement anxiety

   **0**  C. Generalized seizures

   **0**  D. Middle ear barotrauma

**25.** Effects of aircraft vibration on humans include:

   **0**  A. Enhanced performance effectiveness

   **0**  B. Increased accuracy of ECG monitors

   **0**  C. Decreased patient discomfort

   **0**  D. Nausea, vomiting, and fatigue

## ANSWERS

1. **C. Intervention.** Crew members and patients may become incapacitated within seconds of a rapid decompression. The individual crew members must first supply supplemental oxygen to themselves to assure that they will be able to assist other crew members and patients in obtaining emergency oxygen supplies.[1,2]

2. **D. Assessment.** Areas of the body affected by changes in barometric pressure include the teeth, the middle ear, the sinuses, the lungs, and the gastrointestinal tract.[1]

3. **D. Analysis.** TUC at 25,000 feet is 3 to 5 minutes.[1]

4. **A. Evaluation.** The development of hypoxia is affected by the altitude; rate of ascent; individual tolerance; physical fitness; and physical activity. Altitude of 0 to 10,000 feet is stage of normal operations.[1]

5. **B. Intervention.** Increasing movement and applying heat packs to the knee would accelerate bubble formation and cause existing bubbles to expand (Charles' law). Splinting the affected limb would help decrease bubble size and formation in the joint, resulting in decreased tissue ischemia. Supplemental oxygen will reduce stagnant hypoxia in tissue affected by bubble formation.[1,2]

6. **C. Evaluation.** Henry's law explains that as the pressure of a gas over a liquid drops, the amount of that gas dissolved in the liquid also drops. This leads to gas bubble evolution within the fluid. If we apply Henry's law to the human body, we can say that nitrogen bubbles form in body tissues in response to decreased pressure of nitrogen above alveolar capillary membrane.[1-3]

7. **B. Evaluation.** Charles' law describes the relationship between gas volume and gas temperature. During a rapid decompression, the gas volume within an aircraft cabin is expanding rapidly as it escapes into the outside atmosphere. This rapid volume expansion causes a reciprocal drop in temperature. As the temperature drops, water vapor suspended in the cabin atmosphere forms a fine mist or fog.[1]

8. **D. Assessment.** Histotoxic hypoxia is caused by the cells' inability to accept and utilize oxygen. Causes of histotoxic hypoxia include cyanide poisoning, alcohol ingestion, narcotic overdose, and carbon monoxide poisoning.[1]

9. **A. Evaluation.** As altitude increases, the partial pressure of oxygen at the alveolar capillary membrane level drops, leading to hypoxic hypoxia.[1-3]

10. **A. Assessment.** The driving force behind volume expansion is estimated to be 25 mm Hg for every 1000 ft of altitude at altitudes under 10,000 ft.[1]

11. **C. Evaluation.** The accuracy of pulse oximetry is affected by hypothermia, extraneous light, low perfusion states, and motion.[4]

12. **A. Evaluation.** Boyle's law explains the relationship between the volume of gases trapped in the MAST and changes in barometric pressure.[2]

13. **B. Evaluation.** Charles' law describes the relationship of gas volume and temperature. When atmospheric gases are cooled they settle and become more concentrated near the surface of the earth. Therefore, altitude changes in cold environments result in larger barometric pressure changes. As a result, signs and symptoms associated barometric pressure change increase in colder conditions.[1,2]

14. **D. Evaluation.** Barometric pressure changes are greatest at lower altitudes. Because of the relationships between the anatomy of the middle ear, barometric pressure change, and gas volume, barotitis media occurs much more frequently on descent rather than ascent.[1,2]

15. **D. Assessment.** Noise levels within many aircraft can cause temporary or permanent hearing loss within a relatively short period of time.[1,2]

16. **D. Evaluation.** When two noise attenuation devices are worn together, the attenuation levels are additive.[1,2]

17. **C. Assessment.** Vasoconstriction decreases heat loss by restricting the flow of warm blood to the skin and extremities.[1,5]

18. **D. Evaluation.** The humidity inside a pressurized cabin falls rapidly as an aircraft ascends into the cold dry air present at higher altitudes. Exposure to decreased humidity increases as the length of the flight and the altitude increase.[1,2]

19. **B. Evaluation.** The percentage of oxygen in the atmosphere remains constant at 21%. Even though the percentage of oxygen remains constant, the partial pressure of oxygen drops rapidly with increases in altitude (Dalton's law). Decreased partial pressure of oxygen at higher altitudes contributes to hypoxia for crewmembers and patients.[1-3]

20. **B. Evaluation.** Although hypoxia may begin to affect some physiological functions at only a few thousand feet, actual signs and symptoms of hypoxia are not perceivable in most healthy adults until altitudes of 10,000 ft are reached.[1-3]

21. **D. Assessment.** Factors that contribute to the development of hypothermia during transport include the type of warming devices used to maintain the patient's temperature; the length of exposure; the age of the patient; the injury or illness; hypothermia before transport, and the use of neuromuscular blocking agents, which block the patient's ability to maintain his temperature.[6]

22. **B. Intervention.** Methods to decrease motion sickness include eating a small meal before flying; high-flow oxygen; limiting head movement; visual fixation on a point outside of the aircraft; medications such as scopolamine; and relaxing, which can be accomplished by slow deep breathing. One study actually found that slow, deep breathing prevented the development of the gastric dysrhythmia that accompanies motion sickness.[1,7]

23. **A. Assessment.** Positive G forces cause blood pooling in the lower extremities, increased intravascular pressures, and stagnant hypoxia.[1]

24. **C. Evaluation.** A serious complication of hyperbaric oxygen therapy is generalized seizure. Other less serious complications include middle ear barotrauma resulting in pain and discomfort; confinement anxiety; and occasional dry cough.[8]

25. **D. Evaluation.** The effects of aircraft vibration include nausea, vomiting, and fatigue; increased patient discomfort; interference with the accuracy of patient monitoring equipment; and decrease in crew performance effectiveness.[9]

## REFERENCES

1. Krupa DT, editor: *Flight nursing core curriculum,* Park Ridge, MD, 1997, Road Runner Press.
2. National Flight Nurses Association: Flight physiology. In NFNA: *flight nurse advanced trauma course,* Thorofare, NJ, 1994, NFNA.
3. Waggoner RR: Flight physiology. In Semonin-Holleran R, editor: *Flight nursing principles and practice,* St. Louis, 1996, Mosby.
4. Thomas F, Blumen I: Assessing oxygenation in the transport environment. *Air Med J* 18(2):79-86, 1999.
5. Browne-Wagner L, Bodenstedt R: Flight physiology. In Department of Transportation: *Air medical crew national standard curriculum,* Pasadena, CA, 1988, ASHBEAMS.
6. Fiege A, Rutherford W, Nelson D: Factors influencing in flight. *Air Med J* 15(1):18-23, 1996.
7. Jokerst M, Fazio R, Stern R, Kock K: Slow deep breathing prevents the development of tachygastria and symptoms of motion sickness, *Aviation Space, Environ Med* 27(12):1189-1192, 1999.
8. Plafki C, Peters P, Almeling M, and others: Complications and side effects of hyperbaric oxygen therapy. *Aviation Space Environ Med* 71(2):119-124, 2000.
9. Topley DK: Whole body vibration, *AirMed* 5(1):32-37, 1999.

# Chapter 27

# Transport Safety

## REVIEW OUTLINE

I. Safety: definition
   A. Practices incorporated into daily operations with the purpose of reducing or eliminating the chance of severe injury or death to members of the transport team, patients, or other ancillary persons operating around or near the transport vehicle

II. Safety responsibilities
   A. Safety responsibility shared by all members of the air transport program
      1. Administrators
      2. Pilots/drivers
      3. Mechanics
      4. Communications specialists
      5. Nursing/medical personnel
   B. Safety is strengthened by
      1. Teamwork
      2. Training
      3. Communication
      4. Crew resource management
      5. Recognizing that people you are working with and people you transport are individuals with worth and dignity[1]
   C. Comprehensive safety program evaluates
      1. Training
      2. Equipment
      3. Policies and procedures
      4. Reporting and examination of incidents or concerns
      5. Communication

III. Safety regulations
   A. Government
      1. Federal Aviation Regulations (FARs): written and enforced by the Federal Aviation Administration (FAA)
      2. FARs address
         a. Flight operations
         b. Aircraft and equipment operating limitations
         c. Weather requirements
         d. Pilot flight time limitations and rest requirements
         e. Pilot testing and training requirements
         f. Maintenance requirements
      3. FAR Part 91: general operating and flight rules for aircraft operating within U.S. airspace
      4. FAR Part 135: specifies rules for air taxi and commercial operators. Most air medical programs are regulated under this FAR
      5. Ground transport
         a. General Services Administration
         b. State and local agency regulations

IV. Safety voluntary guidelines
   A. Association of Air Medical Services (AAMS)
   B. State EMS agencies
      1. State ambulance regulations
      2. Association of Air and Surface Transport Nurses Transport Guidelines
      3. Association of Air and Surface Transport Nurses Safety Paper

V. Safety risks in the transport environment
   A. Type of mission
      1. Medical
      2. Search and rescue (SAR)
      3. Trauma
   B. Environmental factors
      1. Terrain
      2. Climate
      3. Population density
   C. Air medical environment
      1. Type of aircraft
         a. Rotary wing
         b. Fixed wing
      2. Single vs. multiple engines
      3. Service area of program
      4. Aircraft equipment
         a. Skid height
         b. Flotation devices
         c. Pressurized cabin
         d. Communication equipment
         e. Wire cutters

D. Ground transport environment
1. Type of vehicle
2. Experience of the driver
3. Equipment
    a. Motor
    b. Headlights
    c. Fluids
    d. Siren
    e. Horn
    f. Radios
    g. Suction
    h. Climate control
    i. Generator
VI. Aircraft safety equipment
A. Seat belts and restraints
B. Energy-attenuating seats
C. Clear head strike area
D. Flush mounted or recessed wall equipment
E. Halon fire extinguisher
F. Survival kit
G. Lighting (cabin and outside of aircraft)
VII. Ground transport safety equipment
A. Scene lights
B. Fog lights
C. Fire extinguishers
D. Maps
E. Generator
F. Ground transport vehicle maintenance
1. Fluids levels
2. Visual inspection
3. Audio inspection
4. Equipment inspection
5. Routine maintenance record
VIII. Personal safety
A. Helmets
1. Lightweight
2. Custom fitted
3. Noise reducing
B. Uniforms
1. Flame retardant
2. Cotton underwear
3. Boots
4. Gloves
C. Physical fitness
1. Yearly audiometric examinations
2. No alcohol, tobacco, drug use while on duty
3. Good physical health and agility
D. Safety knowledge
1. Use of fire extinguisher
2. Location of on-board survival kit
3. Use of flotation devices
4. Emergency egress procedures

5. Emergency locator transmitter (ELT) location and activation
6. Fuel shut-off
7. Battery disconnect
8. Fuel spillage
E. Personal survival
1. Mental and physical preparation
2. Shelter building
3. Fire building
4. Signaling
5. Obtaining water
6. Map reading/direction finding
7. Post accident/incident plan (PAIP)
    a. When to activate the PAIP
    b. List of personnel to notify in order of priority
    c. Guidelines to follow in attempts to:
        (1) Communicate with aircraft or ambulance
        (2) Initiate search and rescue or ground support
        (3) Back-up plan for transporting the patient
    d. Procedure to secure all documents
    e. Procedure to release information
IX. Infection control
A. Occupational Safety and Health Administration (OSHA) guidelines
B. Exposure to communicable diseases
C. Methods to prevent contamination and spread of disease
1. Standard precautions
2. BSI (body substance isolation)
3. Vaccinations
4. Testing and follow-up
D. Exposure procedures
1. Reports
2. Testing
3. Treatments for exposures
E. Right-to-know issues
1. Federal guidelines
2. State guidelines
F. Nursing diagnoses
1. Anxiety
2. Fear
3. Knowledge deficit
4. Infection, high risk for
5. Injury, high risk for
X. Scene safety
A. Violent situations
1. Patient(s)
2. Crowds
3. Families

B. Landing zone set-up
  1. Adequate space
  2. Free of debris
  3. Appropriate marking
C. Loading and unloading safety

XI. Patient safety
  A. Securing patient in the aircraft
  B. Securing of medical equipment
  C. Sources of patient discomfort and fear
    1. Fear of flying
    2. Motion
    3. Vibration
    4. Temperature variations
    5. Noise
    6. Atmospheric pressures
    7. Humidity
    8. Confinement
  D. Specific patient populations
    1. Neonates: transport isolettes
    2. Pediatrics: child-restraint systems
    3. Combative or confused patients
      a. Physical restraints
      b. Chemical restraints
    4. Prisoners

XII. Ancillary staff safety
  A. Ancillary staff
    1. Public safety personnel
    2. Hospital staffs
  B. Helicopter safety education
    1. Helicopter safety
    2. Hazardous areas
    3. Selection and preparation of a landing area
    4. Communications
    5. "Hot" loading and unloading
    6. Crowd control
  C. Fixed-wing safety education
    1. Avoiding intake and exhaust areas that may still be hot following landing
    2. Avoiding contact with or close proximity to propellers even when shut down
    3. Ambulance safety while on taxiway or airport ramps
  D. Flight teams must assist the pilot when landing in unfamiliar areas by surveying the landing area from above and looking for any unusual circumstances that may cause injury to those on the ground

XIII. Transport vehicle following
  A. Performed by a trained, dedicated communication specialist
  B. Communication specialists' roles
    1. Tracking the aircraft
    2. Monitoring for overdue aircraft
    3. Instituting downed aircraft procedures

XIV. Quality management programs for safety
  A. Essential element of a safety program
  B. Documentation of safety issues
  C. Documentation of compliance

XV. Accreditation of medical transport systems
  A. General standards
    1. Medical
    2. Aircraft/ambulance
    3. Management and administration
  B. Rotary wing standards
  C. Fixed wing standards
  D. Ground interfacility standards

Transport nurses must recognize the unique hazards found in the hectic and potentially life-threatening environment in which they practice. They must not only recognize hazardous situations but also possess the skills and knowledge to react decisively to prevent these situations from escalating beyond control. The first step of safety management is prevention.[1,8]

The role of the transport nurse related to safety is twofold. The transport nurse's primary role is to provide the most optimal nursing care possible, given the environment in which she functions, to critically ill or injured patients by combining nursing skills with advanced technology. The secondary role of the transport nurse is to function as safety advocate and maintain a secure and protected environment for patients, other transport team members, ancillary staff, public service personnel, bystanders, and all other persons who interact with the transport service. The major concern of every transport service must be safety.

Regardless of the complexities or diverse responsibilities of the transport team, good communication skills, a thorough understanding of vehicle safety and the environment in which the vehicle operates, and knowledge of personal survival skills are essential to providing a safe work environment for the practice of transport.

## REVIEW QUESTIONS

1. Transport program safety is the responsibility of:
  0  A. The program or administrative director
  0  B. The designated safety officer
  0  C. All members of the transport team
  0  D. The pilot or driver in command

2. A comprehensive safety program evaluates all phases of the transport program except:
   - O  A. Training and retraining of the transport team
   - O  B. Policies and procedures related to vehicle safety
   - O  C. Equipment used during air and ground transport
   - O  D. The status of the patient's health insurance

3. Which of the following government agencies regulates flight operations?
   - O  A. The National Transportation Safety Board (NTSB)
   - O  B. The Federal Aviation Administration (FAA)
   - O  C. Occupational Safety and Health Administration (OSHA)
   - O  D. National Institute of Aviation and Health (NIAH)

4. An example of voluntary guidelines for flight safety is:
   - O  A. AAMS guidelines for weather minimums
   - O  B. FAA guidelines for weather minimums
   - O  C. OSHA guidelines for the disinfection of equipment
   - O  D. National Transportation Safety Board (NTSB) reporting guidelines for accident investigation

5. "Sterile cockpit" is defined as:
   - O  A. Assurance that all patient care equipment has been appropriately disinfected
   - O  B. A conversation of a social nature occurring during initial aircraft approach
   - O  C. Conversation with the communication center during the transport process
   - O  D. Conversation kept to an absolute minimum on all approaches and landings

*The Air Care Flight Program was en route to pick up a patient when the aircraft experienced an in-flight emergency requiring an immediate landing. The pilot alerted the medical team to prepare for a hard landing.*

6. Immediate actions that should be performed by the flight team include all of the following except:
   - O  A. Turn the oxygen supply to the OFF position
   - O  B. Secure the patient and any loose medical equipment
   - O  C. Ask the pilot what is wrong and if there is anything you can do
   - O  D. Sit with head up against the headrest and feet flat on the floor

7. The pilot has brought the aircraft to a full stop, but has sustained injuries that render him unconscious. Both medical crewmembers are unharmed. Of the following, which is the greatest danger immediately following impact?
   - O  A. Damage to the radio that may complicate rescue efforts and keep the helicopter from being found sooner
   - O  B. The impact may not have been great enough to activate the Emergency Locator Transmitter (ELT)
   - O  C. The outside temperature of minus 10° F may cause hypothermia to the crew before rescue
   - O  D. The possibility of fire because of the presence of fuel and oxygen in rotary-wing aircraft

8. Following the forced landing, what course of action should be taken by the flight team members?
   - O  A. Immediately evacuate the aircraft and meet at a safe distance from the aircraft until it stops running
   - O  B. Shut off the fuel and battery switches, evacuate the aircraft, and meet at a safe distance
   - O  C. Attempt to remove the injured pilot from the aircraft to a safe distance from the aircraft
   - O  D. Ensure that the Emergency Locator Transmitter (ELT) is transmitting, then evacuate the aircraft and meet at a safe distance

9. The number one killer of people in survival situations is:
   - O  A. Hunger
   - O  B. Thirst
   - O  C. Fatigue
   - O  D. Cold

10. The decision by the flight team to stay at the present site or attempt to hike the estimated 40 miles to a known town would likely be made on the strength of the following information:
   - O  A. The appropriately dressed flight team has an adequate survival kit, including a compass, and poor visibility is moving in, making aerial search and rescue difficult. The flight team should begin moving away from the crash site.
   - O  B. The flight team has an adequate survival kit, but has no flares or signaling devices, and no fresh water. Poor visibility is moving in, making an aerial search and

rescue difficult. The flight team should begin moving away from the crash site.
- 0  C.  The flight team has adequate shelter, water in the form of IV fluids, but no food. Poor visibility is moving in. Staying near the crash site may be the best option.
- 0  D.  The flight team has no survival kit and one member did not dress properly for the cold weather. The pilot is injured and may not survive the night. The flight team should begin moving away from the crash site.

11. When making an emergency landing in the water, the flight team must:
- 0  A.  Inflate their Personal Flotation Device (PFD) before they exit the aircraft
- 0  B.  Swim away from other team members so rescuers can have more to spot
- 0  C.  Leave all equipment inside of the aircraft since it may cause them to sink
- 0  D.  Let the aircraft fill with water to equalize internal and external pressure

12. A basic skill that all flight team members who are employed by programs that operate or fly over large bodies of water should have is:
- 0  A.  The ability to swim
- 0  B.  A knowledge of personal flotation devices
- 0  C.  Open sea survival skills
- 0  D.  The ability to inflate a survival raft

13. Choosing a site for a temporary shelter requires careful consideration. Which of the following sites would make the best choice for a temporary shelter?
- 0  A.  A site below a rocky bluff
- 0  B.  A site near some tall dead trees
- 0  C.  A site at the edge of a stream
- 0  D.  A site near the edge of a clearing of trees

14. Following the forced landing of an aircraft, attempts should be made to contact the hospital base, air traffic control, or flight service on the aircraft radio. If attempts fail, the emergency VHF frequency should be used. This frequency is:
- 0  A.  121.5
- 0  B.  151.2
- 0  C.  125.0
- 0  D.  555.5

15. The most important mental conditioning in a survival situation is:
- 0  A.  A variety of life experiences, including survival training
- 0  B.  The individual's sense of well-being

- 0  C.  Practicing survival principles
- 0  D.  The individual's will to live

16. Protecting the body from hypothermia is essential for flight personnel working in cold weather conditions. Basic protection begins with the knowledge that most heat is lost through:
- 0  A.  Arms and hands
- 0  B.  Feet and legs
- 0  C.  Head and neck
- 0  D.  Chest and back

17. The greatest advantage of conducting a missing/overdue aircraft drill is:
- 0  A.  The drill approximates the stress that the communication specialist may experience if a real incident would ever occur
- 0  B.  Commission on Accreditation of Medical Transport Systems (CAMTS) accreditation requires it for program accreditation of air and ground
- 0  C.  The drill allows the program administration an opportunity to see how their personnel would react, especially when they do not know it's a drill
- 0  D.  That the drill can be completed without performing a critique to identify any deficiencies or problems

18. The primary role of a civilian hospital-based air medical transport team in search and rescue (SAR) is:
- 0  A.  Use their helicopter to perform the rescue before the SAR team arrives
- 0  B.  To communicate only with their home base communication specialist
- 0  C.  Transport the rescued patient to definitive care from a safe landing area
- 0  D.  Not to participate in the SAR debriefing since they are not official members

19. A protocol addressing the response to a hazardous material incident would most likely not contain which of the following statements?
- 0  A.  Patients exposed to a hazardous material (HAZMAT) incident must be flown to a center capable of handling HAZMAT emergencies for primary decontamination
- 0  B.  A relationship with a local HAZMAT resource person/center must be established to ensure quick access to information as needed

0   C. Annual training for air medical personnel and communications specialists must be included in the program's continuing education program

0   D. Extreme saturation with gasoline or diesel fuel should be handled as a HAZMAT incident

20. The most important principle in guiding the actions of the transport nurse while working near a HAZMAT accident area is:

0   A. Quick evacuation and treatment of contaminated individuals

0   B. The need to contain the contamination to a designated area for safe disposal

0   C. The need to evacuate the surrounding area to prevent further contamination

0   D. The individual flight nurse's safety is paramount

21. What is considered a significant exposure to blood?

0   A. Touching a piece of equipment with dried blood on without gloves

0   B. Potentially infectious fluid that comes in contact with a mucous membrane

0   C. Needle stick through a glove in the palm of the transport nurse's hand

0   D. Blood splash on goggles being worn during an intubation procedure

22. The risk for infection after an exposure to blood is determined by:

0   A. The pathogen involved

0   B. The amount of virus in the patient's blood at the time of the exposure

0   C. The type of the exposure

0   D. All of the above

23. Which of the following are examples of appropriate personal protective equipment (PPE) to have available in a transport vehicle?

0   A. Gloves, face shields, masks, gowns

0   B. Gloves, impermeable sheets, and aprons

0   C. Eye protection, masks, gowns

0   D. A spray bottle with bleach for spills

24. When cleaning used patient care equipment, the transport nurse should wear:

0   A. Gloves, goggles, and a gown

0   B. Gloves and goggles only

0   C. No PPE is needed to clean equipment

0   D. Goggles and a gown or an apron

25. What type of cleaning procedure should the transport nurse employ to clean reusable patient care items?

0   A. Reusable items should never be used in the prehospital care environment because of the risk of infection

0   B. Reusable items should be disinfected on a regular basis, which is recorded and documented

0   C. Reusable items need only to be cleaned when they come in contact with a potentially infectious substance

0   D. Reusable items do not require routine cleaning because they pose no threat of exposing patients to disease

26. Can any type of disinfectant be used to clean blood and body fluids out of a helicopter?

0   A. The chance of disease exposure from fluids in a helicopter is minimal

0   B. Any solution can be used as long as it will disinfect all the potential organisms

0   C. Care must be taken with some disinfectants because they may cause corrosion

0   D. There are no disinfectants that may be used to clean body fluids from a helicopter

27. The transport team responded to a motor vehicle crash. The patient required a surgical cricothyrotomy and there is large amount of blood on the road. The transport team should instruct the prehospital providers to:

0   A. Spills do not need to be removed because the sun and the rain will dissipate any infectious agents that may be in the fluid

0   B. Ask the fire service to spray the area with a fire hose and dissipate the blood with a spray of water

0   C. Instruct the personnel to use a 1:100 household bleach solution or approved germicide to clean the fluid

0   D. Instruct the personnel to scrub the area with warm soapy water until the area is clean again

28. The transport nurse suffers a significant exposure to a patient who has been diagnosed with HCV (hepatitis C). Postexposure treatment for this type of exposure includes:

0   A. HBIG and/or hepatitis B vaccination and close monitoring

0   B. 4-week course of zidovudine and lamivudine

0   C. Three to four doses of gamma globulin intramuscularly

0   D. There are no recommended postexposure treatment for HCV

29. Safety evaluation of medical equipment should include all of the following *except:*

0   A. Vibration testing

0   B. Electrical safety testing

0   C. Monitor screen evaluation

0   D. Thermal and humidity conditions

30. Components of scene safety include:

0   A. All patients who are victims of penetrating trauma should be searched or their clothes removed because of the risk of weapons

0   B. Any patient who is under arrest must receive chemical paralysis and intubation before they are transported

0   C. Running to the scene of the crash or injury after exiting the helicopter without your partner

0   D. Not wearing turnout gear if you participate in the extrications because your flight suit will provide all the protection you need

## ANSWERS

1.  **C. Assessment.** Safe program operations require a commitment by all members of the transport program and are strengthened through teamwork, training, and communication. The total safety approach involves developing meaningful measures of safety as well as annual reviews.[2]

2.  **D. Evaluation.** A comprehensive safety program evaluates vehicle safety, equipment safety, team training, safety policies and procedures, and quality-assurance parameters.[2]

3.  **B. Assessment.** The Federal Aviation Administration (FAA) is the federal regulation and enforcement agency that impacts all air medical programs.[3]

4.  **A. Intervention.** The AAMS is a voluntary organization for the providers of air medical transport services. The association encourages and supports its members in maintaining a standard of performance reflecting safe operations and efficient, high-quality patient care; however, it has no power of enforcement over member programs.[3]

5.  **C.** "Sterile cockpit" is defined as minimum conversation from engine start, until air traffic and congestion are cleared and on all approaches and landings.[3]

6.  **C. Intervention.** Immediate actions that the flight team should perform include all of the actions listed except attempting to talk with the pilot. The pilot must not be distracted from concentrating on performing a safe landing and making radio contact.[4]

7.  **D. Assessment.** Fire is the most immediate danger following a forced landing. The aircraft must not be exited until the blades have come to a complete stop.[3,4]

8.  **B. Intervention.** The aircraft must be exited as quickly as possible, pausing only to shut off the fuel and battery switches when possible. Do not attempt to rescue any victims until the danger of fire no longer exists. The crew members should meet at a predesignated rendezvous point near the aircraft.[3,4]

9.  **D. Assessment.** The number one killer of people in survival situations is hypothermia. The prevention of hypothermia begins with the proper selection of clothing.[6]

10. **C. Assessment.** Based on the location of the flight team, the equipment they may have available, and the impending weather, the flight team should stay near the crash site. The priorities of survival include: checking for injuries and administering first aid, building a shelter, providing warmth, obtaining water, signaling, and direction finding.[1]

11. **D.** The flight team should let the aircraft fill with water to equalize the internal and external pressure. Their next step is to unplug, unstrap, exit, and then inflate their life vests.[3]

12. **A. Intervention.** The ability to swim is a basic skill that everyone involved in transport over water must have. Many people have died in survival situations because they could not swim.[1]

13. **D. Assessment.** A temporary shelter situated on the edge of a clearing provides the best visibility. Always scan the site for hazards, which can be found anywhere, and choose a campsite with the fewest hazards. Do not build a shelter beneath rock bluffs because wind and rain may send rocks and debris into the shelter. Do not build a shelter near tall dead trees that can fall or blow down or may be struck by lightning. Shelters built by a stream may be subject to flooding without warning and the noise of running water may deter the people in the shelter from hearing rescuers.[1,6]

14. **A. Intervention.** There are two aeronautical emergency frequencies: 121.5 and 243.0. The Emergency Locator Transmitter (ELT) transmits on the 121.5 frequency.[4]

15. **D. Evaluation.** The most important mental conditioning is the will to live, which cannot be

learned. In many previous survival situations, attitude and sheer willpower were identified as the most important factors in rescued survivors.[1]

16. **C. Assessment.** Most heat is lost through the head and neck. Therefore, protecting these areas is essential. Hands should be protected because they are needed to perform life-saving tasks such as building fire and shelter.[6]

17. **A. Intervention.** The greatest advantage of initiating a PAIP drill is that the communication specialist has the opportunity to experience the stress without a "real" incident. All personnel should always be told that it is a drill, and the drill should be critiqued for deficiencies and problems.[7]

18. **C. Intervention.** Unfortunately, over the years, hospital-based air medical transport team members have died attempting to rescue patients. Without specific SAR training, the primary role of the transport team is to transport the patient to definitive care from a safe landing area.[8]

19. **A. Evaluation.** The primary concern is the safety of the flight team and aircraft in situations where hazardous materials are known to exist. Patients must never be transported prior to decontamination. A HAZMAT resource should be available to all programs, as well as yearly training and updating in HAZMAT responses. Patients contaminated with gasoline or fuel must not be placed in the aircraft until the saturated clothing has been removed.[1]

20. **D. Intervention.** The overriding concern at a HAZMAT incident, as with any dangerous situation, is the safety of the rescuers. Until the properly trained personnel and equipment become available, distance from the accident area is one's greatest ally.[1]

21. **C. Assessment.** A needlestick is considered the most significant exposure to a patient's blood.[9]

22. **D. Assessment.** Most exposures do not result in the health care provider becoming infected, but factors that may determine the risk include:
- The pathogen involved
- The type of exposure
- The amount of blood involved
- The amount of virus in the patient's blood at the time of exposure[9]

23. **A.** The employee must wear personal protective equipment, such as gloves, face shields, masks, eye protection, gowns, and aprons, to prevent the spread of infectious diseases.[10]

24. **A. Intervention.** PPE should be worn when cleaning used patient care equipment. The hepatitis virus can survive for several days in dried blood.[10]

25. **B. Intervention.** Reusable items need to be disinfected on a regular basis, which is recorded and documented on a cleaning schedule. Items need to be cleaned on a scheduled basis so all items are accounted for. The floors and walls typically do not pose a serious threat for spreading infectious diseases unless they come in contact with the infectious substance. A regular schedule is helpful because it can be difficult to be aware of what actually becomes contaminated.[10,11,12]

26. **C. Intervention.** No, some chemicals can interact with the aluminum alloy of the helicopter. The aluminum alloy is attacked by strong corrosives that will decrease the strength of the aluminum. Stress corrosion cracking is rapid and unpredictable.[10,11]

27. **C. Intervention.** The area should be cleaned with 1:100 household bleach or an approved disinfectant in order to protect people from possible exposure.

28. **D. Intervention.** Unfortunately, there are no current recommendations for postexposure treatment for HCV.[9]

29. **C. Assessment.** Safety evaluation of medical equipment includes evaluation of electrical safety, vibration, response to hypobaric and rapid decompression, thermal and humidity conditions; and an in-flight evaluation.[13]

30. **A. Intervention.** Components of scene safety include:
- Wearing appropriate turnout gear to prevent any personal injury
- Conducting a scene survey before exiting the aircraft
- Watching out for your partner
- Searching penetrating trauma victims or remove their close to decrease the risk of weapons
- Establishing protocols related to the transport of prisoners[14]

## REFERENCES

1. North M: Cause factor: human, *Air Med J* 19(1):4-5, 2000.
2. Rouse M: Flight safety and personal survival. In Semonin-Holleran R, editor: *Flight nursing principles and practice,* ed 2, St Louis, 1996, Mosby.
3. Krupa D, editor: *Flight nursing core curriculum,* Park Ridge, MD, 1997, Road Runner Press.
4. Association of Air Medical Services: *Minimum quality standards and safety guidelines,* Pasadena, CA, 1994, AAMS.
5. Semonin-Holleran R, editor: *Flight nursing principles and practice,* ed 2, St Louis, 1996, Mosby.
6. Isaacs SM, Saunders CE, Durrer B: Aeromedical transport. In Auerbach PS, editor: *Wilderness medicine,* St Louis, 1995, Mosby.
7. Rogers L, Fiege A: Missing/overdue aircraft: are you prepared? *AirMed* 5(2):24-26, 1999.

8. Kovacs T: A primer on search and rescue, *AirMed* 6(1):20-24, 2000.

9. CDC: Occupational exposure to blood. Cdc.gov./ncidod/ hp/Blood/Exposure to blood, 1999.

10. Corriere C, Zarro C, Connelly P, Tortella B, and Lavery R: A national survey of air medical infectious disease control practices, *Air Med J* 19(1):8-12, 2000.

11. Semonin-Holleran R, editor: *Prehospital nursing: a collaborative approach,* St Louis, 1994, Mosby.

12. Austin E, Austin H, McKechinie T: The effect of disinfectants on 2024-T3 aluminum in the air medical helicopter, *Air Med J* 1:57-64, 1993.

13. Hale J, Hade E: Safety evaluation of medical equipment before flight certification, *AirMed* 3(3):42-46, 1997.

14. High K, Yeatmann J: Safety: Ground rules for flight crews, *AirMed* 4(6):28-30, 1998.

# Chapter 28
# Patient Care During Transport

**REVIEW OUTLINE**

I. History
  A. Florence Nightingale
  B. Clara Barton
  C. Military service
    1. World War I
    2. World War II
    3. Korean War
    4. Vietnam War
    5. Operation Desert Storm
  D. Laurette Schimmoler
  E. First hospital-based helicopter program—St. Anthony's Hospital
II. Indications for patient transport
  A. Trauma
    1. Recommendations for helicopter transport of trauma patients
      a. Transport time to trauma center >15 minutes
      b. Ambulance transport impeded because of access
      c. Multiple victims
      d. Time to local hospital by ambulance is greater than time to trauma center by helicopter
      e. Wilderness rescue
    2. Mechanism of injury
      a. Accident speeds >55 miles per hour
      b. Patient entrapment
      c. Death of another occupant
      d. Falls >15 feet
      e. Penetrating injuries
    3. Scoring systems
      a. Trauma score <12
      b. Glasgow Coma Scale (GCS) <10
      c. Baxt's Trauma Triage Rule
    4. Specific injuries
      a. Spinal cord injury, or injury producing neurological deficits
      b. Two or more long bone fractures, major pelvic fracture
      c. Major burns
    5. Patient with multiple injuries >55 years of age or patients <12 years of age
  B. Cardiovascular
    1. Need for cardiac intensive care
    2. Need for cardiac catheterization
    3. Need for surgical procedure, e.g., angioplasty or cardiopulmonary bypass
    4. Need for a specific treatment
      a. Experimental
      b. Medications
      c. Mechanical assist devices
    5. Need for organ transport
  C. Maternal
    1. Placenta previa or placenta abruptio
    2. Fetal distress
    3. Maternal trauma
    4. Prenatal complications, e.g., diabetes, preeclampsia
    5. Perimortem delivery
  D. Neonatal transport
    1. Age and weight of the infant
    2. Illness
      a. Sepsis
      b. Respiratory distress
      c. Meconium aspiration
    3. Surgical
      a. Omphalocele
      b. Tracheoesophageal fistula
      c. Diaphragmatic hernia
    4. Injury
    5. Near-drowning
  E. Pediatric
    1. Respiratory distress
    2. Respiratory failure
    3. Shock states
    4. Status epilepticus
    5. Metabolic disturbances
    6. Multiple organ system failure
    7. Multiple trauma
    8. Burns
    9. Near-drowning
    10. Poisonings

11. Foreign body aspiration
12. Specialty referrals such as cardiac, oncology

III. Pretransport planning and patient preparation and transport
   A. Care based on flight nursing standards of practice (nursing process)
   B. Care based on adult critical care transport standards
   C. Care based on standards of American Academy of Pediatrics
   D. Assessment
      1. History
      2. Physical assessment
         a. Primary survey
         b. Secondary survey
         c. Illness/injury survey
   E. Related nursing diagnoses
      1. Infection, high risk for
      2. Altered body temperature, high risk for
      3. Hypothermia
      4. Hyperthermia
      5. Ineffective thermoregulation
      6. Altered tissue perfusion (renal, cerebral, GI, peripheral)
      7. Fluid volume excess
      8. Fluid volume deficit
      9. Decreased cardiac output
      10. Impaired gas exchange
      11. Ineffective airway clearance
      12. Inability to sustain spontaneous ventilation
      13. Impaired skin integrity
      14. Impaired physical mobility
      15. High risk for peripheral neurovascular dysfunction
      16. Body image disturbance
      17. Pain
      18. Anxiety
      19. Fear
   F. Outcome identification
      1. Based on the patient's problem
      2. Provide direction for the care the patient is to receive
      3. Outcomes are based on a collaborative approach to the care of the patient
   G. Planning
   H. Implementation
      1. Collaborative care interventions (care is dependent on the age of the patient)
         a. Airway management
            (1) Basic life support
            (2) Advanced life support
            (3) Rapid sequence induction
         b. Cervical spine immobilization for the injured patient
         c. Breathing/ventilation management
            (1) Ventilators
            (2) Sedation
            (3) Decompression
         d. Circulatory management
            (1) Intravenous access
            (2) Intraosseous access
            (3) Monitoring
            (4) MAST/PASG application
            (5) Urinary catheter
         e. Neurological management
            (1) Cervical spine immobilization
            (2) Traction
         f. Illness/injury specific
            (1) Gastric decompression
            (2) Wound care
            (3) Splinting
            (4) Temperature
      2. Equipment (dependent on the age of the patient)
         a. Airway
            (1) Pulse oximeter
            (2) End-tidal $CO_2$
         b. Breathing
            (1) Ventilators
            (2) Decompression equipment
            (3) Apnea monitor
         c. Circulation
            (1) Intravenous devices
            (2) Cardiac devices
            (3) Invasive monitors
            (4) Central venous pressure (CVP)
            (5) Laboratory values
         d. Neurological
            (1) Cervical collar
            (2) Backboard (adult and pediatric)
            (3) Extrication boards
         e. Temperature
            (1) Isolette
            (2) Warming devices
         f. Transport devices
            (1) Stretcher
            (2) Carbed
            (3) Carseat
      3. Medications
         a. Neuromuscular blockade (NMB)
         b. Sedation
         c. Advanced cardiac life support and/or pediatric/neonatal advanced life support

d. Medical
   (1) Cardiovascular
   (2) Gastrointestinal
   (3) Pulmonary
   (4) Disease-related
   (5) Other
e. Injury
   (1) Head injury
   (2) Spinal cord injury
   (3) Abdominal injury
   (4) Orthopedic injury
   (5) Other
4. Pain management
  a. Level of pain
  b. Medications
  c. Alternative care methods
5. Family care
  a. Information
  b. Additional passengers
  c. Safety

I. Invasive monitoring
  1. Arterial monitoring
    a. Systolic phase
      (1) Valves opening
      (2) Correlation with ECG
      (3) Dicrotic arch
    b. Equipment set-up
      (1) Leveling of transducer
      (2) Zeroing of transducer
    c. Troubleshooting
      (1) Dampened waveforms
      (2) High digital pressure
      (3) Low flow states
  2. Pulmonary artery (PA) catheters
    a. Waveform patterns
      (1) Right ventricle
      (2) PA overwedged
    b. Equipment set-up
      (1) Leveling of transducer
      (2) Zeroing of transducer
      (3) Catheter position
      (4) Inflating PA balloon
    c. Troubleshooting
      (1) Right ventricular position and ectopy
      (2) Dampened waveforms
      (3) High PA digital readings
      (4) Treatment of low PA wedge pressure readings
      (5) Flight transport issues
J. Intraaortic balloon pump (IABP)
  1. Rationale for use

2. Timing of IABP
  a. Triggering
  b. Inflation
  c. Deflation
3. Transport issues
  a. Loss of vacuum
  b. Positioning the patient
4. Complications
  a. Emboli
  b. Thrombus
K. Left ventricular assist device (LVAD)
L. Delayed transport
  1. Prolonged patient entrapment
  2. Wilderness rescue
  3. Limited equipment
  4. Inaccurate assessment of illness or injury
  5. Development of complications from illness or injury that require transport to another facility
M. Evaluation
  1. On-going assessment
  2. Documentation of care effectiveness
  3. Follow-up information

IV. Quality management
  A. National Flight Nurses Association standards
  B. Commission on Accreditation of Medical Transport Systems (CAMTS)
  C. Documentation of care
  D. Identification of care
  E. Initiation of change

V. Challenges in transport nursing practice
  A. Ethical issues (see Chapter 23)
  B. Legal issues (see Chapter 23)
  C. Stress and stress management
    1. Sources of stress
      a. Work environment
      b. Equipment
      c. Age of the patient
      d. Death of patient
      e. Death of co-worker
    2. Reactions to stress
      a. Acute
      b. Chronic
    3. Stress management
      a. Exercise
      b. Diet
      c. Emotional care
    4. Critical incident stress
      a. Hostage situations
      b. Excessive violence
      c. Suicide or unexpected death of a co-worker

d. Incidents attracting media attention
e. Pediatric patients
5. Critical incident stress management
   a. Defusing
   b. Debriefing
   c. Follow-up debriefing

Accc ording to the *Standards of Flight Nursing Practice*[1] and *The Standards for Adult Critical Care Transport*[2] "transport nursing practice involves the nursing process: assessment, diagnosis, outcome identification, planning, implementation, and evaluation." The care of patients begins with obtaining patient information, performing a primary and sometimes a secondary assessment, planning and implementing patient care, and finally evaluating the care provided.

The types of patients encountered depend on the mission of the transport program. Some transport nurses are generalists transporting a variety of patients, where others perform specialty transports such as neonatal or pediatric. In addition, transport nurses collaborate with a variety of different team members, including physicians, respiratory therapists, and paramedics. The educational preparation for transport nursing is discussed in Chapter 1.

A key component of transport nursing care is anticipation. Transport nurses need to always expect the unexpected. The present and potential patient condition requires the transport nurse to have the appropriate equipment and medications available and functioning to prevent any further complication or injury during the transport process.

The family of the ill or injured patient has important needs that the transport nurse must consider. The stresses of transport on the family include complete separation of the patient and their family, transport to an unfamiliar place, the potential risks associated with the transport, and the stress of the transport itself.[3] Most of the time family members cannot accompany the patient because of the transport vehicle size, weight limits, and the condition of the patient.

Other issues involved in patient transport include quality management, ethical and legal issues (see Chapter 23), and stress. Stress and stress management are vital concerns in transport nursing practice. There are multiple sources of stress in the transport nursing environment, including limited space in which to care for patients, equipment malfunctioning, and the age, illness, or injury of the patient. Learning to manage one's stress keeps transport nurses in the prehospital, hospital, and interhospital environments.

This chapter contains some additional review questions that involve issues encountered by transport and prehospital nurses in the care of their patients.

## REVIEW QUESTIONS

1. A very low birth weight infant weighs less than:
   O   A. 2500 g
   O   B. 1500 g
   O   C. 1000 g
   O   D. 2000 g

2. Risk factors associated with an increased risk for neonatal resuscitation include all of the following *except:*
   O   A. History of maternal substance abuse
   O   B. Previous fetal or neonatal death
   O   C. History of normal labor and delivery
   O   D. Prolonged rupture of membranes

3. Indications for intubation in the neonate include:
   O   A. A heart rate greater than 100 beats per minute immediately after delivery of the neonate
   O   B. Effective bag-valve-mask ventilation with an appropriate-sized bag-valve-mask, which results in an increase in the neonate's heart rate
   O   C. The absence of meconium in the neonate's trachea after administration of oxygen by mask
   O   D. The need for prolonged positive-pressure ventilation during transport of the infant to a neonatal intensive care unit

4. During transport of a 28-week-old infant, the child's heart rate begins to decrease. When should the transport nurse initiate cardiac compressions?
   O   A. When the heart rate increases above 100 beats per minute when the child is stimulated
   O   B. When a change in ventilation is initiated and is effective in increasing the child's heart rate
   O   C. If the infant's heart rate falls below 60 to 80 beats per minute and does not increase despite effective ventilations
   O   D. After the flight nurse checks the infants DNR status to determine whether the infant should be resuscitated

5. The transport nurse is able to determine that the umbilical catheter is correctly placed by:
   - 0  A. Obtaining a good blood return after the catheter is inserted
   - 0  B. Inserting the catheter until it can no longer be threaded into the umbilical vein
   - 0  C. Observing there is no return of free blood once the catheter has been inserted
   - 0  D. Inserting the catheter into the thickest-walled vessel that can be visualized

*The transport team has been called to transport a 30-week-old infant who is having severe respiratory distress and has been diagnosed with respiratory distress syndrome. Upon arrival at the referring facility, the transport nurse finds a 3500 g child with rapid grunting respirations, flaring, and sternal retractions. The child has circumoral cyanosis and an oxygen saturation rate of 88% on 100% oxygen by mask.*

6. Preparation of this neonate for transport would include:
   - 0  A. Maintaining the child's airway with 100% oxygen by mask
   - 0  B. Endotracheal intubation to increase the neonate's oxygenation
   - 0  C. Initiating effective bag-valve-mask ventilation for transport
   - 0  D. Obtaining a chest radiograph to confirm the referring physician's diagnosis

7. To determine which size endotracheal tube this child would require, the flight nurse could use which of the following?
   - 0  A. 16 + the infant's age/4
   - 0  B. The infant's nares
   - 0  C. Width of the infant
   - 0  D. Weight of the infant

*A 32-week-old infant is being transported to the neonatal intensive care unit after delivery because the mother had prolonged rupture of her membranes. The neonate is febrile, has a heart rate of 200, and delayed capillary refill >4 seconds. She is maintaining her airway and has oxygen at 100% by mask. The baby weighs 4.5 g.*

8. The transport nurse would administer a fluid bolus of:
   - 0  A. 45 ml of O negative blood
   - 0  B. 45 ml of normal saline
   - 0  C. 90 ml of normal saline
   - 0  D. 45 ml of dextrose and water

9. In order to evaluate the effectiveness of this neonate's resuscitation, the transport nurse would monitor:
   - 0  A. The neonate's brachial and pedal pulses
   - 0  B. The neonate's radial and pedal pulses
   - 0  C. The neonate's rhythm on the cardiac monitor
   - 0  D. The number of diapers the neonate uses

10. The neonatalogist with the transport team speaks to the mother and tells her of the gravity of her child's condition. Which nursing diagnosis would be appropriate to plan the care of this infant's mother?
    - 0  A. Ineffective breastfeeding, related to the infant being transferred to the neonatal intensive care unit
    - 0  B. Ineffective family coping, related to the infant being transferred to the neonatal intensive care unit
    - 0  C. Fear, related to the infant being transferred to the neonatal unit and the seriousness of the baby's condition
    - 0  D. High risk for caregiver role strain, related to the neonate being transferred to the intensive care unit

11. The transport team has been called to transport a set of conjoined twins who are joined at the thorax. Both infants are full term and experiencing no distress. Preparation for the transport of these infants should include:
    - 0  A. Assuring that there is one functioning intravenous line because the infants would share the intravenous fluids
    - 0  B. Administering any sedative needed for transport to the stronger of the twins to evaluate the effectiveness of the medication
    - 0  C. Placing the conjoined infants as different levels in the isolette to ensure that they do not become hypovolemic
    - 0  D. Calculating their fluid needs based on their total body weight and administering the total fluids divided between both infants

12. The advantages of "hands-off" defibrillation during air medical transport include all of the following *except:*
    - 0  A. Arcing of the current during defibrillation
    - 0  B. Preapplication of defibrillation pads
    - 0  C. Safe distance from the patient during the procedure
    - 0  D. Decreased incidence of pads slipping during the procedure

13. Electromagnetic interference (EMI) during air transport may affect which of the following patients?
    - 0  A. A patient who is being paced with an external pacemaker
    - 0  B. A patient being monitored with a portable cardiac monitor
    - 0  C. A patient with a permanent internal pacemaker
    - 0  D. A patient with an arterial line on a portable monitor

*A 5-year-old child is involved in a motor vehicle accident. The child has suffered a severe head injury and is to be transported by helicopter to the children's hospital. The parents would like to accompany the child to the hospital on the helicopter.*

14. The transport team must consider which of the following when making the decision about whether the parents may accompany the child?
    - 0  A. Whether the parents can pay for the child's transport
    - 0  B. Whether the referring hospital will assume liability for the parents' transport
    - 0  C. Whether the pilot and the other crew members like the parents
    - 0  D. What affect the parents' presence may have on the child during the transport

15. The transport team is unable to let the child's parents accompany them during the transport. What interventions could the transport nurse implement to meet the needs of the parents?
    - 0  A. Do not allow the family to see the child before transport because it may upset them to see his injuries
    - 0  B. Explain to the family that a fixed-wing aircraft is more likely to crash than a helicopter

- 0  C. Allow the family to talk to and touch the child before leaving the referring facility for the receiving facility
- 0  D. Tell the family to call information for directions to the receiving hospital once the transport vehicle and team have left the hospital

16. A common complication of manual ventilation during air transport is:
    - 0  A. Hypercapnia from excessive ventilation
    - 0  B. No change in the patient's metabolic status
    - 0  C. Adequate and consistent tidal volumes ($V_t$)
    - 0  D. Reexpansion of a deflated lung after intubation

17. The effects of mivacurium may be increased with the use of:
    - 0  A. Nitroglycerin
    - 0  B. Ceftriaxone
    - 0  C. Gentamicin
    - 0  D. Heparin

*A 3-year-old girl with a history of status epilepticus is being transferred to another facility for care. The child has been intubated with a 4.5 ETT according to the Pediatric Advanced Life Support Guidelines and has a peripheral IV running normal saline.*

18. What additional interventions should the transport nurse consider in order to prepare this child for transport?
    - 0  A. Insert a gastric tube to decompress the child's stomach and prevent possibility of aspiration during transport
    - 0  B. Change the intravenous fluid to dextrose in water to prevent the development of hypoglycemia during transport
    - 0  C. Change the air in the endotracheal cuff to normal saline so that altitude changes will not affect it
    - 0  D. Insert an intraosseous needle so that the child has additional intravenous access during the transport

19. Delayed transport of a critically ill patient may occur because:
    - 0  A. The patient was not appropriately insured, so the transport team needed to wait for assurance of payment
    - 0  B. The acuity of the patient's illness was not initially recognized by the referring facility

C. The referring facility was tired of the patient and referred him to another facility for further care

D. The patient refused to be transferred despite his altered mental status and the referring facility had to wait until he was no longer responsive

20. An 18-year-old man diagnosed with meningococcal meningitis is to be transferred to another intensive care unit by helicopter. He is currently intubated and on a ventilator. His oxygen saturation is 88% on 100% oxygen. His vital signs are 86/50; HR 110R with assisted ventilations. He has already received a 500 ml fluid bolus. Which of the following nursing diagnoses would be most appropriate for the flight nurse to base care on?

A. Gas exchange, impaired, related to altered oxygen supply as evidenced by his low oxygen saturation

B. Infection, high risk for, related to his medical diagnosis of meningitis evidenced by his low oxygen saturation

C. Injury, high risk for, related to moving the patient out of the referring hospital evidenced by his low oxygen saturation

D. Fluid volume overload, related to the patient's medical diagnosis of meningitis evidenced by his low oxygen saturation

21. In order to improve this patient's oxygen saturation during transport, the flight nurse would:

A. Extubate the patient and bag-valve-mask him until he could be reintubated at the receiving facility

B. Start a dopamine drip at 2-5 μg/kg to increase the patient's blood pressure and improve his perfusion

C. Place the patient on a cardiosynchronous pulse oximeter to monitor his oxygen saturation during transport

D. Manually hyperventilate the patient to increase his $pO_2$ and thus increase his oxygen saturation

22. Information that should be communicated to a receiving facility so that a transport decision can be made includes all of the following *except:*

A. Patient's age, weight, and sex

B. The type of insurance the patient has

C. Pertinent patient medical history

D. Diagnosis and current vital signs

23. A source of stress in the transport nursing environment is:

A. Appropriate and functioning equipment in the transport vehicle

B. Good working relationships with one's co-workers and hospital personnel

C. Ample space in the aircraft for patient care and resuscitation during transport

D. Expected death of a pediatric patient during transport

24. An acute reaction to stress is:

A. Chronic illness

B. Anomia

C. Powerlessness

D. Anger

25. An example of stress management after a critical incident would be:

A. Drinking a bottle of beer

B. Taking a brisk walk

C. Smoking a pack of cigarettes

D. Going to a bar for a beer

26. Potential side effects of succinylcholine include all of the following *except:*

A. Increased intragastric pressure

B. Increase in serum potassium

C. Decreased intraocular pressure

D. Triggering malignant hyperthermia

27. Which of the following is an intubating dose of a nondepolarizing neuromuscular blocking agent?

A. Mivacurium 0.15 mg/kg rapid IVP

B. Mivacurium 0.25 mg/kg slow IVP

C. Vecuronium 0.05 mg/kg IVP—adult

D. Vecuronium 0.25 mg/kg IVP—child

28. High-dose methylprednisolone, if administered within 8 hours of injury, has been shown to improve the outcome of spinal cord injury. Some actions of the drug that are thought to facilitate this process include all of the following *except:*

A. Decreased nerve excitability

B. Restoration of extracellular $CA^{++}$

○    C. Inhibition of tissue lipid peroxidation

○    D. Repression of the release of free fatty acids

29. A relative contraindication to the administration of methylprednisolone after spinal cord injury includes:

○    A. Blunt injury to the spinal cord

○    B. Spinal cord lesion at the Cl level

○    C. A positive PPD within the last 7 days

○    D. History of gastrointestinal bleeding

30. Cyanide toxicity is a potentially lethal side effect of nitroprusside infusion. An acute symptom that should alert the transport nurse to the possibility of cyanide poisoning would be:

○    A. A GCS of 15

○    B. Hypertension

○    C. Seizures

○    D. ECG changes

31. Current dosage recommendations for the peripheral vasodilator and potent antihypertensive, sodium nitroprusside (Nipride), ranges from 0.5 to 8 µg/kg/min for parenteral administration. If your patient weighed 74 kg, the rate of nipride infusion in ml/h at a dilution of 50 mg in 250 ml D5W would range from:

○    A. 11 to 178

○    B. 5 to 89

○    C. 9 to 142

○    D. 5 to 71

32. A 78-year-old patient has suffered an acute inferior myocardial infarction that has failed fibrinolytic therapy. He is to be transferred to another facility for rescue angioplasty. However, he has never flown before and is quite anxious. The referring physician is considering midazolam 2 mg intravenously. A potential adverse effect of this drug the flight nurse must consider before administration is:

○    A. It will increase the patient's respiratory rate requiring that a non-rebreather mask be placed on the patient during transport

○    B. It will increase his systemic vascular resistance, placing him at risk of increasing his cardiac output and causing bradycardia

○    C. Midazolam has analgesic effects that will enhance the effects of nitroglycerin and decrease the patient's need for additional morphine for his chest pain

○    D. Midazolam decreases peripheral vascular resistance, lowering the patient's blood pressure and resulting in hypotension

33. The following statements are true regarding the administration of benzodiazepines *except:*

○    A. A potential side effect of IV midazolam (Versed) is bronchospasm and laryngospasm

○    B. All benzodiazepines must be administered with caution in elderly, debilitated patients

○    C. Sedative and hypnotic effects are diminished when benzodiazepines are administered along with narcotics

○    D. Midazolam is a water-soluble benzodiazepine that is two to three times more potent than diazepam

34. Flumazenil is to be used with great caution in which type of scenario?

○    A. Benzodiazepine overdose with respiratory depression

○    B. Diazepam overdose with alcohol intoxication

○    C. Midazolam overdose with tricyclic antidepressant ingestion

○    D. Lorazepam overdose with drug-induced coma

35. Patient anxiety related to air medical transport may be managed by:

○    A. Administering phenothiazines to decrease the symptoms related to the patient's anxiety about flying

○    B. Asking the patient about previous flight experience and past reactions to news stories about plane crashes

○    C. Telling the patient that she is an adult and must learn to cope with these types of stresses because there is no other way to get there

○    D. Explaining to the patient that he must fly in the smaller aircraft, which is the most difficult one to manage a patient in

*The transport team is called to transport a 2-year-old near-drowning victim. The child is currently undergoing full CPR. The referring rescue squad has administered the first dose of epinephrine through an intraosseous needle.*

36. The second and subsequent epinephrine dosages recommended for asystolic or pulseless arrest in children, per American Heart Association recommendations, involve:
    - O   A. 0.1 mg/kg of 1:10,000 solution IV or IO
    - O   B. 0.01 mg/kg of 1:1,000 solution IV or IO
    - O   C. 0.1 mg/kg of 1:1,000 solution IV, IO, or ETT
    - O   D. 0.01 mg/kg of 1:10,000 solution ETT

37. High-dose epinephrine provides both alpha- and beta-adrenergic agonist effects. Which action is thought to be of primary benefit with attempts at cardiopulmonary resuscitation?
    - O   A. Alpha-agonist effect
    - O   B. Beta-agonist effect
    - O   C. Both alpha- and beta-agonist effects
    - O   D. Neither alpha- nor beta-agonist effects

Questions 38 through 40 are to be answered using information from the following patient scenario:

*During the resuscitation of an elderly female (100 kg) who suffered a cardiac arrest during transport, the following sequence of events ensued: She arrived at the landing zone per basic life squad, with bag-valve-mask ventilations, cardiac compressions, and no IV in place. Her initial rhythm upon placement of the cardiac monitor was ventricular fibrillation. She was immediately defibrillated with 200, 300, then 360 joules, with no apparent change in her cardiac rhythm.*

38. She was immediately intubated by the transport nurse. How much epinephrine should be administered through the endotracheal tube?
    - O   A. Epinephrine 1 mg (1:1,000) ETT
    - O   B. Epinephrine 2 mg (1:1,000) ETT
    - O   C. Epinephrine 2 mg (1:10,000) ETT
    - O   D. Epinephrine 0.1 mg/kg (1:1,000) ETT

*CPR was continued and IV access was obtained. Defibrillation was promptly repeated with 360 joules, again with no change in her cardiac rhythm.*

39. The transport nurse administered 100 mg of lidocaine without any affect. What other drug may be considered for treatment of this patient's ventricular arrhythmia?

- O   A. Adenosine 12 mg IVP
- O   B. Atropine 3 mg IVP
- O   C. Bretylium 50 mg/kg IVP
- O   D. Procainamide 30 mg/min IVP

40. The patient develops a pulse at a rate of 56 beats per minute and blood pressure of 88/50. What interventions should the transport nurse consider next?
    - O   A. Administration of atropine 3 mg IVP
    - O   B. 200 ml fluid bolus of normal saline
    - O   C. Epinephrine infusion at 2-10 μg/h
    - O   D. Dopamine infusion at 2-10 μg/h

41. Indications for the administration of sodium bicarbonate during resuscitation include:
    - O   A. Uncorrected hypoxic metabolic acidosis
    - O   B. Known overdose of tricyclic antidepressants
    - O   C. Post arrest on return of spontaneous circulation
    - O   D. To make the urine acidic in drug overdoses

42. Administration of $D_{50}$ is indicated when:
    - O   A. Prehospital adult resuscitation exceeds 30 minutes
    - O   B. A whole blood glucose demonstrates hypoglycemia
    - O   C. The patient with an altered mental state may have had a stroke
    - O   D. A whole blood glucose assay demonstrates hyperglycemia

43. Adenosine:
    - O   A. Should be the first drug administered in wide complex tachycardia
    - O   B. May be used safely in patients with poor left ventricular function
    - O   C. Should be administered quickly and followed by a saline flush
    - O   D. Is effective in terminating arrhythmias such as atrial fibrillation or flutter

44. A potential adverse effect of adenosine administration is:
    - O   A. Persistent first-, second-, or third-degree AV block
    - O   B. Arrhythmias such as ventricular tachycardia
    - O   C. Facial flushing, shortness of breath, and dyspnea
    - O   D. Hypoventilation and systolic hypertension

**45.** Amiodarone facilitates the termination of sustained ventricular tachycardia by:

0   A. Causing coronary artery vasoconstriction and decreasing coronary blood flow

0   B. Causing peripheral vasoconstriction and increasing systemic vascular resistance

0   C. Shortening infranodal conduction and lengthening the sinus cycle

0   D. Prolonging the action potential and retarding the refractory period

**46.** Serious adverse affects following mannitol administration may include which of the following:

1. Paradoxical increased ICP
2. Seizures
3. Pulmonary edema and heart failure
4. Acute renal failure

0   A. 1 and 2

0   B. 2 and 3

0   C. 1, 2, and 3

0   D. All of the above

**47.** The transport nurse is caring for a 55-year-old man, weighing approximately 80 kg, who was involved in a serious motor vehicle accident and suffers severe head injuries. His neurological examination reveals decerebrate posturing of his extremities and a unilaterally dilated pupil. After initial resuscitation is completed involving immobilization, intubation, and oxygenation, as well as intravenous access, medical direction orders mannitol to be administered.

0   A. Mannitol administration involves a dosage of .25g to 2g/kg of a 20% solution

0   B. Mannitol administration involves a 50% solution at a dose of 20 to 160 g

0   C. Mannitol should be administered with an electrolyte solution

0   D. Mannitol may be administered with fresh frozen plasma

**48.** Magnesium sulfate may be used to treat which of the following:

0   A. Third-degree heart block with hypotension

0   B. Torsades de pointes or refractory VT

0   C. Seizures due to severe head injury

0   D. Second-degree heart block in an acute MI

**49.** Nursing assessment parameters during the infusion of magnesium for preeclampsia/eclampsia should include which of the following:

1. Fetal heart rate and reactivity
2. Intake and output
3. Deep tendon reflexes
4. Respiratory rate and function

0   A. 1, 2, and 4

0   B. 1, 3, and 4

0   C. All of the above

0   D. None of the above

**50.** The transport team is called to transport a 65-year-old female who has been involved in a motor vehicle accident. She has suffered a pulmonary contusion and a moderate head injury. Upon arrival at the referring facility, the transport team finds a patient in severe respiratory distress being treated with a nonrebreather mask. Her oxygen saturation is 80%. The transport team prepares to intubate the patient when her family doctor states that she has cancer and has given him verbal DNR orders. He states that the patient must be transported without intubation. The transport team may:

0   A. Refuse to transport this patient because she has cancer and does want to be resuscitated

0   B. Transport the patient because she has a medical problem other than cancer that may be treated and reversed

0   C. Refuse to transport because the physician has given them a verbal order that the patient is a DNR patient

0   D. Attempt to contact the patient's family and wait to see if they will reverse the doctor's verbal order

**51.** Visualization of only the corniculate cartilages is what grade on the Cormak and Lehane Airway Classification System?

0   A. Grade II

0   B. Grade I

0   C. Grade III

0   D. Grade IV

**52.** Potential adverse reactions associated with the IV administration of fentanyl (sublimaze) include:
   1. Diaphoresis
   2. Hypotension
   3. Muscle rigidity
   4. Tachycardia
   0   A. 1, 2, and 3
   0   B. 1, 2, and 4
   0   C. 2, 3, and 4
   0   D. All of the above

**53.** During the active resuscitation phase of a patient exhibiting signs and symptoms of neurogenic shock, hemodynamic effects of phenylephrine (Neo-Synephrine) that may prove beneficial include:
   0   A. Alpha, beta$_1$-, and beta$_2$-agonist effects
   0   B. Alpha-agonist effects, with an increase in HR
   0   C. Alpha-agonist effects, with an increase in systemic resistance
   0   D. Alpha and beta$_1$-agonist effects, with an increase in cardiac output

**54.** Side effects of terbutaline sulfate (Brethine) when used as a tocolytic agent are:
   0   A. Hyperkalemia
   0   B. Bradycardia
   0   C. Hypoglycemia
   0   D. Palpitations

**55.** Information needed to calculate IV medication infusion rates include:
   0   A. Dose to be infused/concentration of medication in solution/patient's weight
   0   B. Amount of fluid to be infused and patient's weight
   0   C. Concentration in medicine solution and amount of IV fluid
   0   D. Dose to be infused and patient's weight

**56.** If you were asked to start a dopamine infusion at 8 $\mu$g/kg/min (concentration of 1,600 $\mu$g/ml) on a patient weighing 72 kg, the flow rate in drops per minute that you would infuse equals:
   0   A. 27 gtt/min
   0   B. 25.2 gtt/min
   0   C. 21.6 gtt/min
   0   D. 20 gtt/min

**57.** A 28-year-old male has been involved in a motor vehicle crash. He has sustained a severe head injury requiring intubation and oxygenation.

Which of the following agents may be used to sedate this patient for safe transport?
   0   A. Vecuronium 10 mg every 20 minutes
   0   B. Propofol infusion 3 to 5 mg/kg
   0   C. Ketamine 1 to 2 mg/kg as an infusion
   0   D. Etomidate 0.3 mg/kg every 15 to 20 minutes

**58.** When preparing an obstetrical patient for transport, the transport team should:
   0   A. Place the patient in a right lateral recumbent position
   0   B. Always perform a vaginal examination before transport
   0   C. Place the patient in a left lateral recumbent position
   0   D. Place a stretcher restraint directly over the patient's abdomen

**59.** Which of the following statements is true regarding the administration of heparin?
   1. Low-dose heparin is effective in prophylaxis against thrombosis
   2. High-dose heparin (0.3 U/Ml and above) is required once clotting is established
   3. Vitamin K is the antidote for heparin overdose
   4. Heparin slows the incorporation of new fibrin, preventing clot extension
   0   A. 1 and 2 only
   0   B. 1, 2, and 4
   0   C. 2, 3, and 4
   0   D. All of the above

**60.** The flight nurse receives a report about a cardiac patient who is presently on a nitroglycerin (NTG) infusion. The nurse reports that this patient is on a drip at 32 ml/h and she is uncertain what this converts to in $\mu$g/min. The concentration of NTG is 150 mg in 500 ml D5W. What is the actual dose of NTG in $\mu$g/min that the patient is receiving?
   0   A. 40 $\mu$g/min
   0   B. 107 $\mu$g/min
   0   C. 150 $\mu$g/min
   0   D. 160 $\mu$g/min

**61.** Which action is not characteristic of the intravenous infusion of nitroglycerin?
   0   A. Decreases afterload
   0   B. Relaxes smooth muscles
   0   C. Increases cardiac output
   0   D. Decreases preload

62. Which of the following actions are characteristic to *both* the administration of dopamine and dobutamine?
    1. Vasoconstriction
    2. Positive inotrope
    3. Alpha stimulation
    4. Increased peripheral perfusion
    5. Increased cardiac output
    6. Tachycardia
    7. Beta$_1$ stimulation
    8. Increased myocardial contractility
    0  A. 1, 2, 4, and 5
    0  B. 3, 4, 5, and 6
    0  C. 2, 3, and 5
    0  D. 2, 5, and 7

63. Which of the following shock states would be a potential indication for the administration of norepinephrine (Levophed)?
    1. Cardiogenic shock
    2. Hypovolemic shock
    3. Septic shock
    4. Anaphylactic shock
    0  A. 1 and 2 only
    0  B. 3 and 4 only
    0  C. 1, 2, and 4
    0  D. All of the above

64. Advantages of using the laryngeal mask airway (LMA) include:
    0  A. Advanced airway skills are required to use this type of airway
    0  B. Blind insertion can only be accomplished from the front of the patient
    0  C. Endotracheal intubation can be accomplished through the LMA
    0  D. All laryngeal tracheal masks are made from latex

65. The flight team is transporting a man who has suffered 90% total body surface area (TBSA) full-thickness burns of his trunk, arms, legs, and groin, exhibiting significant hypotension. Which alternative site to place an oximetry probe is least affected by poor perfusion?
    0  A. Index finger
    0  B. Chest wall
    0  C. Earlobe
    0  D. Great toe

66. Which of the following will *not* cause changes in the pulse oximetry readings?
    0  A. CO poison
    0  B. Anemia

0  C. Hypovolemia
0  D. Patient motion

67. All of the following statements are true regarding the accuracy of the pulse oximetry measurements *except:*
    0  A. You can avoid performing ABG sticks in acute patient conditions with the use of pulse oximetry
    0  B. You may verify the reading by observing the pulse waveform display
    0  C. Comparing the heart rate displayed on the oximeter and the patient's pulse is a reliable check for accuracy
    0  D. Pulse oximeters are unreliable during cardiac arrest states because there is no pulse

68. In which of the following clinical situations would ETCO$_2$ readings be beneficial in determining ETT placement?
    1. A near-drowning victim with a palpable pulse and blood pressure
    2. A patient who has been under CPR for approximately 15 minutes
    3. A trauma victim with extensive facial injuries and extensive blood in the airway
    4. A patient who has suffered a massive pulmonary embolus
    0  A. 1 and 3
    0  B. 1 and 4
    0  C. 3 and 4
    0  D. All of the above

69. Which of the following is *not* a common cause of low end-tidal CO$_2$ readings?
    0  A. Esophageal intubation
    0  B. Pulseless electrical activity
    0  C. Inadequate chest compressions
    0  D. Tension pneumothorax

70. Which of the following circumstances may cause an inaccurate ETCO$_2$ reading when determining tube placement?
    1. Administration of drugs via endotracheal route
    2. ETCO$_2$ concentrations during profound shock or CPR
    3. Esophageal intubation of a patient who has been drinking beer
    4. Use on a victim who has aspirated a large amount of blood
    0  A. 1, 2, and 4
    0  B. 1, 3, and 4

0 C. 1, 2, and 3
0 D. All of the above

71. A disadvantage of ventilator use during transport is:
0 A. Frees an additional pair of hands during transport
0 B. Aids in preventing barotrauma during transport
0 C. Delivers consistent tidal volumes during transport
0 D. Loss of the ability to feel lung compliance

72. You are asked to place a patient suffering from a severe closed head injury on a ventilator, postintubation. Which of the following settings would be appropriate for this patient weighing 185 lbs?
0 A. 100% $FiO_2$, 700 cc TV, rate 12
0 B. 100% $FiO_2$, 700 cc TV, rate 18
0 C. 100% $FiO_2$, 1.0 L TV, rate 16
0 D. 100% $FiO_2$, 1.5 L TV, rate 14

73. Which of the following is a relative contraindication to the use of transcutaneous pacing during transport?
0 A. Unstable drug-induced bradycardia
0 B. Hypotension due to hypovolemia
0 C. Prolonged cardiac arrest prior to pacing
0 D. Symptomatic bradycardia due to hypothermia

74. Which of the following are acceptable methods of determining "capture" of the transcutaneous pacer?
1. Observe a pacer spike followed by a wide QRS complex
2. Hear blood flow with a doppler
3. Improved level of consciousness
4. Involuntary arm muscle contraction
0 A. 1 and 2
0 B. 1, 2, and 3
0 C. 2 and 3
0 D. All of the above

75. Which of the following pad placement positions are recommended for transcutaneous pacing?
0 A. Apply the anterior electrode to the right lateral aspect of the patient's chest and the posterior electrode over the right scapula

0 B. Apply the anterior electrode over the right side of the sternum at the fourth intercostal space
0 C. Apply the posterior pad to the left lateral aspect of the spine at approximately heart level
0 D. Apply the posterior pad on the left chest in the subclavicular area when using the anterior-anterior position

76. A potential complication associated with the use of a transcutaneous pacemaker during transport that may have lethal complications is:
0 A. Minor local skin burns from poor, dried electrodes, outdated pads
0 B. Battery failure in the pacing unit without an alternate power source
0 C. Continuous capture through multi-use pads
0 D. Development of transient hypertension from pacing

77. The transport nurse is caring for a patient in complete heart block. The patient has received a total of 3 mg of atropine IVP with no change in heart rate or rhythm. You notice that the patient suddenly has a decrease in mental status and becomes hemodynamically unstable with a B/P of 60/systolic, HR 30. Which of the following settings would be appropriate to utilize when *initiating* transcutaneous pacing?
0 A. Demand mode, highest output titrating down, rate 60
0 B. Demand mode, lowest output titrating up, rate 70
0 C. Asynchronous mode, highest output titrating down, rate 70
0 D. Asynchronous mode, lowest output titrating up, rate 120

78. Arterial systole begins with the opening of:
0 A. Mitral valve
0 B. Tricuspid valve
0 C. Aortic valve
0 D. Bicuspid valve

79. Onset of systole correlates with what segment of the ECG complex?
0 A. T-wave
0 B. Slightly after QRS complex
0 C. QRS complex
0 D. PR interval

80. Following a sharp rise on the arterial pressure waveform, a small dip occurs on the down slope (see figure below). This dip, which marks the onset of diastole and closure of the aortic valves, is called:

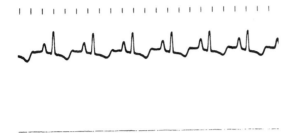

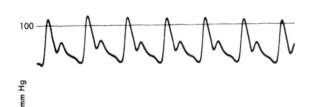

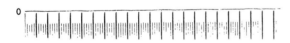

    0   A. Peak systolic pressure
    0   B. Dicrotic notch
    0   C. Diastole
    0   D. Secondary waves

81. Arterial waveforms in the elderly have all the following characteristics *except:*
    0   A. Dampened dicrotic notch
    0   B. Absent secondary diastolic waves
    0   C. Increased pulse pressure
    0   D. Sharpened dicrotic notch

82. Before any hemodynamic pressure measurements can be obtained, the transport nurse must position the patient in which manner?
    0   A. Flat supine position without a pillow
    0   B. Head of the bed elevated at 90°

    0   C. Head of the bed elevated to 60°
    0   D. In a position where the reference point is midchest

83. Upon arrival at the referring facility the transport nurse's assessment findings reveal a dampened arterial waveform and mottling of the extremity that is distal to the radial arterial line site. Immediate interventions include all the following *except:*
    0   A. Assess collateral artery for blood flow
    0   B. Flush catheter with saline fluid syringe
    0   C. Assess IV pressure bag for heparin
    0   D. Immediately remove arterial catheter

84. During flight (altitude 8000 ft) the patient's arterial waveform begins to *dampen.* There are no clinical symptoms, and the patient's vital signs are stable. Which of the following would not contribute to a dampened waveform?
    0   A. A cannula lodged against the arterial vessel wall
    0   B. Air trapped between the transducer and dome diaphragms
    0   C. Stopcocks inadvertently turned in the wrong direction
    0   D. Kinking of the arterial catheter

85. A transport nurse's assessment of the accuracy of an arterial waveform is performed by initially obtaining a cuff blood pressure. A slight difference between the cuff and arterial blood pressure is normally:
    0   A. 5 to 10 mm Hg
    0   B. 11 to 15 mm Hg
    0   C. 16 to 20 mm Hg
    0   D. >20 mm Hg

86. During transport, the nurse notes an increasing heart rate despite the mean arterial pressure (MAP) remaining constant. Which of the following may contribute to these changes?
    0   A. Improper calibration of the equipment
    0   B. Kinked arterial monitoring lines
    0   C. Insufficient pressure in the pressure bag
    0   D. Patient's status deterioration

**87.** Ensuring consistency of hemodynamic readings during transport is achieved by taping the transducer to the phlebostatic axis reference point. Which of the following locations serves as this reference point?

0   A. Second intercostal space/midaxillary line

0   B. Second intercostal space/anterior axillary line

0   C. Fourth intercostal space/midaxillary line

0   D. Fourth intercostal space/anterior axillary line

**88.** Once the transducer is level to the phlebostatic axis, the transducer must be "zeroed." Prior to pushing and releasing the auto zero function button, the stopcock on the transducer must first be open to which port:

0   A. Patient

0   B. Flush

0   C. Air

0   D. Monitor

**89.** During flight (altitude 3500 ft), the patient becomes slightly restless. The transport nurse observes abnormally high digital pressures; however, the waveform remains normal. Troubleshooting focuses on:

0   A. Ensuring transducer at phlebostatic axis

0   B. Checking stopcock's positions

0   C. Aspirating the line for patency

0   D. Flushing the system

**90.** Preventing inadvertent tubing separation and accidental blood loss from an arterial line during transport is best achieved with all the following interventions *except:*

0   A. Set alarm systems

0   B. Use Luer-Lok connections

0   C. Keep connections visible

0   D. Monitor the MAP

Questions 91 through 93 are to be answered using the following patient scenario:

*Upon arrival at the referring facility, the transport nurse assesses a cardiac patient with a pulmonary artery catheter. The patient is secured to the transport stretcher and the pulmonary artery pressure monitoring system has been zeroed, leveled, and calibrated. The system has no air bubbles, and the transducer is set up correctly.*

**91.** When the patient has been placed on the transport stretcher and the monitoring equipment secured and calibrated, the transport nurse observes the following. This waveform is indicative of:

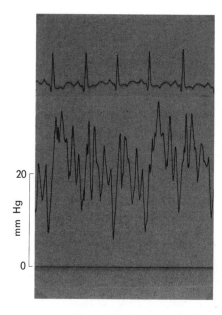

0   A. A normal pulmonary artery (PA) waveform without interference

0   B. A pattern of elevated (PA) pressure

0   C. A waveform demonstrating excessive catheter movement

0   D. Normal (PA) wedge pressure waveform

**92.** The patient simultaneously develops ventricular ectopy during this period. The first intervention the flight nurse should do is:

0   A. Administer an antiarrhythmic medication

0   B. Inflate the PA balloon

0   C. Flush the hemodynamic line setup system

0   D. Deflate the PA balloon

**93.** The transport nurse inflates the PA balloon with 2.0 ml of air, and the following pattern occurs:

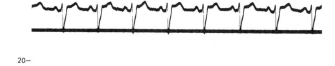

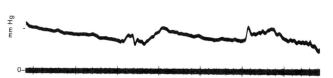

The following immediate action should be taken:

0   A. Deflate balloon

0   B. Withdraw PA catheter 5 cm

0   C. Activate quick-flush device

0   D. Check stopcocks

94. The transport team is requested to transport a 66-year-old diagnosed with an acute anterior wall myocardial infarction. During flight, the patient's clinical status deteriorates. The systolic pressure falls to 70 mm Hg. The PA wedge pressure reading has increased to 20 mm Hg. Which of the following interventions would best assist the patient's hemodynamic status?

0   A. Administer 500 ml normal saline bolus

0   B. Administer dopamine infusion

0   C. Administer 500 ml lactated Ringer's bolus

0   D. Administer nitroglycerine infusion

Questions 95 through 97 are to be answered utilizing the following patient scenario:

*The patient at the referring facility was diagnosed with an acute inferior wall myocardial infarction. Nitroglycerine and dopamine infusions were initiated for hemodynamic support. The referring nurse stated that the arterial line correlates with BP cuff, and the PA wedge pressures correlates with the PA end-diastolic pressure. Initial assessment revealed ECG-sinus rhythm with ST elevation in leads II, III, and AVF. Patient denies chest pain or discomfort. The patient is secured to transport stretcher, and the arterial and PA catheters are properly zeroed.*

95. During flight, the patient develops chest pain, diaphoresis, and hypotension. The transport nurse is unable to obtain a PA wedge waveform. An alternate method to assess the patient's fluid volume status is best accomplished by:

0   A. Arterial diastolic blood pressure

0   B. PA systolic pressure

0   C. PA end-diastolic pressure

0   D. Arterial systolic pressure

96. The patient continues to experience chest pain, diaphoresis, and hypotension. The PA end-diastolic pressure is 4 mm Hg. Which of the following interventions may best assist the patient's hemodynamic condition?

0   A. Increase dopamine infusion

0   B. Increase nitroglycerine infusion

0   C. Administer morphine IVP

0   D. Administer normal saline bolus

97. Upon arrival at the receiving hospital, the patient states his neck feels "wet." In assessing the area, the transport nurse finds fluid leaking from the catheter. Three small black bands are noted at the point the PA catheter inserts into the subclavian introducer. Immediate intervention includes:

0   A. Flushing the catheter to determine patency

0   B. Inflating PA balloon to see if the monitor works

0   C. Advancing PA catheter until the lines disappear

0   D. Administering the IV medications at another site

98. Upon arrival at the referring facility, the transport nurse is unable to obtain a normal PA waveform pattern. The waveform appears dampened. In assessing the flush system, the flush bag device has insufficient pressure. A clot in the catheter is suspected. Corrective measures include:

0   A. Gentle aspiration followed by gentle flushing

0   B. Instill 1000 units heparin in catheter

0   C. Discontinue and change flush set-up device

0   D. Reposition catheter to assess waveform changes

99. The transport team is requested to transport a patient diagnosed with an anterior wall myocardial infarction. The vital signs have been stable. Cuff blood pressures correlate well with the arterial line. Pulmonary artery (PA) pressure is 25/10 mm Hg, and PA wedge pressure is 11 mm Hg. Due to equipment failure, only one invasive pressure channel is available. Which of the following parameters should be monitored during transport?

0   A. Central venous pressures

0   B. Arterial line pressures

0   C. Pulmonary artery wedge pressures

0   D. Pulmonary artery pressures

100. Inflating a pulmonary artery balloon requires how much air?

0   A. Less than 0.5 cc

0   B. 0.5 to 1.0 cc

0   C. 1.25 to 1.5 cc

0   D. 1.6 to 2.0 cc

101. Intraaortic balloon pump (IABP) therapy is indicated to:
    0  A. Decrease cardiac afterload
    0  B. Decrease systemic perfusion
    0  C. Increase myocardial oxygen demands
    0  D. Decrease coronary artery perfusion

102. The most commonly used reference point, or "trigger," for inflation and deflation of the intraaortic balloon pump (IABP) is the patient's:
    0  A. T wave of ECG
    0  B. R wave of ECG
    0  C. Slightly prior QRS complex
    0  D. Slightly after QRS complex

103. Adjusting the inflation time of the IABP corresponds to which segment of the arterial waveform?
    0  A. Peak systole pressure
    0  B. End diastole pressure
    0  C. Systole upstroke
    0  D. Dicrotic notch

104. Optimal deflation of the intraaortic balloon pump (IABP) occurs:
    0  A. At peak systole pressure
    0  B. At mid-diastole pressure
    0  C. Prior to systolic upstroke
    0  D. At dicrotic notch

105. During transport, the patient with an IABP requests to "sit up a bit" so she can "see the scenery." The patient's vital signs have been stable. Which of the following responses should the flight nurse give the patient?
    0  A. You'll have to lie flat to prevent kinking of the catheter
    0  B. You'll have to lie flat to prevent the catheter from migrating
    0  C. You can only have your head raised with pillows
    0  D. You can have your head raised less than 15°

106. The transport team has been requested to transport a patient with an IABP. The transport nurse can prevent a serious complication of IABP by assessing which of the following?
    0  A. Monitoring the insertion site for infection
    0  B. Preventing complications from immobility

    0  C. Monitoring for signs of improved cardiac function
    0  D. Monitoring the patient's left radial pulse

107. During transport, your assessment of the IABP reveals a loss of vacuum. Indicate the amount of air needed to manually inflate and deflate the balloon every 5 minutes in order to prevent clot formation.
    0  A. 10 cc of air in a 20 cc syringe
    0  B. Half the total amount of the balloon volume
    0  C. Total amount of the balloon volume
    0  D. Inflation/deflation not necessary due to administration of anticoagulant therapy

*A 19-year-old man is the victim of a drive-by shooting. The patient is lying supine on a lawn and is moaning. The patient's skin is pale, cool, and diaphoretic. He has a weak radial B/P of 110 and a respiratory rate of 36. Gunshot wounds are noted to the right upper chest, approximately 2 cm below the clavicle and to the right upper quadrant.*

108. What is the first priority of the transport nurse when entering the scene?
    0  A. Check the patient's airway for patency
    0  B. Obtain report from the first responders
    0  C. Evaluate the scene for potential hazards
    0  D. Complete a primary assessment in 60 seconds

109. During the primary survey, you note that the patient's respiratory rate is 36 per minute. At what rate should the transport nurse be concerned about respiratory compromise?
    0  A. 28 to 30
    0  B. 24 to 26
    0  C. 18 to 20
    0  D. 22 to 26

110. During the primary survey, the transport nurse discovers that the gunshot wound has caused an open pneumothorax (sucking chest wound). At this point the transport nurse would administer oxygen and:
    0  A. Decompress the left chest with a 14-gauge needle
    0  B. Decompress the right chest with a 10-gauge needle
    0  C. Apply a sterile occlusive dressing to the wound
    0  D. Apply a pulse oximetry probe to monitor the $SaO_2$

111. During the primary survey, which three observations will assist in determining the patient's hemodynamic stability?
    1. Skin color
    2. Blood pressure
    3. Pulse
    4. Level of consciousness
    0   A. 1, 2, and 3
    0   B. 1, 3, and 4
    0   C. 2, 3, and 4
    0   D. 1, 2, and 4

112. The patient is combative and uncooperative, requiring restraint for safe transport. The most common type of chemical restraint used by most air medical transport programs is:
    0   A. Leather restraints or police handcuffs attached to the transport stretcher
    0   B. Neuromuscular blockade with concomitant benzodiazepine administration
    0   C. Haloperidol or droperidol intravenously or intramuscularly
    0   D. Morphine or fentanyl intravenously every 60 minutes

*A 24-year-old woman was a passenger on a motorcycle that broadsided an automobile at a high rate of speed. The patient was found approximately 40 ft from the accident site. She was not wearing a helmet. Upon initial assessment, she is unresponsive to verbal stimuli, does not open her eyes, withdraws to pain, and is moaning.*

113. From the description of this patient, what would her GCS be?
    0   A. 7
    0   B. 8
    0   C. 6
    0   D. 9

114. Oxygenation and ventilation should be accomplished by what method?
    0   A. $O_2$ at 15 L/minute per nonrebreather mask
    0   B. $O_2$ at 5 L/minute per nasal cannula
    0   C. Endotracheal intubation with 100% $O_2$
    0   D. Bag-valve-mask ventilation with room air

115. When securing the airway of a multiply injured patient, which additional intervention should be performed?
    0   A. The head should be placed in the "sniffing" position for better tube placement
    0   B. An additional caregiver is needed to perform spinal immobilization

    0   C. Blow-by oxygen should be administered during the entire procedure
    0   D. An intravenous line should always be inserted before intubation is attempted

116. During transport, the patient's GCS remained 7. Her pulse rate is 64 and her respirations are being assisted at a rate of 24. Her B/P decreases to 88/40. The transport nurse should:
    0   A. Increase her ventilation rate to 30 to decrease her intracranial pressure
    0   B. Initiate a vasoactive medication until her systolic is 100 ml/Hg
    0   C. Place the patient in Trendelenburg position to increase her blood pressure
    0   D. Administer isotonic IV fluids until an adequate blood pressure is obtained

*A 15-year-old male patient dove from a rock approximately 15 feet into a shallow river, hitting his head on the river bottom. Since the dive, he has been unable to move his extremities and has no sensation from the nipple line down.*

117. During the primary survey, it is important to expose the patient to:
    0   A. Avoid missing any obvious injuries such as a protruding object or other injuries that may have been missed
    0   B. Obtain intravenous access to administer pain medication during the transport process
    0   C. Mark on the patient the level of sensation that he is able to perceive
    0   D. Induce mild hypothermia, which may protect the spinal cord from swelling and additional injury

118. When securing this injured patient to a backboard, the patient's head should be secured:
    0   A. First before his trunk and extremities
    0   B. Last after his trunk and extremities
    0   C. At the same time as the trunk and extremities
    0   D. Not at all because he is already paralyzed

119. The patient asks if he will ever move again. The transport nurse should:
    0   A. Tell the patient that everything is going to be fine because he is being transported to a level I trauma center
    0   B. Tell the patient that you will take very good care of him but that he has a serious injury and may never move again

C. Tell him not to worry about it because there are other things he should be concerned about at this time

D. Change the subject by pointing out what equipment is used inside of the aircraft and how rapidly you will get him to the hospital

*You arrive at the scene of a motor vehicle accident to find a 68-year-old woman who was the unrestrained front-seat passenger in a truck/auto accident as seen in the figure below.*

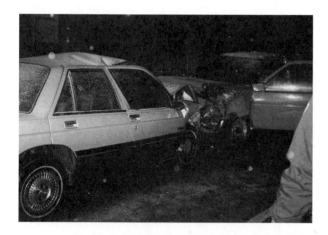

**120.** From the transport nurse's observation of the crash scene, which injuries would the transport nurse anticipate based on the mechanism of injury?

A. Fractured ribs

B. Spinal injury

C. Pelvic fracture

D. All of the above

**121.** The patient is extricated from the car. Her airway is patent, high-flow oxygen is applied. She has equal breath sounds, but no peripheral pulses are palpated. The patient has received 2 L of normal saline, and the transport team decides to infuse the patient with O-negative packed red blood cells. Advantages of transport programs administering blood during transport include:

A. Delaying the launch of the transport because the blood bank is located some distance from the transport vehicle

B. Clinical evaluation of the amount of significant blood loss is difficult in the transport environment, so deciding when to administer the blood may be difficult

C. Blood resuscitation is indicated after a 2 L bolus of crystalloid in patients with ongoing blood loss to increase oxygen carrying capacity

D. Not all transport teams employ personnel who are familiar with blood transfusion procedures, and patients may be placed at grave risk

**122.** During transport, the patient is complaining of severe dyspnea. She has no palpable radial pulse, the monitor shows a heart rate of 140, and upon auscultation, breath sounds are found to be absent on the right side. Her neck veins are slightly distended. The transport nurse should suspect (a):

A. Cardiac tamponade

B. Simple pneumothorax

C. Tension pneumothorax

D. Hypovolemic shock

**123.** Predisposing factors to empyema include all of the following *except:*

A. Multiple chest tube placement

B. Prehospital tube placement

C. Underlying pulmonary damage

D. Persistent pleural effusion

*You respond to a construction accident. You arrive to find a 28-year-old male patient who has sustained a traumatic amputation of his right thumb and a partial amputation of the right index finger by a table saw.*

124. An important determinant in the success of reimplantation is:
    0  A. The general health of the patient before the injury
    0  B. The amount of time the amputated part is ischemic
    0  C. How contaminated the amputated part has become
    0  D. The amount of tissue that has been amputated

125. How many hours after injury may cooled fingers be successfully reimplanted?
    0  A. 10 to 28 hours
    0  B. 4 to 6 hours
    0  C. 2 to 4 hours
    0  D. 8 to 10 hours

126. How should the amputated fingers be transported?
    0  A. Immersed in cold, sterile water, sealed in a plastic bag
    0  B. Placed in a bag of ice, wrapped in a moistened dressing, and placed in a basin
    0  C. Wrapped in a moistened gauze, sealed in a plastic bag, and placed in melting ice
    0  D. Wrapped in a dry sterile dressing and placed dry in a plastic bag

127. During the transport, management of severe head injury includes:
    0  A. Administering high-dose glucocorticoids intravenously as soon as possible
    0  B. Hyperventilating the patient at a rate of 30 to decrease the pCO$_2$ to 30
    0  C. Administering mannitol prophylactically to prevent an increase in ICP
    0  D. Maintaining an adequate blood pressure to maintain adequate CPP

*Your rotary-wing aircraft has been called to a rural facility to transport a 19-year-old male patient who was involved in an assault. He is approximately 2 hours post injury and has been diagnosed with a probable diffuse axonal injury. His GCS is 5 (E-1, V-1, M-3). Pupils are midsize and nonreactive to light. The patient has been intubated and is being manually oxygenated, has two peripheral IVs at a keep open rate (TKO), and remains in full spinal immobilization.*

128. In preparation for transport, the transport nurse should:
    0  A. Remove the patient's cervical collar and raise the head of the bed to 30° to facilitate intracranial blood flow
    0  B. Insert a gastric tube to decompress the patient's stomach and decrease the risk of aspiration
    0  C. Increase the patient's intravenous fluid rate to 100 ml/h for fluid maintenance and to decrease the patient's intracranial blood flow
    0  D. Decrease the assisted ventilatory rate to 16 breaths per minute to decrease the risk of pulmonary edema

129. The referring facility shows the transport nurse the patient's C-spine film. After reviewing the film, the flight nurse should consider all of the following *except:*
    0  A. The film shows all seven vertebrae without deformity. The patient may be removed from spinal immobilization.
    0  B. The film does not show all seven vertebrae. The patient should remain in spinal immobilization.
    0  C. The film shows all seven vertebrae without deformity. The patient should remain in spinal immobilization.
    0  D. The film shows deformity. The patient should remain in spinal immobilization until he arrives at the receiving hospital.

130. Subcutaneous emphysema on a chest radiograph:
    0  A. Is a uniform density collection of blood
    0  B. Is defined as fluid collection in the pleural space
    0  C. Is noted as radiolucent pockets or spongy areas
    0  D. Ill-defined, saucer-shaped, nonvascular densities

## ANSWERS

1. **B. Assessment.** A very low birth weight infant weighs less than 1500 g. A low birth weight infant weighs less than 2500 g, and a very, very low birth weight infant weighs less than 1000 g.[4]

2. **C. Assessment.** Risk factors associated with an increased risk for neonatal resuscitation include age >35 years, diabetes, hemorrhage, no prenatal care, infection, premature rupture of membranes, and a prolonged labor.[5]

3. **D. Assessment.** Indications for endotracheal intubation of the neonate include the need for tracheal suctioning for the presence of meconium, ineffective bag-valve-mask ventilation, and, when there is a need, prolonged positive-pressure ventilation, which may be required during transport.[5]

4. **C. Intervention.** Chest compressions should be initiated in the neonate if the child's heart rate decreases below 60 beats per minute or is 60 to 80 beats per minute and is not improving with ventilation and oxygenation.[5]

5. **A. Evaluation.** The flight nurse should obtain a good blood return to indicate that the umbilical catheter is appropriately inserted. The catheter should only be inserted 1 to 4 cm and should be inserted in the umbilical vein. The umbilical vein is a thin-walled single vessel compared with umbilical arteries, which are thick walled and are paired.[5]

6. **B. Intervention.** Preparation for the transport of this child should include definitive airway management. Based on the child's clinical findings and oxygen saturation, endotracheal intubation before transport would afford the best method of managing this child's airway.[5-7]

7. **D. Intervention.** In order to determine the size of the endotracheal tube of this neonate, the flight nurse could use the length of the infant, the weight of the infant, or the formula: postconceptual age in weeks/10.[7]

8. **B. Intervention.** The infant should receive 45 ml of normal saline.[5]

9. **A. Evaluation.** The neonate's central and peripheral pulses should be monitored to evaluate the effectiveness of fluid resuscitation.[6,7]

10. **C. Analysis.** Based on the gravity of the child's condition, the mother is probably fearful of whether the child will survive. Many neonatal transport teams carry a camera so that they can leave a picture of the child with the mother, as well as calling the mother when arriving at the receiving facility to help decrease her fear about her child.[5]

11. **D. Intervention.** The intravenous fluids should be calculated based on the total weight of the twins and then divided and given to each infant. Each infant should have her own intravenous access. Medication should be given to the weaker or smaller of the twins first so that its effects can be evaluated. Positioning of the infants in the isolette should ensure that both twins are at the same level to prevent hypovolemia.[4,8]

12. **A. Assessment.** A disadvantage of any defibrillation procedure is arcing of the current, especially during air transport, because of the potential of igniting a fire. There has been a recent report of a fire that resulted from arcing of the current during patient defibrillation with a "hands-off" defibrillator. The current ignited the blankets in which the patient was wrapped.[9,10]

13. **C. Assessment.** Electromagnetic interference (EMI) has been reported to trigger or inhibit pacemaker output, cause inappropriate programming, and cause permanent function disruption.[11]

14. **D. Assessment/Intervention.** When deciding whether family members should accompany a child during transport, the flight team needs to consider the size of the transport vehicle, the condition of the child, if the flight program has a protocol to allow ride-along, and what effect the presence of the parents would have on the child.[12]

15. **C. Intervention.** Nursing interventions for families include speaking to the family before transport, allowing the family to see the child before transport; and providing them with written material about the transport, how to get to the receiving facility, and who to contact on their arrival.[3,12]

16. **A. Assessment.** Research has shown that bag ventilation contributes to either hypocapnia or hypercapnia because of interruption of ventilation, limited crewmembers, and the need to interrupt ventilation to perform other treatment modalities.[13,14,15]

17. **C. Assessment.** The administration of aminoglycosides to the patient receiving mivicurium will increase the length of time of the neuromuscular blockade. Additional medications that will increase neuromuscular blockade include quinidine, local anesthetics, halothane, procainamide, and lithium.[16]

18. **A. Intervention.** Inserting a nasogastric tube will decompress the child's abdomen and decrease the possibility of aspiration. Since the child was intubated using PALS guidelines, the endotracheal tube will not have a cuff.[5]

19. **B. Assessment.** Transport of a critically ill or injured patient may be delayed because of prolonged entrapment, lack of rescue equipment and personnel, bad weather conditions, and inaccurate assessment of the acuity of the patient's illness or injury.[13]

20. **A. Analysis.** The most appropriate nursing diagnosis on which to base this patient's care would be gas exchange, impaired, related to his medical diagnosis as evidenced by his oxygen saturation.

21. **B. Intervention.** Initiation of a vasocative drug such as dopamine once fluid resuscitation has failed may help enhance organ perfusion and oxygenation.[17]

22. **B. Assessment.** The insurance status of the patient should not factor into the decision to transport a patient to the appropriate receiving facility for care.[13]

23. **D. Assessment.** Sources of stress in the flight and prehospital care nursing environment include lack of adequate space, malfunctioning equipment, difficult work relationships, age of the patient, and death of the patient (expected or unexpected).[18,19]

24. **D. Assessment.** Stress reactions are classified as either acute or long-term. Examples of acute stress reactions include exhaustion, headaches, nightmares, and anger. Long-term stress reactions include chronic illness, alteration in personal finances, anomia, and negative patient interactions.[18,19]

25. **B. Intervention.** Stress management after being exposed to a critical incident would include eating an appropriate diet, particularly one high in vitamin B, cutting back on alcohol and cigarettes, and exercise such as a brisk walk.[20,21]

26. **C. Assessment.** An adverse reaction involving the administration of succinylcholine is increased intraocular pressure. Relative contraindications for use should therefore include penetrating eye wounds, eye surgery, and glaucoma.[22] Complications involving increased intracranial pressure, muscle fasciculations, and cardiac dysrhythmia can be greatly reduced with premedication of lidocaine 1 mg/kg IVP.[22]

27. **B. Intervention.** The recommended intubating dose of mivacurium chloride is 0.25 mg/kg (0.15 mg/kg over 1 to 2 minutes, followed in 60 seconds by 0.10 mg/kg). This regimen speeds the onset of action, producing intubating conditions in approximately 90 seconds.[23] The recommended paralyzing dosage of vecuronium (Norcuron) ranges from 0.04 mg/kg to 0.1 mg/kg in the child and 0.1 mg/kg in the adult patient.[23]

28. **A. Intervention.** Methylprednisolone is a synthetic glucocorticoid that is thought to limit secondary injury to the spinal cord by inhibiting lipid peroxidation. This, in turn, helps to limit formation and release of the various deleterious chemicals (i.e., prostaglandins), maintain spinal cord blood flow, decrease nerve degradation, and enhance nerve excitability.[24]

29. **D. Assessment.** GI bleeding is a relative *complication* associated with glucocorticoid use, but was not found to worsen with administration of this drug. A contraindication to the initiation of treatment is a spinal cord lesion below L-2. Special considerations in methylprednisolone administration do include pregnancy, age less than 13 years, penetrating wounds to the spinal cord, fulminant infection or TB, HIV infection, and severe diabetes.[24] Administration of methylprednisone, which can cause immunosuppression, may worsen these conditions.

30. **B. Assessment.** Although the first clinical indicators of cyanide toxicity may be behavioral, these changes are often attributed to "ICU psychosis" in the critically ill. A good warning sign of impending toxicity may be the presence of hypertension. Unfortunately, this will often trigger staff to increase the nipride infusion to control the rising blood pressure, and rapidly compound the cyanide accumulation and resultant life-threatening complications.[25]

31. **A. Intervention.** When determining any infusion rate, one must first calculate the concentration of the solution. This solution was made with a dilution of 50 mg of Nipride in 250 ml $D_5W$. After dividing 50 mg by 250 ml, a concentration of 0.2 mg/ml or 200 μg (0.2 ¥ 1,000) per ml was determined. To further calculate the dosage rate in μg/kg/min, you must simply multiply the appropriate numbers. (Example: 8 μg ¥ 74 kg ¥ 60 min) (60 minutes will convert the product to the rate of ml/hour.) Lastly, this total must be divided by the concentration; i.e., 200 μg in this example. The entire formula written out would appear as: 8 ¥ 74 ¥ 60 = 35,520 divided by 200 = 177.6.

32. **D. Assessment.** The side effects of midazolam include respiratory depression and decrease in peripheral vascular resistance, which results in hypotension.[23]

33. **C. Assessment.** You may get prolonged respiratory depression when these drugs are combined with other CNS depressants, alcohol, or barbiturates. There is also an increased sedative and hypnotic effect when combined with fentanyl, narcotic agonists, or analgesics. Benzodiazepines will demonstrate a shorter onset of action and a longer duration of sedation when used in combination therapy.[23]

34. **C. Evaluation.** Flumazenil has a specific warning label against its use in multiple drug ingestion, especially if a tricyclic antidepressant (TCA) is suspected. This warning is secondary to the adverse effect of seizures brought about in patients treated with flumazenil and the fact that life-threatening seizures can occur in TCA overdose.[26]

35. **B. Intervention.** Research has found that the most effective methods to manage patient anxiety related to flying include:

    - Most patients are more concerned about their medical condition than the flight
    - Asking patients about their previous flight experience and their reactions to plane crashes can help predict their level of anxiety
    - Patients' anxiety levels decrease as the flight progresses
    - Educating patients about the transport environment[27]

36. **C. Intervention.** For asystolic, or pulseless, arrest in children, the recommended *first dose* is: IV/IO: 0.01 mg/kg (1:10,000) ETT: 0.1 mg/kg (1:1,000) *subsequent doses:* IV/IO/ETT: 0.1 mg/kg (1:1,000)[5]

37. **A. Assessment.** The effects of the beta agonist are increased heart rate, increased force of contraction (both of these lead to an increase in myocardial oxygen consumption), and bronchodilation. The alpha-agonist action results in vasoconstriction, leading to an increase in B/P. Several investigators have established that increasing the alpha-agonist effect (by increasing the dose of epinephrine) results in improved coronary blood flow, improved cerebral blood flow, and improved rate of resuscitation.[28]

38. **C. Intervention.** The recommended dose of epinephrine is 1 mg IVP every 3 to 5 mins.[31]

39. **D. Intervention.** Recent research has demonstrated that procainamide may be more effective than lidocaine in terminating spontaneously occurring monomorphic ventricular tachycardia. Procainamide is administered 30 mg/min until 17 mg/kg; widened QRS, hypotension, or cessation of the dysrhythmia.[29,30]

40. **B. Intervention.** When bradyarrhythmias occur, the cause should be first evaluated. Causes of bradyarrhythmias include hypoxia, hypovolemia, and hypothermia. A fluid bolus should be tried first, then atropine or vasocative drugs considered.[29]

41. **B. Evaluation.** Sodium bicarbonate is indicated if a tricyclic overdose has occurred to alkalinize the urine. Sodium bicarbonate is considered possibly helpful in cases of *documented* metabolic acidosis after return of spontaneous circulation.[31]

42. **B. Intervention/Evaluation.** Clinical findings classically associated with hypoglycemia are not adequately specific to guide the use of the use of glucose in resuscitation. However, research has demonstrated that glucose actually increases in long-term adult resuscitation. Because the research continues to be unclear, it is recommended that $D_{50}$ be administered if the patient is hypoglycemic.[30]

43. **C. Intervention.** The starting dosage of adenosine is 6 mg, given rapid IV push over 1 to 3 seconds. Because of its extremely short elimination half-life in blood, adenosine must be given very quickly and *followed* with a saline solution flush to ensure that the drug reaches the AV node. If the first dose is not effective within 1 to 2 minutes, a follow-up dose of 12 mg may be administered.[31]

44. **C. Assessment.** The adverse effects associated with a bolus of adenosine are transient and generally do not require intervention. These side effects have been attributed to a complex interplay of direct effects on organ adenosine receptors, vascular chemoreceptors, and autonomically mediated responses. These side effects have an average duration of less than 60 seconds, and none last more than 2 minutes.[31]

45. **D. Intervention.** Amiodarone reduces membrane excitability and facilitates the termination of ventricular arrhythmia by prolonging the action potential, retarding the refractory period of the myocardial conduction system.[29,30]

46. **D. Evaluation.** All are potential adverse effects following mannitol administration. Paradoxical increased ICP and further deterioration of patient status may be seen, especially if the blood-brain barrier is not intact. Seizures may be secondary to electrolyte imbalances. Pulmonary edema and heart failure can ensue from fluid overload.[16]

47. **A. Intervention.** Mannitol should be dosed between .25 g/kg to 2 g/kg as a 15%, 20% or 25% solution and infused over 10 to 60 minutes. When using the higher concentrations, an in-line filter may help to prevent unnoticed crystals from infusing into the patient. Concentrated mannitol is incompatible with both electrolyte solutions and blood products.[16]

48. **B. Intervention.** Magnesium is considered a treatment of choice in patients with torsades de pointes. Hypomagnesemia can precipitate refractory VF and can hinder the replenishment of intracellular potassium. Magnesium sulfate, 1 to 2 g,

is diluted in 100 ml $D_5W$ and administered over 1 to 2 minutes in VF/VT. Magnesium is also used to control seizures in pregnancy-induced hypertension. Magnesium decreases acetylcholine in motor nerve terminals, providing the anticonvulsant property.[16]

49. **C. Assessment.** Fetal heart rate and reactivity may decrease with this drug if using it during labor. Intake and output should remain at 30 ml/h or more, whereby its use is contraindicated in patients with renal disease. A decrease in knee jerk or patellar reflex may signal $Mg^{++}$ toxicity. Lastly, respiratory status must be continuously evaluated and the drug held if the RR is < 16/min. (Also, the respiratory rate and rhythm of the newborn should be monitored closely if $Mg^{++}$ was administered 24 hours or less before delivery.)[16,19]

50. **B. Intervention.** The transport team should transport the patient because there are only verbal and no written DNR orders. The patient is unable to confirm or deny what her physician has stated. When uncertain, the team should always act in the best interest of the patient.[32]

51. **C. Assessment.** The Cormak and Lehane Classification System is based on four grades.
    - Grade I: Glottis, including anterior and posterior commissures, can be fully exposed
    - Grade II: Glottis can be partially exposed
    - Grade III: Glottis cannot be exposed, only corniculate cartilages can be visualized
    - Grade IV: Glottis, including corniculate cartilage, cannot be exposed[33]

52. **A. Assessment.** Circulatory responses associated with the IV administration of fentanyl may involve bradycardia, hypotension, circulatory depression, and cardiac arrest. Potential adverse reactions involving respiratory functions may include muscle rigidity (especially muscles of respiration) following rapid IV infusion, laryngospasm, bronchoconstriction, respiratory depression, and respiratory arrest.[16]

53. **C. Evaluation.** Hemodynamic effects of Neo-Synephrine IV include: A strong alpha-adrenergic effect, causing vasoconstriction, *no* beta$_1$ or beta$_2$ stimulation; no change in heart rate; a slight decrease or no change in cardiac output; and an essential increase in systemic vascular resistance.[16]

54. **D. Assessment.** Side effects of terbutaline include tachycardia, palpitations, transient hyperglycemia, nausea and vomiting, and pulmonary edema.[34]

55. **A. Intervention.**[16,35]

56. **C. Intervention.** To determine the flow rate in drops per minute, you would multiply 8 (μg) ¥

72 (kg) ¥ 60 (min)—and then divide this total by 1600 (μg/ml—concentration).

57. **D. Intervention.** Vecuronium is a neuromuscular blocking agent, not a sedative. Propofol can cause hypotension, and ketamine may increase ICP. Etomidate decreases cerebral oxygen consumption and ICP.[36]

58. **C. Intervention.** The patient should be placed in a left lateral recumbent position to displace the gravid uterus from the inferior vena cava and increase cardiac output.[19,34]

59. **B. Intervention.** Protamine sulfate is an antidote to heparin.[16]

60. **D. Assessment.** When calculating this dose, one must first determine the concentration of the NTG solution,[16] then multiply the concentration times the rate and divide this total by 60 (to determine/per minute).[35]

61. **C. Evaluation.** NTG infusion relaxes all smooth muscles by direct action, with the most prominent effect on vascular smooth muscle. Resulting vasodilation produces lowered peripheral resistance (decreasing afterload), fall in B/P, and *decreased* cardiac output due to reduced venous return to the heart (decreasing preload).[16]

62. **C. Assessment.** Both dopamine and dobutamine are positive inotropic agents, increasing cardiac output. Dopamine exerts alpha stimulation, and dobutamine exhibits both alpha and beta$_1$ stimulation. *Only* dopamine causes vasoconstriction, as well as frequently precipitating tachycardia. Dobutamine *itself* enhances peripheral perfusion and increases myocardial contractility.[16]

63. **D. Assessment.** Norepinephrine is one of the most powerful vasoconstrictors because of its potent action on alpha$_1$ receptors. Norepinephrine can be useful in severely hypotensive patients, especially when other agents have failed. It may be particularly helpful in septic shock, when systemic vascular resistance is greatly decreased, as well as in situations with loss of venous tone.[16]

64. **C. Intervention.** The advantages of the laryngeal mask airway (LMA) include:
    - Minimal training is needed to use the LMA
    - No manipulation of the cervical spine is necessary for insertion
    - LMAs are not made out of latex
    - Endotracheal intubation can be performed through the LMA[37]

65. **C. Intervention.** In vasoconstricted patients, the earlobe is the site least affected by poor perfusion. The bridge of the nose would also be a viable choice in this instance. (The side of the foot is

usually reserved for a small infant.) The important goals are to select a highly vascular site that is rich in arterial blood and to ensure correct sensor placement on the patient so that the light-emitting sensor and light-receiving sensor are opposite each other.[38,39,40]

66. **B. Assessment.** Abnormal hemoglobins such as carboxyhemoglobin (CO poison) or methemoglobin cannot be distinguished from oxyhemoglobin by pulse oximeters that use two wavelengths of red light. Anemia itself should not affect oximetric $SaO_2$ readings. However, hypotensive conditions or other conditions that affect peripheral vascular and tissue perfusion (i.e., hypothermia, vasocative drug therapy) do adversely affect the accuracy of the pulse oximetry measurement. Motion artifact interferes with the pulsatile signal and results in either false $SaO_2$ measurements or complete loss of a pulse signal.[38,39,40]

67. **A. Evaluation.** Although it may be adequately used as a screening tool for evaluating patient oxygenation, take care in placing too much reliance on pulse oximetry when a more inclusive arterial blood sample is indicated. Pulse oximetry alone does not provide information on ventilatory status, as measured by $CO_2$ tension and acid-base balance. ABG analysis is the most reliable test for determining the adequacy of respiratory gas exchange.[38,39,40]

68. **A. Assessment/Intervention.** $ETCO_2$ can be used to confirm ETT placement with virtual certainty in the *nonarrested* patient who has a pulse and adequate perfusion. Disorders that cause significant ventilation/perfusion mismatch (e.g., massive PE) or that decrease $CO_2$ production (e.g., hypothermia) are accompanied by a low $ETCO_2$ concentration. The $ETCO_2$ readings, in these cases, would therefore be of no use to aid with determination of ETT placement.[41]

69. **B. Assessment.** Causes of low $ETCO_2$ readings may involve situations prohibiting adequate ventilation, adequate blood flow (e.g., tension pneumothorax, pericardial tamponade) or mismatch between ventilation and perfusion. Pulseless electrical activity (PEA) in itself is not a cause of low $ETCO_2$ concentrations. Furthermore, if a patient exhibits PEA with an $ETCO_2$ concentration of more than 3%, it is highly likely that the patient has an adequate cardiac output but that the pulse is not palpable due to arterial vasoconstriction.[41]

70. **C. Assessment.** Colormetric $ETCO_2$ devices contain a Ph-sensitive membrane that can be altered by administration of certain drugs via the ETT. If the ETT is positioned properly in the trachea but the blood flow is severely reduced, as during profound shock or CPR, less $CO_2$ will be carried to the lungs, which will result in a low $ETCO_2$ reading. Adversely, when an ETT has been inserted into the esophagus of a patient who has recently ingested a carbonated beverage, such as beer or soda, the initial $ETCO_2$ reading may appear falsely normal or even high.[41]

71. **D. Intervention.** When using a ventilator, the flight nurse loses the ability to feel the compliance of the patient's lungs. One advantage of using a ventilator is that ventilator settings during transport can remain consistent. Studies have shown that manual ventilation with self-inflating bags during transport can lead to unintentional hyperventilation and respiratory alkalosis, resulting in hypotension and cardiac dysrhythmia. This will also aid greatly in preventing barotrauma, especially in the pediatric patient, as a result of too-aggressive resuscitation.[42]

72. **C. Intervention.** The fraction of inspired oxygen ($FiO_2$) is often initiated at 100% in the acutely injured patient and later weaned according to blood gas determination. Tidal volume is the volume of air inspired or expired during a normal breath. During mechanical ventilation, tidal volume is calculated as 10 to 15 cc/kg.[42]

73. **C. Intervention.** External pacing is *not* indicated in cases where a prolonged period of time has elapsed between cardiac arrest and treatment. Pacing here is often ineffective due to the heart muscle's limited response to the electrical stimulation of the pacer. External cardiac pacing should not be attempted in patients with hypotension as a result of hypovolemia. Pacing is frequently beneficial only when the symptoms are the result of cardiac disturbance.[43,44]

74. **B. Assessment.** When you have obtained capture through the myocardium, you should see a wide QRS complex and a tall, broad T-wave appearing with the spike and at the rate set by the pacer. During external pacing, you are applying an external electrical source, which is capable of contracting not only heart muscle but also skeletal muscle. This contraction of skeletal muscle, in and of itself, is not evidence of capture. Effective pacing is best determined by the patient's clinical response: an elevation of blood pressure, a palpable pulse, improved LOC, and improved skin color and temperature.[44]

75. **C. Intervention.** The anterior electrode should be applied over the apex of the heart, avoiding di-

rect placement over the sternum. The posterior pad is placed on the patient's back, avoiding both the spine and the scapula. (These bony protrusions increase transthoracic resistance and make pacer capture harder to obtain). If you are unable to utilize the anterior-posterior placement of the electrodes, the anterior-anterior position may be used. The anterior electrode should be placed on the left side of the chest, midaxillary over the fourth intercostal space, and the posterior pad should be placed on the right chest in the subclavicular area.[44]

76. **B. Evaluation.** Battery failure or general equipment failure can have lethal consequences for the patient who is pacemaker dependent. Skin burns may occur due to poor or dried electrode contact. The battery life of each unit varies somewhat, but in all cases the pacer should be plugged into an external power source with prolonged pacing. Failure to capture can be due to numerous factors: the current MA may need to be increased, the electrodes may be improperly placed, or during prolonged pacing the myocardium may become desensitized to the current and subsequently may need more current supplied to the muscle. Lastly, during the initial phases of pacing, there may be a transient amount of hypotension until the body begins to compensate to the new rate and rhythm. If this occurs, it may be beneficial to give a fluid bolus and evaluate the response.[19,44]

77. **B. Intervention.** The pacing mode may be demand or asynchronous. The demand mode allows the pacer to sense the patient's own rhythm and fire only if the rate falls below the selected pacing rate. The output is usually in milliamps or voltage. Use the lowest setting possible to obtain capture of the pacer. If no ventricular capture occurs, the output should be sequentially increased until capture does occur. The pacing rate is usually set anywhere between 60 to 80 beats per minute. This rate is selected to ensure adequate cardiac output without the increased myocardial oxygen demands that higher rates would require.[43]

78. **C. Assessment.** Arterial systole begins with the opening of the aortic valve and rapid ejection of blood into the aorta. This period is indicated on the arterial waveform as rapid upstroke phase.[45]

79. **B. Assessment.** Onset of systole occurs immediately after ventricular depolarization, which corresponds to slightly after the QRS complex on the ECG.[45,46]

80. **B. Assessment.** The dicrotic notch represents the small dip on the downslope of an arterial pressure waveform and marks the end of the ejection pe-

riod. The dicrotic notch occurs after the T wave on the ECG.[45,46]

81. **D. Assessment.** Answers A, B, and C reflect normal changes in the elderly due to arterial stiffening with increased pulse wave velocity.[46]

82. **D. Intervention.** It is not required that the patient be kept in a flat position when obtaining measurements. *As long as the air-reference port is level to the patient's midchest level,* the patient may be elevated up to 45°, or in a lateral recumbent position.[46]

83. **B. Intervention.** A clot in the catheter is suspected if a patient has dampened waveform and absent or weakened pulses. Initially flushing the catheter may result in dislodging the clot. Interventions consist of *gentle aspiration* of the line using a small syringe, then flushing the line with the inline flush device.[17]

84. **C. Evaluation.** Stopcocks inadvertently turned will result in *loss of waveform.* Troubleshooting consists of checking line set-up: adequate pressure in flush bag, absence of bubbles and kinks in the tubing, quick rise to the top of the scale, and a "square" off of pattern when triggering the fast-flush device.[17,46,47]

85. **A. Assessment.** A slight difference between arterial and cuff pressures is 5 to 10 mm Hg in the normovolemic patient. Abnormal low readings occur due to decreased flow state, use of pressor drugs, improper calibration, and incorrect transducer placement.[17]

86. **D. Assessment.** Clinical findings such as increasing heart rate and consistent mean anterior pressure (MAP) are physiological attempts to compensate for an altered perfusion status. If hemorrhagic conditions exist, or cardiac output decreases, the body compensates by constricting peripheral vessels to maintain blood pressure. In hemorrhagic situations, the MAP may remain constant, while the pulse pressure narrows. Monitoring both systolic and diastolic pressures aides in assessing changes in perfusion.[17]

87. **C. Assessment.** The fourth intercostal space/midaxillary line serves as the reference point for the level of the transducer, which ensures consistency of hemodynamic readings. For each inch the transducer is away from this point, the difference in values is approximately 2 mm Hg.[47,48]

88. **C. Intervention.** The stopcock located on the transducer must be open to air in order to negate the effects of atmospheric pressure so that the only pressure values that are measured are the ones within the blood vessels or within the heart. Once the digital monitor reading falls to "zero," turn the stopcock back to the open position.[48,49]

89. **A. Intervention.** Abnormally high digital pressures with normal waveforms are caused when the transducer falls below the phlebostatic axis reference point. Patients that are diaphoretic and/or restless may cause the transducer to slip posteriorly and thereby produce abnormally high digital readings.[47,48,49]

90. **D. Intervention.** In hemorrhagic situations, the MAP may remain constant, while the pulse pressure narrows. Monitoring both systolic and diastolic pressures aides in assessing blood loss.[48]

91. **C. Assessment.** This is a waveform that demonstrates catheter fling that is caused by excessive catheter movement, which could have occurred during transfer or movement of the patient. This will interfere with the transport nurse's ability to monitor the patient.[45]

92. **B. Intervention.** Initial action consists of inflating the PA balloon. This serves two functions: it assists decreasing myocardial irritability and subsequently decreases ventricular dysrhythmia, and assists the catheter to float with the flow of blood from the right ventricle into the pulmonary artery. It is not uncommon for ventricular ectopy to occur when the catheter tip is in the right ventricle.[17,47]

93. **A. Intervention.** The pulmonary artery (PA) catheter is in an overwedge pattern. The balloon has been overinflated, and the PA vessel may rupture from overinflating the balloon. Corrective measures consist of deflating the balloon, and re-inflating slowly, with enough air to obtain PA wedge pressure. Flushing of the catheter in a wedge position is associated with PA rupture and hemorrhage.[49,50]

94. **B. Intervention.** Normal PA wedge pressure is 8 to 12 mm Hg. Administering a fluid bolus (answers A and C) would only increase a high PA wedge pressure and further compromise the hemodynamic status. Administering a nitroglycerine infusion (answer D) could potentially decrease the patient's systolic blood pressure. Initiating dopamine infusion (answer B) will assist in increasing the patient's cardiac output.[45]

95. **C. Assessment.** In the absence of mitral valve and pulmonary disease, the PA end-diastolic pressure value corresponds closely to the PA wedge pressure. If PA end-diastolic (PAD) and PA wedge pressures are similar, then PAD can be substituted for PA wedge pressure.[45]

96. **D. Intervention.** The patient's PAD pressure is abnormally low. Normal PAD pressures are 8 to 12 mm Hg. Administering a fluid bolus may increase filling pressures and improve cardiac output.[45,48]

97. **D. Intervention.** The PA catheter has black bands on the catheter that indicate length of insertion. Narrow black bands represent 10 cm lengths, and wide black bands indicate 50 cm lengths. The normal subclavian insertion site markings are approximately 45 to 50 cm. It appears that during transport the catheter was inadvertently pulled out (catheter marking showing three narrow bands at subclavian insertion site).[47,51,52]

98. **A. Intervention.** Most often fibrin at the tip of the catheter is the cause for pressures to become dampened. The incident of thrombus formation is increased in patients with low cardiac outputs. Careful aspiration, followed by gentle flushing, usually corrects this problem.[47]

99. **D. Assessment.** Spontaneous migration of the PA catheter toward the periphery pulmonary bed may occur. Migration of catheter into a wedge position will result in pulmonary infarct. Continuous monitoring of PA pressures is important to detect a PA wedge waveform.[47,52,53]

100. **C. Intervention.** It should take 1.25 to 1.5 cc of air to wedge a pulmonary artery catheter. Any amount less than this indicates that the catheter is too far into the pulmonary artery.[17]

101. **A. Intervention.** IABP therapy actually *decreases* afterload. Prior to systolic, the deflation of the balloon creates a vacuum-like effect in the aorta, thereby increasing forward propulsion and decreasing afterload.[17]

102. **B. Assessment.** The most commonly used reference point or "trigger" for inflation and deflation of the intraaortic balloon pump (IABP) is the R wave of the patient's ECG.[54,55]

103. **D. Assessment/Intervention.** Intraaortic balloon pump (IABP) inflation is an ideally timed small box on the ECG paper before the dicrotic notch. This results in changing the typical U-shaped dicrotic notch to a sharp V shape (see below).[17,54]

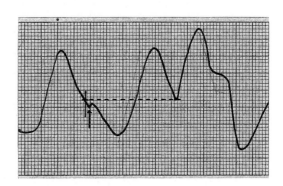

104. **C. Assessment.** Intraaortic balloon pump (IABP) deflation occurs just before the aortic valve opens. This period of time is immediately before the upstroke on the arterial waveform. See the figure below for safe and unsafe timing for counterpulsation.[17,54]

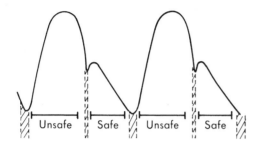

From Quaal, S: *Comprehensive intraaortic balloon counterpulsation,* ed 2, St. Louis, 1993, Mosby.

105. **D. Intervention.** For patient comfort, the head of bed can be elevated to less than 45°. This prevents kinking of the intraaortic balloon pump catheter and migration of the catheter.[17]

106. **D. Assessment.** A *major complication* of IABP is ischemia of limb or renal circulation. The catheter may trigger thrombus formation, occluding the femoral artery. Migration proximally occludes the subclavian artery, or distally the renal circulation. Arrhythmia can affect timing of IABP; however, it is not a major complication.[17]

107. **B. Intervention.** To prevent clot formation along the dormant balloon, it is necessary to inflate/deflate with half of the total amount of the balloon volume. Assess for causes of loss of vacuum: large leak-loose connections, loss of power source, or empty $CO_2$/helium tank.[48,55]

108. **C. Assessment.** An important aspect of assessment in the prehospital setting includes the scene itself. The nurse can gather many important clues from the scene that may influence the entire assessment. It is also the first priority to protect the emergency responders and the patient from further injury. The flight nurse should evaluate the scene and, if necessary, move the patient to a safe area before initiating treatment.[19]

109. **A. Assessment.** The patient's chest should be exposed and visually inspected to assess ventilatory exchange. Airway patency does not ensure adequate ventilation. The nurse should suspect respiratory compromise if the patient's respiratory rate is greater than 28 to 30 breaths per minute.[19]

110. **C. Intervention.** With a sucking chest wound, air passes from the atmosphere, through the chest wall, into the pleural space, and out again with a loss of thoracic pressure. If the diameter of the hole is greater than two thirds of the diameter of the trachea, there is preferential flow of air through the chest wall defect, which is the path of least resistance. The occlusive dressing prevents the atmospheric air from passing through the chest wall.[19]

111. **B. Assessment.** Three initial observations can give the nurse information regarding the patient's hemodynamic stability.
    1. *Level of consciousness.* As a person's blood volume decreases, cerebral perfusion is impaired, affecting level of consciousness.
    2. *Skin color.* In persons of fair skin color, an ashen, gray face and pale, white extremities are ominous signs of hypovolemia. In persons of color, paleness of the mucous membranes is a sign of shock.
    3. *Pulse.* As the shock state progresses, the peripheral pulses become weak and thready.[19]

112. **B. Intervention.** The most common chemical restraints used by air medical transport programs are paralytics, intubation, and concomitant benzodiazepine administration. Narcotics are infrequently used because of potential vital sign effects.[56]

113. **A. Assessment.** The GCS provides a means to quantitatively measure the patient's best response in three areas:
*Eye opening*
Spontaneously   4
To verbal stimuli   3
To pain   2
No response   1
*Best verbal response*
Oriented and converses   5
Disoriented and converses   4
Inappropriate words   3
Incomprehensible sounds   2
No response   1
*Best motor response*
Obeys commands   6
Localizes to pain   5
Withdrawal   4
Flexion-abnormal   3
Extension   2
No response   1
TOTAL   (3 to 15 points)[19]

114. **C. Intervention.** A patient with a GCS of 8 is considered to be in coma and should have his or her airway protected. Also, emergency treatment of the patient with a serious head injury is aimed at protecting the brain from further insults by

maintaining adequate cerebral oxygenation and preventing systemic hypotension.[13,19,61]

115. **B. Intervention.** The potential for concomitant cervical spine injury is a major concern for the patient requiring an airway procedure. For orotracheal intubation, the two-person in-line manual cervical immobilization should be used.[19]

116. **D. Intervention.** At no time should fluids be withheld from a hypotensive, head-injured patient. If the mean arterial pressure is allowed to drop, a resultant drop in cerebral blood flow will occur, leading to cerebral anoxia.[19,61]

117. **A. Assessment.** Due to lack of sensation, which resulted from the spinal cord injury, the patient will be unable to know if he is injured below his spinal cord injury. The flight nurse must expose the patient in order to do a thorough assessment.[13,19]

118. **B. Intervention.** The trunk of the body and the extremities should be secured to the board first with manual stabilization of the head, as tightening of straps may cause movement of the body. Secure the head last using a towel roll or commercial device to control lateral movement of the head.[57]

119. **B. Intervention.** A spinal cord injury, which causes a permanent disability, is extremely frightening to the patient and his or her support group, and has a profound impact on their lives. If there is a deficit present, caregivers should provide positive support, but not offer false hope.[13,19]

120. **D. Assessment.** Autopsy findings, observations by trauma surgeons, and data collected through crash tests with anthropomorphic dummies, have provided a correlation between mechanisms of injury and groups of common injuries. Patterns found with side impacts include clavicle fractures, rib fractures, flail chest, pulmonary contusions, lacerated liver/spleen, cervical spine fracture, cerebral contusion/hemorrhage, femur fracture, and pelvic fracture.[19]

121. **C. Intervention.** An important advantage of the use of blood during transport is the early administration of a resuscitation fluid that increases the patient's oxygen-carrying capacity, unlike crystalloids. However, administration of blood by untrained personnel or delay in transport to obtain the blood are not advantages to its use.[58,59,60]

122. **C. Assessment.** Tension pneumothorax is a clinical diagnosis. It is characterized by respiratory distress, tachycardia, hypotension, tracheal deviation, unilateral absence of breath sounds,

neck vein distention, and cyanosis as a late manifestation.[60]

123. **B. Assessment.** Risk factors for the development of empyema include pneumonia, wound infection, and effusion.[60]

124. **B. Evaluation.** The time the severed part is without blood flow is an important determinant in the likelihood of successful reimplantation. Fingers contain no muscles and are more resistant to ischemia than muscular tissue.[19]

125. **A. Evaluation.** Cooled tissue is more resistant to ischemia because of decreased metabolism.[19]

126. **C. Intervention.** Cooled tissue is more resistant to ischemia because of decreased metabolism. Freezing the amputated part should be avoided because the expansion associated with the formation of ice crystals results in cellular damage.[19]

127. **D. Intervention.** Maintaining an adequate blood pressure to maintain adequate cerebral perfusion pressure is critical in the head-injured patient.[61]

128. **B. Intervention.** Vomiting in a fully immobilized patient will increase the possibility of aspiration. Gastric decompression may reduce the chances of vomiting and improve ventilation.[19]

129. **A. Assessment and Intervention.** A lateral C-spine film in and of itself is not conclusive to rule out a spinal injury in a head-injured patient.[34]

130. **C. Assessment.** Subcutaneous emphysema is noted on the radiograph as radiolucent pockets or spongy areas in the soft tissue.[34,161]

## REFERENCES

1. Hepp H: *Standards of flight nursing practice,* St Louis, 1995, Mosby.
2. Air and Surface Transport Nurses Association (ASTNA): *Standards for Adult Critical Care Transport,* Des Plaines, IL, Author.
3. Fulz J, and others: Air medical transport: what the family wants to know, *J Air Med Transport* 12:431-435, 1993.
4. Behrman R, Kleigman R, Jenson H, editors: *Nelson textbook of pediatrics,* ed 16, Philadelphia, 2000, WB Saunders.
5. Chameides L, Hazinski M, editors: *Pediatric advanced life support 1997-1999,* Dallas, American Heart Association.
6. Aoki B, McCloskey K: *Evaluation, stabilization, and transport of the critically ill child,* St Louis, 1992, Mosby.
7. McClosky K: *Guidelines for air and ground transport of neonatal and pediatric patients,* Elk Grove Village, IL, 1993, American Academy of Pediatrics.
8. DeBoer S, Jaracz G, Lass N: Did you bring two isolettes? Transport of conjoined twins, *Air Med J* 18(1):35-37, 1999.
9. Waggoner R, and others: Airborne defibrillation . . . the sequel, *J Air Med Transport* 10:19-21, 1991.

10. National Flight Nurses Association: Report of an on-board fire post hands-off defibrillation, *Concern Network,* 1994.

11. Gordon R, O'Dell K: Permanent internal pacemaker safety in air medical transport, *J Air Med Transport* 11:22-23, 1991.

12. Brown J, Tompkins K, Chancy E, Donovan R: Family member ride-alongs during interfacility transport, *Air Med J* 17(4):169-173, 1998.

13. DeJarnette R, editor: *Flight nursing advanced trauma course,* ed 2, Park Ridge, MD, 1994, National Flight Nurses Association.

14. Erler C, Rutherford W, Fiege A, and others: Monitored arterial and end-tidal carbon dioxide during in-flight mechanical ventilation, *Air Med J* 15(4):171-176, 1996.

15. Martin S, Agudelo W, Oshsner M: Monitoring hyperventilation in patients with closed head injury during air transport, *Air Med Transport* 16(1):15-18, 1997.

16. McKernry L, Salerno E: *Pharmacology in nursing,* St Louis, 1998, Mosby.

17. Alspach JG, editor: *AACN Core curriculum for critical care nursing,* ed 5, Philadelphia, 1998, WB Saunders.

18. Semonin-Holleran R, editor: *Prehospital nursing: a collaborative approach,* St Louis, 1994, Mosby.

19. Semonin-Holleran R, editor: *Flight nursing principles and practice,* ed 2, St Louis, 1996, Mosby.

20. Mitchell J: Comprehensive traumatic stress management in the emergency department, *Leadership Manag* 1:3-14, 1991.

21. Kalaine S: Critical incident stress management: taking care of our own, *AirMed* 5(6):34-36, 1999.

22. Munford B: Practical pharmacology of neuromuscular blockade, *Air Med J* 17(4):149-156, 1998.

23. Stoelting RK: *Pharmacology and physiology in anesthetic practice,* Philadelphia, 1999, Lippincott-Raven.

24. Nayduch D, Lee A, Butler D: High-dose methylprednisolone after acute spinal cord injury, *Crit Care Nurs* 69-78, August 1994.

25. Hall VA, Guest JM: Sodium nitroprusside-induced cyanide intoxication and prevention with sodium thiosulfate prophylaxis, *Am J Crit Car* 2:19-27, 1992.

26. Kriegsman W, Peppers M: Flumazenil for benzodiazepine overdose, *Emergency* 1:21-26, 1994.

27. Demmons L, Cook E: Anxiety in adult fixed-wing air transport patients. *Air Med J* 16(3):77-80, 1997.

28. Rutherford W: High-dose epinephrine in cardiac arrest: a brief review, *J Air Med Transport* 12:9-11, April 1992.

29. Kloeck W, Cummins R, Chamberlain D, and others: ILCOR Advisory statements: special resuscitation situations, Dallas, 1999, American Heart Association.

30. Dries D: Recent progress in adult cardiac life support, *Air Med J* 19(2):36-46, 2000.

31. Cummins R, editor: *Advanced life support,* Dallas, 1997, American Heart Association.

32. Williams A: The dilemma of DNR orders, *AirMed* 4(4):9-10, 1998.

33. Duchynski R, Brauer K, Hutton K, and others: The quick look airway classification, *Air Med J* 17(2):46-50, 1998.

34. Krupa D: *Flight nursing core curriculum,* Park Ridge, MD, 1997, Roadrunner Press.

35. Means BA, Taplett LC: Quick reference to critical care nursing, Gaithersburg, MD, 1986, Aspen Publishers.

36. Bobek E, Zinc B: Airway management of neurologic emergencies, *Air Med J* 18(2):68-72, 1999.

37. Martin S, Ochsner M, Jarman R: The LMA: A viable alternative for securing the airway, *Air Med J* 18(2):89-92, 1999.

38. DeJarnette R, and others: Pulse oximetry during helicopter transport, *Air Med J* 12:93-96, 1993.

39. Meade D, Farrell K: Pulse oximetry in the field, *J Emerg Med Serv* 3:50-57, 1994.

40. Thomas F, Blumen I: Assessing oxygenation in the transport environment, *Air Med J* 18(2):79-86, 1999.

41. Ornato JP, Peberdy MA: Prehospital end-tidal carbon dioxide monitoring, *J Emerg Med Serv* 8:140-148, 1993.

42. Rouse MJ, Branson R, Semonin Holleran R: Mechanical ventilation during air medical transport: techniques and devices, *J Air Med Transport* 12:5-8, 1992.

43. Wertz E: External cardiac pacing, *Emergency* 4:53-56, 1994.

44. Haught J: Catching up with cardiac pacing, *Emergency* 4:40-43, 1993.

45. Dailey E, Schroeder JS: *Techniques in bedside hemodynamic monitoring,* ed 5, St Louis, 1994, Mosby.

46. Ahrens TS: *Hemodynamic waveform recognition,* Philadelphia, 1993, WB Saunders.

47. Proehl J, editor: *Emergency nursing procedures,* ed 2, Philadelphia, 2000, WB Saunders.

48. Logston Boggs R, Wooldridge-King M, editors: *AACN Procedure Manual for Critical Care,* ed 2, Philadelphia, 1993, WB Saunders.

49. Woods SL, Mansfield L: Effect of patient position upon the pulmonary artery wedge pressures in nonacutely ill patients, *Heart Lung* 5(1):83-90, 1976.

50. Baele PL, and others: Continuous monitoring of mixed venous oxygen saturation in critically ill patients, *Anesthesia Analg* 61(6):513-517, 1982.

51. Hardy J, Ward DR, Gilliliau R: Fatal pulmonary hemorrhage complicating Swan-Ganz catheterization, *Surgery* 91:24, 1982.

52. Bongard FS, Sue D: *Current critical care diagnosis and treatment,* Norwalk, CN, 1994, Appleton & Lange.

53. Visalli F, Evans P: The Swan-Ganz catheter: a program for teaching safe, effective use, *Nursing* 11(1), 1981.

54. Wojner AW: Assessing the five points of the intraaortic balloon pump waveform, *Crit Care Nurs* 14(3):48-52, 1994.

55. Quall SJ: *Comprehensive intraaortic balloon pumping,* ed 2, St Louis, 1993, Mosby.

56. Brauer K, Hutton K: Chemical restraints in the air medical transport environment, *Air Med J* 16(4):105-107, 1997.

57. Jacobs BB, Hoyt S, editors: *Trauma nursing core course,* Park Ridge, MD, 1995, Des Plaines, IL, Emergency Nurses Association, 2000.

58. Berns K, Zietlow S: Blood usage in rotor-wing transport, *Air Med J* 17(3):105-110, 1998.

59. Macnab A, Pattman B, Wadsworth L: Potentially fatal hemolysis of crossmatched blood during interfacility transport: standards of practice for safe transport of stored blood products, *Air Med J* 15(2):69-72, 1996.

60. Snow N: Tube thoracostomy in the air medical setting, *Air Med J* 5(3):54-57, 1999.

61. Letarte P, Shea J, Dries D: Management of head injury in the field environment, *Air Med J* 18(2):73-78, 1999.

# Index

# NOTES

# NOTES

# NOTES

# NOTES